Spectacle Frames
and their Dispensing

HENRI OBSTFELD

M.Phil., F.C.Optom., F.B.O.A;H.D., D.C.L.P.

Senior Lecturer in Ophthalmic Lenses and Dispensing
City University, London, UK

W.B. Saunders Company Ltd

London • Philadelphia • Toronto • Sydney • Tokyo

W. B. Saunders Company Ltd   24–28 Oval Road
London NW1 7DX

The Curtis Center
Independence Square West
Philadelphia, PA 19106–3399, USA

Harcourt Brace & Company
55 Horner Avenue
Toronto, Ontario M8Z 4X6, Canada

Harcourt Brace & Company, Australia
30-52 Smidmore Street
Marrickville, NSW 2204, Australia

Harcourt Brace & Company, Japan
Ichibancho Central Building, 22-1 Ichibancho
Chiyoda-ku, Tokyo 102, Japan

Extracts from British Standards are reproduced with the permission of BSI. Complete copies
can be obtained from BSI Sales, 389 Chiswick High Road, London W4 4AL, UK.

A catalogue record for this book is available from the British Library

ISBN 0-7020-1928-3

Typeset by Paston Press Ltd., Loddon, Norfolk
Printed in Great Britain by The Bath Press, Bath

CONTENTS

FOREWORD

Technological change has affected the ophthalmics industry of the 1990s to the same extent as many others. The dispenser must now be prepared to deal with many frame and lens materials, many of which are not compatible with traditional methods of preparation and adjustment. At the same time, it is a common problem within both small and large ophthalmic practices that many of the 'tricks of the trade' are rapidly disappearing as the older generation of dispensers retires. Both dispensing opticians and optometrists are facing new challenges as the scope of practice of both dispensing professionals expands further into contact lens fitting on the one hand, and therapeutic optometry on the other. Traditional spectacle dispensing has given way in both instances.

While there have been many books written on the optics and prescribing of ophthalmic lenses, relatively little attention has been paid to the art and science of spectacle frames. Whether one considers principles of frame design, the considerations of frame selection, or the problems of adjusting or repairing a frame, there is almost nothing in the practitioner's library that brings all of these aspects of spectacle frames together under one cover. Henri Obstfeld has done an admirable job of doing just that. The student will find basic information on spectacle frame technology and illustrated descriptions of adjustment and repair techniques suitable for all ophthalmic frame materials. The experienced practitioner will be reminded of the repair techniques which are rarely, if ever, taught to today's students of opticianry or optometry. I hope that readers of this book will find it as informative and enjoyable as I did.

B. Ralph Chou, Msc, OD, FAAO
Associate Professor, School of Optometry,
University of Waterloo, Waterloo, Ontario, Canada

INTRODUCTION

I believe that dispensing is just as important as refracting as it is, after all, by the final product, the pair of spectacles, by which you will most frequently be judged. Most of my patients who complain of their glasses are dissatisfied with the dispensing rather than the refraction. One group of dispensing problems comprises ill-fitting frames. . . .

The cure . . . . is to improve standards of dispensing . . . and it could be argued that in not offering the client the best dispensing advice you are failing in your professional duty.

Prof. John Weatherill,
Owen Aves Memorial Lecture, 1988

The number of textbooks on this subject is very limited, and many have not been updated. There is a wealth of information on dispensing matters scattered about. Unfortunately, much is not in book-form and not easily accessible, a large quantity of material having been published in languages other than English.

In writing this text I have tried to provide a comprehensive account of the many aspects that play a part in the production as well as the dispensing of spectacle frames. I have avoided writing about spectacle lenses as such. That subject is already adequately covered and regularly updated. Owing to the diversity of aspects and background information associated with spectacle frames, there was no obvious order in which to write. Readers may well prefer to select their own sequence.

The foundation of my interest in spectacle frames was laid by W.J. Biessels and P.J. Tierolf at the Christiaan Huygensschool, now Zadkin College, in Rotterdam. Over the years I have learned a great deal from colleagues in practice as well as in academic life. I must mention here Charles Batson, now retired, and particularly John Campbell whose assistance with the photography, and recall of 'what', 'where' and 'how to' dating back to the days of my predecessor, the late Paul Fairbanks, has been most valuable.

In compiling this book I have had a great deal of support from friends and acquaintances in the spectacle frame and associated industries, both here and abroad. By listing the names of Gerhard Balder, the late Arthur Bennett, the late Neville Chappell, Ralph Chou, Jacques Dessallais, Dieter Fahrner, Angela Fuller, A. Oliver Goldsmith, Rocky Goldfoot, Roy Goodwin, Shelagh Hardy, Terry Joyce, Frank Norville, Joel Obstfeld, Malcolm Polley, Peter Price, G. Roebuck, Angela Rossi, Angela Sandler, Keith Sheffield, Peter Viner, Leslie Walther, Ivan Wilson and the librarians of City University and the (British) College of Optometrists, I have failed to mention *everybody* to whom my thanks are due. A very different type of support and encouragement was given by my wife Dorothy and by my sons; theirs was equally valuable.

Acknowledgement is made to the British Standards Institution for its consent to quote from their publications without which it would have been practically impossible to write this text. Let me take this opportunity to remind readers that, at present, many Standards are in the process of being replaced by European Standards (European Norms – EN) and International Standards which are issued by the International Standards Organization (ISO). Unfortunately, this continuing process prevents the contents of any book of this nature to be up-to-date.

During a dozen years or so students have asked me to recommend a textbook on 'dispensing' and I have disappointed them. I can only hope that I will not disappoint them again.

Suggestions for improvements will be very welcome.

Henri Obstfeld

Note: North American English equivalent terms taken from the ANSI Z80.5 and the International Standard ISO 7998, (1984), as appended to BS 3521: Part 2 (1991), are frequently given in the text and printed in *italics*.

REFERENCES

BS 3521: Part 2 (1991). *Terms Relating to Ophthalmic Optics and Spectacle Frames. Part 2: Glossary of Terms Relating to Spectacle Frames.* London: British Standards Institution.

ISO 7998 (1984). *Optics and Optical Instruments – Spectacle Frames – Vocabulary and Lists of Equivalent Terms.* Genève: International Standards Organization.

Weatherill, J. (1989). The Owen Aves Memorial Lecture, 1988 – the future of optometry. *Optom. Today,* 12–14, Jan. 14.

ANSI Z80.5 (1979). American Nat. Standard requirements for dress ophthalmic frames. New York: Am. Nat. Standards Institute, Inc.

CHAPTER 1

Basic Terminology

1.1 Introduction

Unless we speak the same language, we will be unable to understand each other: when we discuss a particular subject, it is necessary to use the same words in connection with that subject. 'Spectacle frames' is the subject under discussion, and standardized terminology on this subject has been available since the introduction of British Standard BS 3521 in 1962. It was produced 'to assist the mutual understanding' of all concerned with spectacle frames.

The international community has recognized that different terminology is used even in countries where, in principle, the same language is in use. A prime example is British and North American English; hence, the issue by the International Organization for Standardization of Standard ISO 7998 in 1984 which lists equivalent terms in no less than six languages, together with the two versions of English referred to above. In this text the North American English terms will be printed in *italics*.

1.2 General Terms

Some of the general terms set out in BS 3521 (Part 2) of 1991, applying to spectacle frames in general, are defined in Table 1.1, and those describing their major parts, are defined in Table 1.2.

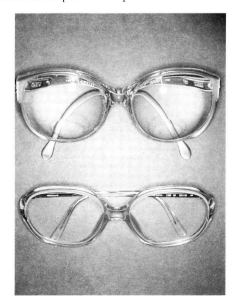

Fig. 1.1 *Upper: spectacles fitted with bifocal lenses. Lower: an 'empty', plastics frame*

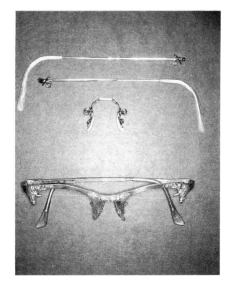

Fig. 1.2 *Upper: 'three piece' mount consisting of two sides and a bridge. Lower: a metal mount with fancy decorations*

Spectacle frames and their dispensing

TABLE 1.1. Terms and definitions: spectacle frames

Term	Definition
Spectacles (Fig. 1.1)	Optical appliances comprising lenses and a frame or mount with sides extending towards or over the ears. Synonyms: eyeglass frames, eyeglasses, glasses, spectacle frame
Frame (Fig. 1.1)	Spectacles or eyeglasses, considered without the lenses, having rims which will substantially or completely surround the lenses
Mount (Fig. 1.2)	Spectacles or eyeglasses, considered without the lenses, having no rims or with rims that do not substantially surround the lenses
Plastics frame (Fig. 1.1)	Frame of which the essential parts of the front are made of a plastics material or of a natural material of similar properties

TABLE 1.2 Terms and definitions: spectacle frame parts

Term	Definition
Front (Fig. 1.3)	The part of the frame or mount comprising the bridge, rims (if any), joints and/or lugs
Bridge (Figs 1.2 and 1.3)	That part of the front which forms the main connection between the lenses or rims. The bridge assembly is generally taken to include the pads, if any
Rim (Fig. 1.3) *Eyewire**	That part of the frame or mount which partly or completely surrounds the lens
Pad (Fig. 1.3)	An extension of, or attachment to, the bridge or the rim to bear on the nose. Synonym: nose pad
Joint (Fig. 1.4) *Hinge*	The hinge linking the side and the front
Lug (Fig. 1.3) *End-piece*	An extension at each end of the front to which the joint or side is attached
Side (Figs 1.2 and 1.4) *Temple*	An extension of, or attachment to, the front passing towards or over the ear
Eyewire*	Material in the form of rolled or drawn metal strip from which rims are made

*The word has a different meaning in **UK** and **North American** English.

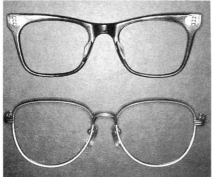

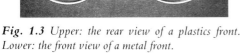

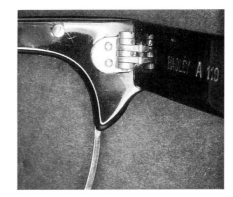

Fig. 1.3 *Upper: the rear view of a plastics front. Lower: the front view of a metal front.*

Fig. 1.4 *The joint or hinge (centre) links the side (on the rightnt) to the front (on the left)*

Armed with the basic terminology, the exploration can begin. Note that in the following chapters terms that have not yet been defined will sometimes be used.

REFERENCES

BS 3521: Part 2 (1991). *Terms Relating to Ophthalmic Optics and Spectacle Frames. Part 2: Glossary of Terms Relating to Spectacle Frames.* London: British Standards Institution.

ISO 7998 (1984). *Optics and Optical Instruments – Spectacle Frames – Vocabulary and Lists of Equivalent Terms.* Genève: International Standards Organization.

CHAPTER 2

History

2.1 Introduction

I do not claim that this summary represents a comprehensive or accurate history of the development of spectacle frames. However, it does cover the significant developments. The dates should be considered as advisory and not necessarily as the actual year of introduction of any particular item, although the more recent dates are accurate. The illustrations shown represent the type of front or frame described. However, they were not necessarily made during the period chronicled.

2.2 Chronological Review

1270 'Manokel' was the term used for a positive lens set in a rim attached to a handle (Fig. 2.1). It appears on a statue in the cathedral of Konstanz (southern Germany) and probably predates spectacle frames proper.

1286 Spectacles were probably invented by a glass worker in Pisa (Italy).

1300 The first reference to spectacles is found in Venice (Italy).

'Rivet' frames are the oldest known type of frames. They consist of two manokels, with an iron rivet connecting the handles.

1350 Wooden rivet frames dated around this period were found in the choir of the monastery of Wienhausen (Lower Saxony, Germany). They are the oldest known samples of spectacle frames (Fig. 2.2).

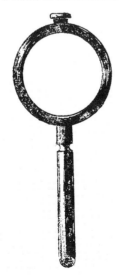

Fig. 2.1 *The manokel was probably the forerunner of the spectacle frame*

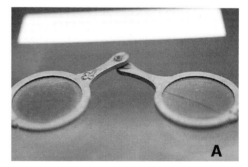

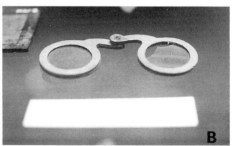

Fig. 2.2 *Two rivet frames on display in the museum of the monastery of Wienhausen (northern Germany). A, box wood, type I; B, lind (lime) wood, type II (courtesy T. Finkelstein)*

1400 Watermarks in Spanish paper, in the form of rivet frames. 'Bow' frames (Fig. 2.3), so called because of their curved bridge, appear. They were made of iron, bronze, wood, horn or bone.

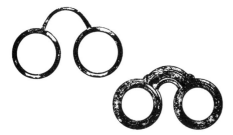

Fig. 2.3 *Bow frame*

1430 'Bonnet' frames (Fig. 2.4) were suspended from a bonnet or cap. Others were tied with a ribbon to the ears.

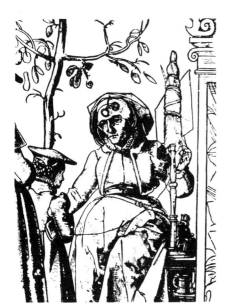

Fig. 2.4 *Bonnet frame. After a woodcut by Tobias Stimmer (1539–1584)*

1440 A rivet frame of about this date was excavated at Trig Lane in the City of London, UK. It was made of bone from a bull. Its probable origin was the Low Countries.

1450 'Thread' frames (Fig. 2.5), probably developed in Spain, had one or two holes pierced in the temporal side of each rim. A thread passed from the holes around the ears and this kept the frames in place. Spanish missionaries introduced thread frames to China from where they found their way to Japan.

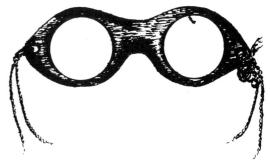

Fig. 2.5 *Thread frame*

1460 Paul van (de) Bessen, the earliest recorded spectacle maker in Britain, immigrated from the Netherlands. Evidence of spectacle makers in France.

1478 Decree of the town council of Nürnberg (Germany) concerning spectacle makers. J. Pfuhlmaier is the earliest recorded German spectacle maker (Nürnberg).

1485 Spyke Dowd: earliest recorded English spectacle maker. Earliest mention of concave lenses.

1500 'Leather' frames (Fig. 2.6) were made out of one piece of sole leather. The leather was cut

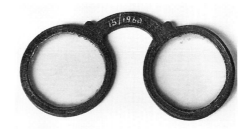

Fig. 2.6 *Leather frame*

into rims connected by a curved bridge. Such a spectacle was found in Boston, Lincolnshire (UK), made at about this time.

In an improved type of rivet frame the distance between the rims was adjustable thanks to the use of flexible material (metal wire, whale bone), so that the frame could be clamped on the nose. Previously, spectacles had been hand-held or suspended. 'Slit' or 'split' frames (Fig. 2.7) could also be clamped on the nose.

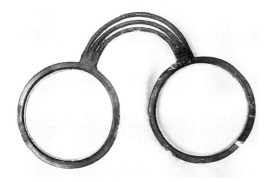

Fig. 2.7 Slit or split frame

Bow frames were now also made of silver, gold and fish bone, and with slits in their bridge which made them somewhat flexible. Some bow frames had a pair of springs on the nasal side of the bridge. The springs would press on the nose and so hold the frame in place (Fig. 2.8).

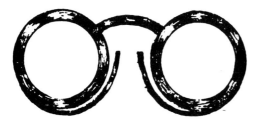

Fig. 2.8 A bow frame with springs which grip the nose

'Hinge' frames (Fig. 2.9) had developed from rivet frames where the rivet had been replaced by a hinge.

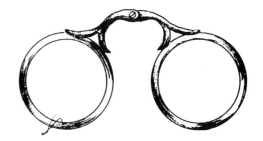

Fig. 2.9 Hinge frame

'Forehead' frames consisted of a front and a stem or handle attached to the bridge. The stem would be clamped between forehead and cap thus suspending the front before the eyes.

Frames were now also made of brass and lead.

1550 'Folding' frames were originally hand-held and looked like a pair of scissors. The lenses were fitted in the 'finger holes' and the 'blades' were held in the hand.

1570 'Headband' frames (Fig. 2.10) consisted of a metal band which surrounded the head. Each lens could be moved separately along the band and suspended before an eye.

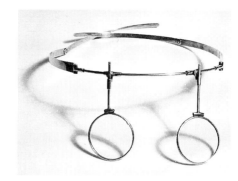

Fig. 2.10 Headband frame

1583 'Belt' frames (Fig. 2.11) were the first that were attached to the head. The lenses, held in horn rims, were fitted into a wide leather belt. The latter was worn around the head, above the

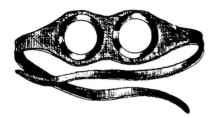

Fig. 2.11 *Belt frame*

ears, and the belt was knotted at the back of the head.

1600 'Wire' frames (Fig. 2.12) were made of one length of flattened, usually copper, wire. Each lens was contained in a rim with a thin looped wire thread that was hooked around one end of the rim and a part of the bridge.

Fig. 2.12 *Wire frame*

1620 The first American colonist to wear glasses was the pilgrim Peter Brown.

1623 First mention of protective spectacles.

1629 The Worshipful Company of Spectacle Makers (London, UK) received its Royal Charter from Charles I.

1650 'Scissors' spectacles (Fig. 2.13) were in the form of two lenses mounted on arms that could be folded into a stem which formed an integral protective case. Tortoise shell used as frame material.

1720 'Quizzing' glasses (Fig. 2.14) were an updated version of the manokel.

1730 'Monocle': this single lens (see Fig. 2.34),

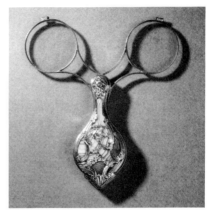

Fig. 2.13 *Scissors frame (courtesy Trustees of the British Optical Association Foundation, London)*

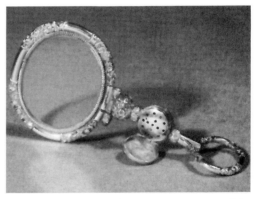

Fig. 2.14 *Quizzing glass (courtesy Trustees of the British Optical Association Foundation, London)*

with or without a frame or mount, was meant to be held between the brow and the cheek while the wearer contracted the orbicularis muscle. It was usually attached to the wearer's clothing with a ribbon, chain or thread.

'Pince-nez' (see Figs 2.29 and 2.31) or nose squasher, consisted of a wire front held on the nose by tension from a spring as bridge which was attached to the rims.

'Temple' frames (Fig. 2.15 and 2.16) probably originated in Britain. They consisted of a front

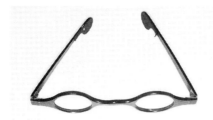

Fig. 2.15 *Temple frame made of tortoise shell, with round-end sides*

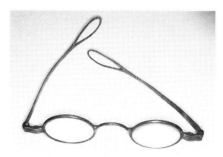

Fig. 2.16 *Temple frame with loop-end sides*

and a pair of sides that did not extend as far as the ears. The latter were often covered by a wig. The sides were made of silver or steel and they ended in a ring or spiral in order to improve the grip.

1740 James Ayscough (London, UK) probably invented the double hinged side (Fig. 2.17) where

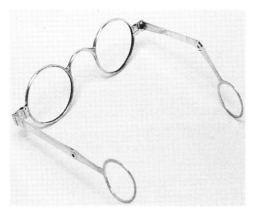

Fig. 2.17 *Frame with double hinged sides. The second hinge is placed near the middle of the side*

the second hinge is placed roughly halfway along the length of the side. When unfolded, they extend beyond the ear or over a wig.

1750 Metal frames were now being mass produced in Germany.

1752 Ayscough modified the double hinged side: the second joint was now placed near the ear point (Fig. 2.18). A variation was a side where the joint let the further portion of the side be rotated downwards so that it could lie behind the ear (like a drop end side).

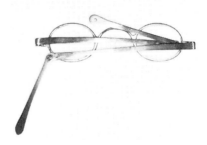

Fig. 2.18 *Frame with double hinged sides. The second hinge is placed at the ear point so that a drop would be formed when the end is rotated downwards*

1780 'Lorgnette' invented by George Adams. This was a hand-held frame (Fig. 2.19), meant for occasional use. It consisted of a handle into which the lenses could be folded when not in use. Later called 'face-à-main'.

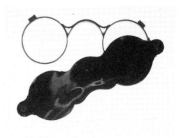

Fig. 2.19 *Lorgnette, later referred to as a 'face-à-main'*

1790 The sliding side (Fig. 2.20) was a side which could be extended, by means of a sliding portion, over the ear.

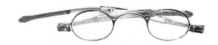

Fig. 2.20 *A frame with sliding sides*

1797 John Richardson fitted a pair of jointed rims behind the front (Fig. 2.21). Each rim contained a positive or a tinted lens and could be rotated to fit behind the front, thus transforming a distance pair of glasses into a reading pair, or into protective glasses. Other devices to assist presbyopes were developed. Until this time lens shapes had been round. Oval and rectangular shapes were patented by Dudley Adams.

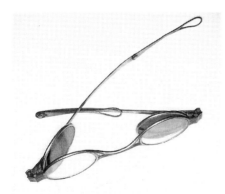

Fig. 2.21 *A frame with jointed rims and double hinged, loop-end sides. The jointed rims contain tinted lenses*

The X-bridge (Fig. 2.22) was introduced by John Richardson. Because the spectacles could be reversed, one eye could be fitted with a distance lens, and the other with a reading lens (for uniocular wearers).

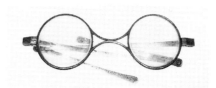

Fig. 2.22 *A frame with an X-bridge*

1800 'Flip up' fronts (Fig. 2.23) were used either for distance and near corrections, or for a correction with additional absorptive lenses.

'Steel-wire' spectacles (Fig. 2.24) had usually undergone a heat treatment which gave them a 'blued' appearance; most had oval lenses and straight sides.

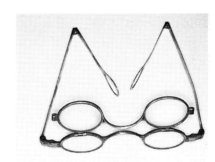

Fig. 2.23 *A frame with flip-up front and double hinged, loop-end sides*

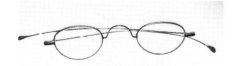

Fig. 2.24 *Steel wire frame*

1817 Rolled gold manufacturing process developed by John Turner.

1818 'Folder': a lorgnette (Fig. 2.25) modified by Lepage (Paris) into an eyeglass of which one lens could be folded in front of the other when not in use.

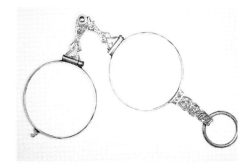

Fig. 2.25 *Folder frame*

1825 The 'unfolding lorgnette' usually had three spring-loaded joints – one on either side of the bridge, and the third between one rim and the handle. One lens could be rotated in front of the other, and they would fold over the handle. (British patent of R. B. Bate.) The K- (Fig. 2.26) and W-bridge (see Fig. 11.5), and curl sides were in use.

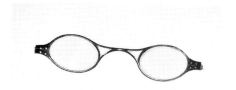

Fig. 2.26 *Frame with a K-bridge (courtesy H. Orr)*

1830 Spring-loaded lorgnette (Fig. 2.27): the joint of the bridge was fitted with a spring which would unfold the front on pressing a small button.

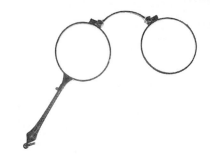

Fig. 2.27 *Unfolding lorgnette*

1836 'Weighted' spectacles were a modification of thread spectacles. The threads hung down over the ears and had a weight attached to their ends thus counterbalancing the weight of the front.

1840 'Rimless' frames (Fig. 2.28) (inventor: Waldstein, Vienna, Austria). The front was fashioned originally out of a single piece of glass into which the lenses were surfaced. Because of its weight, the glass bridge was later replaced by a metal spring.

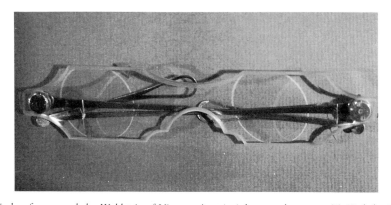

Fig. 2.28 *Rimless frame, made by Waldstein of Vienna, Austria (photograph courtesy T. Finkelstein)*

1846 Modern pince-nez (Fig. 2.29) illustrated in a French patent of Berthiot. In the course of the next 50 years numerous variations were introduced. The most important modification was due to the introduction of cylindrical lenses: in order to keep the axes fixed, the rims had to be made to slide apart along a system of spring-loaded bars.

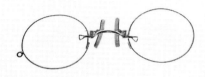

Fig. 2.29 *Pince-nez with rotating 'plaquets' which act as pads, gripping the nose*

1850 Folding frames (Fig. 2.30) were now available with a vertical hinge at the centre of the bridge which allowed the same side of each bridge to be folded together.

'Invisibles' (see Fig. 11.4) were frames with a very thin rim which fitted in a groove in the lens. Viewed from the front, they were almost invisible. Aluminium was a very expensive frame material.

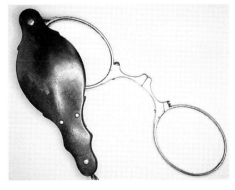

Fig. 2.30 *Folding frame. The bridge includes a vertical hinge*

1894 Seamless gold plating (i.e. gold filled) patented in the USA.

1900 The pince-nez (Fig. 2.31) was at the peak of its popularity and available in great variety. The principal part was the curved, metal bridge which had a post on either side containing a screw. A short bar, with a placquet (pad) on the top, rotated around the screw and was returned by a spring. Pressure, exerted by a finger (hence the name 'finger piece mount') on the bar, opened the placquets whereupon the mount was placed on the nose.

The 'astig clip' (Fig. 2.32) may be considered as a development of the flexible bow frame, for use with cylindrical lenses. The pad resembled the plaquet of the pince-nez, but the bridge was not fixed. Many designs were patented – all aimed at preserving the position of the axes of the lenses while varying the distance between rims; they usually consisted of a spring arrangement between two (or more) parallel bars.

Cellulose nitrate and alloys containing nickel and tin were used for frames.

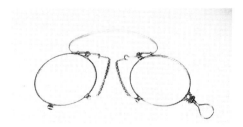

Fig. 2.31 *Pince-nez with spring-loaded plaquets*

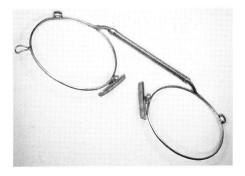

Fig. 2.32 *Astig clip*

1910 The 'Oxford' (Fig. 2.33) may be described as an American modification of a wire folding frame. It introduced the metal pad frame where two rims were connected by a spring as bridge, placed almost at a tangent to the upper part of the rim. A small ring fitted to one rim allowed a chord, chain or wide ribbon to be attached and connected with the wearer's clothing or a hair pin.

Von Rohr introduced telescope spectacles.

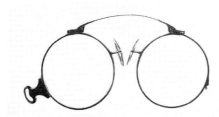

Fig. 2.33 *Oxford frame; one rim of this specimen folds in front of the other rim*

1911 Von Rohr introduced the spectacle magnifier.

1915 Monocles (Fig. 2.34) were now also made of cellulose nitrate and hard rubber.

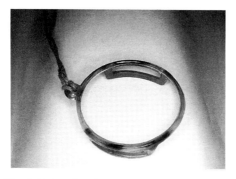

Fig. 2.34 *Hand-made, plastics monocle*

1920 Cellulose acetate, suitable for injection moulding of frames, started to be used.

The 'Windsor' frame (see Fig. 11.5): a nickel frame with cellulose nitrate-clad rims.

'Rimless' frames introduced along with the hockey end or drop end side. Eye shapes were now round, oval, PRO (pantoscopic round oval) and octagonal (see Table 16.1).

'Library' frames (Fig. 2.35) consisted of a heavy front and broad sides and were made of tortoiseshell or plastics.

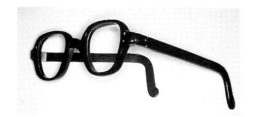

Fig. 2.35 *Library frame*

1925 Casein or galalith used in frame production. Some had bizarre eye shapes.

1932 High joint, metal frame with plastics nose pads and anatomically formed side drop introduced by Carl Zeiss Jena, in Germany.

An American catalogue presents the first children's frames.

1935 The 'Aviator' lens shape (Fig. 2.36) introduced by Bausch & Lomb, in the USA.

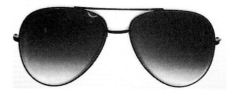

Fig. 2.36 *The aviator lens shape has a similar shape to the visual field*

1937 N. W. Chappell (personal communication, 1989) obtained a patent for metal-combination and suspension ('supra') frames.

1939 As an off-shoot of the supra style, two-tone plastics frame material was created.

Stainless steel used as rim around lenses.

1945 The first polymethyl methacrylate frames produced in the Netherlands from material recovered from crashed fighter planes.

First semi-rimless frame made of stainless steel (Fig. 2.37), the 'Ilford', manufactured by E. Trestain.

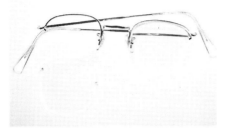

Fig. 2.37 *Ilford stainless steel semi-rimless frame. The lens is held in position by clamps that fit into slots made in the lens edge. As a result of the right lens having been removed, the tension in the stainless steel rim causes the right side to rise*

Semi-rimless frames were available in great variety.

'Upswept' style frames introduced in the United States (Fig. 2.38).

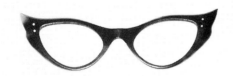

Fig. 2.38 *An upswept lens shape in which the upper edge (and that of the frame) has a marked upward slope towards the temple*

1947 First metal-combination frame (Fig. 2.39) produced by the American Shuron Optical Co.

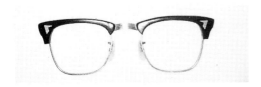

Fig. 2.39 *Metal-combination frame*

1950 Fashion made itself felt in frame design. This included fancy eye shapes and sides, and (metal) decorations on the front and/or sides, and plastics material laminated with textile (Fig. 11.25) and lace, with 'upswept' (Fig. 2.40) or 'harlequin' eye shapes. Plastics coloured other than brown (mottled) and black were used.

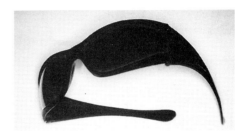

Fig. 2.40 *Wrap-around sunglasses. This specimen is made from polycarbonate material*

'Wrap-around' sunglasses (Fig. 2.40) make their appearance.

'Combination' frames are very popular.

'Phantom' rimless mounts consisted of a three-piece crystal plastics (polymethylmethacrylate) mount to which clear plastics lenses were bonded.

Cellulose acetate butyrate material used for protective frames and goggles.

1951 W. Conway developed a machine that 'shoots' the core into plastics spectacle sides.

1952 M. Birch, the first British professional frame designer, launched the 'Mirage' (Fig. 2.41), an upswept 'nylon supra', made of polymethylmethacrylate.

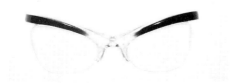

Fig. 2.41 *The 'Mirage' Supra frame. The swept-back lug starts its sweep from the temporal edge of the lens*

1954 The 'Nylor' nylon supra patent, held jointly by N. W. Chappell and Société des Lunetiers, filed.

1955 Polyamide frames (Fig. 2.42) produced.
Anodized aluminium used for fronts and sides (Fig. 2.43).

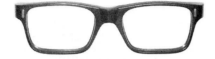

Fig. 2.42 *Polyamide frame*

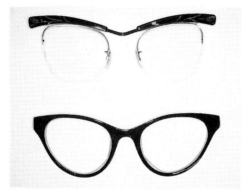

Fig. 2.43 *Above: semi-rimless frame with anodized aluminium browbar; below: anodized aluminium, metal-rimmed frame with plastics lining in the grooves of the rim to prevent glass lenses from breaking*

1958 Nylor frame (see Fig. 11.4) launched.

1965 Optyl introduced as a new frame material, by W. Anger of Austria. Imitation wood (cellulose acetate or nitrate) frames used.

1967 Second-generation Optyl material introduced.

1970 'Square' lens shapes (Fig. 2.44); increasing eye sizes demand larger uncut lens sizes.

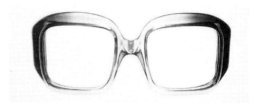

Fig. 2.44 *Square lens shape: frame is made of Optyl material*

1971 Third-generation Optyl introduced.

1975 Rivetted joints replaced by concealed, heat-inserted joints that allow easy angle of side adjustment.
Unconventional (Fig. 2.45) and bespoke frames are available.

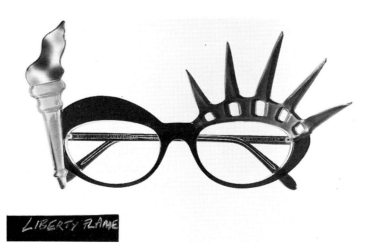

Fig. 2.45 *Unconventional frame (courtesy Anglo American Eyewear Co., London, UK)*

1978 Cellulose propionate frames (Fig. 2.46) produced by injection moulding.

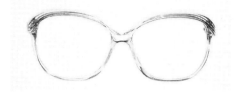

Fig. 2.46 *Cellulose propionate frame*

1985 Carbon fibre reinforced frames (Fig. 2.47) appear.

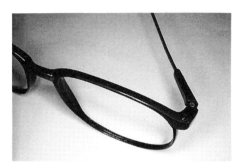

Fig. 2.47 *Carbon fibre reinforced frame. Frames made of this material tend to have sides that show a very distinctive butt. This specimen has also got a closing block as part of the swept-back lug. The lug point lies on the back plane of the front where the lug turns backward*

1987 'Round' lens shapes (Fig. 2.48) with box lens sizes up to 62 mm.

'Eyemetrics' computer-assisted rimless frame design, developed by W. Anger.

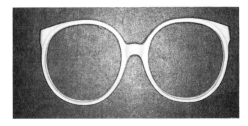

Fig. 2.48 *Round lens shaped frame. The large lens size requires a relatively low bridge*

1989 'Retro' styles: small round/PRO and shallow eye shapes reminiscent of the 1930s to 1950s become fashionable.

1991 Frames with a bar across the front and a minimal rim (Fig. 2.49), if any (Fig. 2.50), around the lenses.

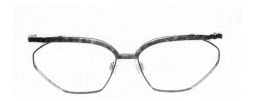

Fig. 2.49 *Frame with an accentuated browbar and minimal rim*

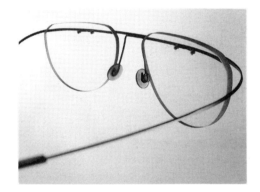

Fig. 2.50 *Minimal, jointless one-piece mount (courtesy Silhouette Eyewear/A. Schmiedt U.K. Ltd.)*

1993 Minimal mounts, resembling three-piece rimless spectacles (Fig. 2.51), sometimes glazed with dissimilar eye shapes.

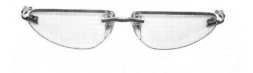

Fig. 2.51 *Minimal, three-piece mount with shallow lens shape*

REFERENCES

The above list was compiled from the following sources.

Andressen, B.M. (1994). *Brillen des 20. Jahrhunderts.* München: Klinkhardt & Biermann.

Anonymous (1991). Orbituary: Walter Conway, *Optician* **202**, 5316. 8, Aug. 30.

Appuhn, H. (1958). Ein gedenkwürdiger Fund. *Zeiss Werkzeitschrift*, **27**, 2–8.

Appuhn, H. (1973). *Der Fund vom Nonnonchor.* Kloster Wienhausen, Band IV, p. 10–16.

Bock, E. (1903). *Die Brille und ihre Geschichte.* Vienna: J. Safar.

Crundall, E. (1989) Flats versus torics. *Dispensing Optics* **4**, 11–14, May.

Bronson, L.D. (1974). *Early American Specs.* Glendale (CA): Occidental Publ. Co.

Chappell, N.W. (1989). Personal communications.

Chappell, N. (1989). A British invention makes history. *Optician* **198**, 13–14. 4, Aug.

Corson, R. (1967). *Fashion in Eyeglasses.* London: Peter Owen.

Court, T.H., & von Rohr, M. (1928–1929). On the development of spectacles in London from the end of the seventeenth century. *Trans. Optical Soc.* **30**(1), 1–21.

Davidson, D.C. (1989). *Spectacles, Lorgnettes and Monocles. Album 227.* Princes Risborough (Bucks): Shire Publications.

Doorn, B. van (1994). De kinderbril van handicap tot mode-item. *Oculus, Holland* **56**, 5, 47–49.

Dreyfus, J. (1988). The invention of spectacles and the advent of printing. *Library* **10**, 2, 93–106.

Frank, A. (1993). *The Seeing Eye.* Jersey (Channel Islands): Arthur Frank (private publication).

Franklin, F. (1992). Letter to the Editor: Trident missile. *Optician* **204**, 5364, 9.

Greef, R. (1948). Die Entwicklung der Formen und Fassungen der Brillengläser. In: Henker, O. *Der Augenoptiker*, Vol. 3, pp. 346–373. Pösneck/ Jena: R. A. Lang.

Greef, R., Hallauer, O., Lundsgaard, K., Pflugk, A. von, Reiss, W., Simon & Weve, H.J.M. (1929). *Katalog einer Bilderausstellung zur Geschichte der Brille.* Amsterdam: A.E. d'Oliveira.

Hamblin, D.J. (1983). What a spectacle! Eyeglasses and how they evolved. *Smithsonian*, March, No. 268, 100–111.

Hardy, S. (1982). Frame materials, part 3. *Manufact. Optician Int.* **35**(8), 31–32.

Hardy, S., & Hardy, W.E. (1982). Frame materials, part 1. *Manufact. Optician Int.* **35**(6), 18–23.

Klotz, A. (1988). *Die Brille.* Stuttgart: Württemburg, Landesbibliothek.

Kortland, K. (1990). *Het oog wil ook wat—optiek door de eeuwen heen.* Rotterdam: K. Kortland (private publication).

Kühn, G., & Roos, W. (1968). Siebenjahrhunderte Brille. *Deutsches Museum, Abhandlungen u. Berichte* **36**(3), 6–28.

Kuisle, A. (1985). *Brillen: Gläser, Fassungen, Herstellung.* München: Deutsches Museum.

MacGregor, R.J.S. (1993). Whalebone spectacles. *Ophth. Antiq. Int. Collectors Club Newsletter*, No. 43, 5–6.

Marley, P., Margolin, J.-C. & Bie'rent, P. (1988). *Spectacles & Spyglasses.* France: Hoebeke.

Orr, H. (1985). *Illustrated History of Early Antique Spectacles.* Beckenham (Kent): Orr.

Pastoor, D.W., & Obstfeld, H. (1990). Perspex frames in post-war Holland. *Optician* **200**(5278), 17–19.

Pistor, H. (1953). Die Brille im Wandel der Zeiten. In: *Über Brillen und über das Brillentragen*, pp. 5–13. Oberkochen (Württ.): Zeiss-Opton.

Poulet, W. (1978). *Atlas on the History of Spectacles.* Bonn–Bad Godesberg: Wayenborgh.

Rasmussen, O.D. (1950). *Chinese Eyesight and Spectacles*, pp. 15–27. Tonbridge (Kent): Rasmussen.

Rhodes, M. (1982). A pair of fifteenth century spectacle frames found in the City of London. *Antiquaries J.* **62**, 57–73.

Rohr, M. von. (1923–1924). The Thomas Young Oration. *Trans. Optical Soc.* **25**, 41–71.

Rohr, M. von. (1924–1925). Additions to our knowledge of old spectacles. *Trans. Optical Soc.* **26**, 175–187.

Rossi, F. (1989). *Brillen: vom Leseglas zum modischen Accessoire.* München: Callwey.

Rosen, E. (1956). The invention of eyeglasses, Part I. *J. Hist. Med.* **11**, 1, 13–46.

Rosen, E. (1956). The invention of eyeglasses, Part II. *J. Hist. Med.* **11**, 2, 183–218.

Turner, G. L'E. (1988). Spectacles over seven hundred years. In: Winkler, W. (ed.) *A Spectacle of Spectacles*, pp. 9–16. Leipzig: Edition Leipzig.

Völcker-Janssens, W. (ed.) (1994). *Da Guckste! Technik- und Kulturgeschichte der Brille.* Koblenz: Landesmuseum.

Wheway, F.H. (1941). Sixty years a frame maker. *Optician* April, 74.

CHAPTER 3

Morphology and Anthropometry

3.1 Introduction

Morphology is the science of form, in particular the outer form and inner structure, and the development of, living organisms and their parts. Anthropometry concerns itself with the measurement of the human body. Both are relevant to the design and fitting of ophthalmic appliances. However, the discussion of morphology and anthropometry will be restricted to the outer form of the human head. For detailed information about the inner structures of the head one should refer to textbooks on human anatomy and physiology.

One is, of course, aware of the many variations in form and position of the different parts of the human head, and how they may even affect one's subjective perception of that person. Also, note that the overall size of the female face is usually about 4/5th of that of the male.

The spectacle frame must be designed in such a manner that both anthropometric and cosmetic demands are satisfied. Psychological factors, as perceived by the spectacle wearer (and his aesthetic adviser, a role often assigned to the dispenser), may prove to be of overriding importance. Mechanical factors are greatly dependent on the anthropometry of the head, although some physiological aspects, in particular those concerning the skin, play an interactive role (Section 13.7).

The leading roles in this complicated interaction of factors must be apportioned to the eyes, nose, eyebrows, cheeks, eyelashes, the temples of the head, and the ears, all supported by the skull. An important aspect that must always be kept in mind, is the intrinsic asymmetry of the face. Darras (1982) demonstrated this most convincingly: the photograph of a perfectly symmetrical face obtained by manipulation so that each half of the face is a mirror of the other, gives the observer a feeling of unease, because it is so abnormal! (See Fig. 14.6).

3.2 Details

The observations made in the following paragraphs are given with respect to Caucasians and may differ in other races (see Section 3.4). Many of the more general facial measurements given are based on those of Mercier (1977).

3.2.1 THE HEAD
Marden (1987) provided measurements of the head of adults, and variations with age and gender (Table 3.1; see Fig. 3.1).

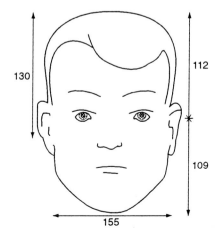

Fig. 3.1 *Average dimensions (in millimetres) of the adult male's head, based on Marden's (1987) figures*

TABLE 3.1 *Measurements of the head (after Marden, 1987)*

	Distance (mm)				
	Maximum		Average		Minimum
Adult males:					
Crown to eyes	140		112		89
Eyes to chin	132		109		97
Temple to temple	168		155		140
Crown to earhole	147		130		112

Variations with age (years) and gender		4	8	12	14	adult
Face to back	Female	170	178	183	185	190
	Male	175	183	185	193	196
Eye above ground	Female	937	1168	1376	1511	1506
	Male	937	1178	1397	1607	1643

3.2.2 THE SKULL

Plan views or horizontal sections through the human skull (Fig. 3.2) reveal many variations. However, there is one outstanding aspect of this sectional view: the anterior part of the head is wedge-shaped. The plane of the face normally represents the narrowest, vertical section through that wedge. This is a most important aspect that should never be forgotten when selecting, fitting and adjusting a spectacle frame. If the frontal width of the frame is narrower than the temple width, or the angles of let-back are too small, the wedge will become operational in that the temples of the head will propel the frame forward (Chapter 13).

The other aspect of importance is that each ear point (defined as the depression between the uppermost external ear and the skull) is not necessarily part of this wedge. It may be situated beyond the widest part of the head where there is another wedge-shaped part of the skull pointing away from the face.

The bones of the skull also determine the shape of the face (see Fig. 14.3), which is equally diverse. An interesting aspect is its height-to-width ratio. If this is equal to 1, the face will be roughly round, but may also be square. Faces are more frequently higher than wide, with a ratio of about 3:2 (Mercier, 1979) and when including the hair, the ratio is about 4:3 (Marden, 1987). This is of consequence to both the spectacle frame designer and the dispenser in that it determines certain cosmetic aspects.

Attention must also be drawn to the shape of the vertical section through the skull from the ear

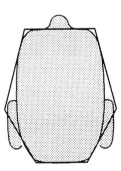

Fig. 3.2 *Horizontal section through the skull showing two wedges pointing away from each other and joined at the level of the ears*

point up to 3 cm behind it. In the plane through the ear point, the bones of the skull usually depart very little from being parallel. Just beyond the ear point, in many people, there is a groove in the mastoid bone. It is situated a little above the level of the auditory meatus (ear opening), and varies in shape and size. Fahrner (1987) showed that its mean depth relative to the ear point, measures 5 ± 5 mm, and wrote that it is present in about 65% of the population.

The inward angle of the mastoid bone is 20° in 19% of subjects, 15° in 28%, 10° in 22% and 5° in 17% (Murrel, 1976). Käpernick (1977) reported having observed mastoid bones forming a wedge pointing upwards. The shape and inclination of the mastoid is of great importance in the fitting and adjustment of spectacle frames (Chapter 14).

3.2.3. EYES

Although this appears to be a simple subject, it encompasses many aspects. The eyeball itself is essentially round, with a diameter of around 25 mm. The palpebral aperture, through which the eye is visible to the onlooker, is traditionally described as being almond-shaped. The horizontal dimension is generally about 30 mm. Its vertical dimension varies somewhat from person to person but is usually about 1 mm smaller than the vertical dimension of the cornea, and measures about 10 mm. It can be a little smaller,

TABLE 3.2 *Variation of facial measurements with age. Mean values, based on Hantman (1978); ranges (where given, between brackets) from Kaye (1969; for age group >15) and from Hantman (1978). Distances in millimetres; angles in degrees*

	Male (years)			Female (years)		
	<15	15–60	>60	<15	15–60	>60
Mean age	8·25	23·6	70·4	8·3	26·0	74·6
N	60	141	7	51	51	23
PD	54·1 S	65·4	66·0	54·3 S	62·2	61·6
Frontal angle	26·0 S	22·4 S	25·9	25·8 S	20·6 S	27·4
	(20/40)	(15/35)	(20/30)	(22/40)	(15/30)	(20/35)
Apical radius	8·8	8·8	9·3	8·4	8·2	8·3
	(7/11)	(7/12)	(8/11)	(8/11)	(5/10)	(7/11)
Bridge height	3·5 S	5·9	5·6	2·8 S	5·1	5·0
	(−2/+6)	(−2/+12)	(+3/10)	(−2/+6)	(−2/+12)	(+1/+8)
Distance	17·4 ?	16·4	19·6	17·3 ?	15·9 ?	17·2
between rims	(17/24)	(12/24)	(15/21)	(16/25)	(11/22)	(10/21)
Head width	134·4 S	150·6	152·4	128·4 S	144·2 ?	140·7
Front to bend	93·9 S	107·4	108·6	91·7 S	101·5	101·5
	(80/110)	(70/125)	(105/120)	(80/105)	(80/120)	(95/110)
Splay angle	30·0	19·0+		28·5	19·9+	
	(15/37)	(5/35)+		(20/50)	(5/40)+	

DBR measured at 10 mm below crest; PD, interpupillary distance.
S, Significant difference between adjacent age groups; ?, could be significant.
+, From Hanford (1970).
Neither the range of PD, nor that of the head width is given: the first is unrelated to frame measurements, and the second can be adjusted.

but if it were equal to or larger than the cornea, the presence of a pathological condition should be considered. Note that the palpebral aperture may be slightly inclined to the horizontal meridian.

The distance between the inner canthi of the palpebral apertures is about equal to their width, that is, 30 mm. The distance between the centres of the pupils of the eyes can vary considerably (see Table 3.2 and Chapter 21), and usually dictates the distance between the optical centres of the spectacle lenses for distance vision. In modern frames any relationship between the interpupillary distance and the distance between the centre of the frame's apertures has been abandoned. The difference in level of a pair of eyes does not normally exceed 2 mm (Spooner, 1951).

3.2.4 NOSE

This organ is arguably the most important structure with respect to a spectacle frame, because their relationship will greatly determine whether the frame will fit comfortably, or not.

The upper portion of the nose is supported by the right and left parts of the nasal bones, and the lower portion by cartilage. Hence, the latter is flexible: it may be compressed and its tip may be displaced by applying a little pressure. Its major parts are the wings and the septum which divides the nasal cavity.

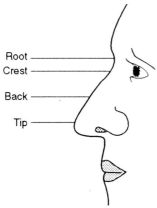

Fig. 3.3 *Parts of the nose*

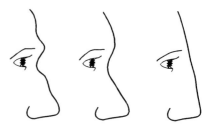

Fig. 3.4 *Various shapes of the root of the nose. Consider the consequences for a well-fitting spectacle frame*

The muscles of the nose receive their motor supply from the facial nerve. The sensory nerves are branches of the trigeminal nerve. The blood supply is through the infra-orbital artery. There is an abundance of lymphatic vessels in the lower part of the nose.

In the median plane (Fig. 3.3), one distinguishes between the root, crest, back and tip of the nose. The root is situated at the junction of the nasal and frontal bones. It may be continuous with the forehead, or offset so that the crest of the nose is parallel to the forehead (Fig. 3.4). The bridge of the nose is the elevation formed by the nasal bones themselves. This is also the area where the bridge of a spectacle front should rest on the nose. The crest may be straight, concave, convex or display a wave-like configuration. Frequently, crest and forehead will be noticeably inclined (Fig. 3.5). The back connects tip and crest (Fig. 3.6) and is the longest portion. The tip may be pointed or round, and point into the air or downwards (Fig. 3.7). It lies about 25 mm in front of the corneal vertex.

The relative levels of the eyes and the bridge of the nose are of major interest when selecting and fitting a spectacle frame (Section 14.3). The distance from the eyes to the nostrils grows steadily through infancy – proportionally much more so than the rest of the face. This distance is about 50 mm in an average adult. The lateral aspects of the nostrils are about 30 mm apart. This is equal to the width of the eye aperture.

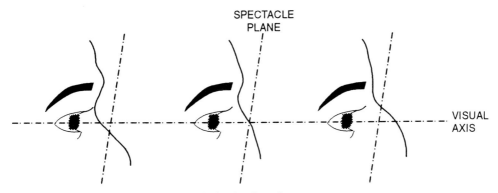

Fig. 3.5 *Various relationships between the forehead and nasal crest*

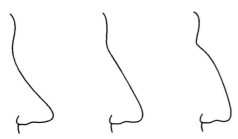

Fig. 3.6 *Various shapes of the back of the nose. Consider the consequences for a well-fitting spectacle frame*

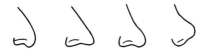

Fig. 3.7 *Various shapes of the tip of the nose*

Of importance to spectacle frame designer and fitter alike is the inclination of the nasal flanks, both in the vertical and horizontal planes. In the horizontal plane, and roughly at level with the lower eyelid, one measures the splay angle of the nose (Fig. 3.8). This will vary somewhat and depends on the extent to which the nasal bone and crest have developed and protrude. The protrusion is usually measured from a line passing through the apexes of the cornea or of the upper lid when the eye is closed (Fig. 3.9).

The frontal view of the nose (Fig. 3.10) may give a good indication of its symmetry. This will help the dispenser to determine which type of bridge would fit that patient's nose best, or whether a special frame that will accommodate a particular irregularity may be needed. The horizontal asymmetries (e.g. the horizontal distance between nasal midline and eye) are usually not

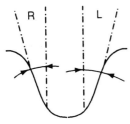

Fig. 3.8 *Horizontal section through the nose level with the horizontal centre line. Note the asymmetry of the right and left splay angles*

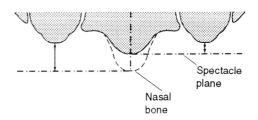

Fig. 3.9 *The extent of the protrusion of the nasal bone governs the distance between the apexes of the cornea or of the upper lid when closed, and the spectacle plane*

greater than 3 mm while vertical asymmetries usually do not exceed 2 mm (Spooner, 1951).

Note that the shape of the baby's nose is markedly different from that of the adult. It is small, wide and its crest is invariably concave, forming a sunken bridge.

The female nose is not only proportionally smaller than that of the male, but it is also proportionally wider. Furthermore, the female nose is more concave and its bridge more depressed.

It is interesting to note that the distinguishing characteristics mentioned above are exactly those that are most pronounced in children.

3.2.5 EYEBROWS

The shape of the eyebrows (Fig. 3.11) is determined by the shape of that part of the frontal bone forming the upper limit of the orbital foramen, together with the growth of the hairs (which may be modified for aesthetic reasons). The female brow is less pronounced, and tends to support scantier hair growth; hairs become thin-

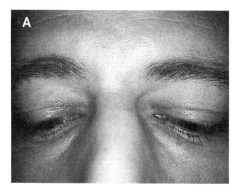

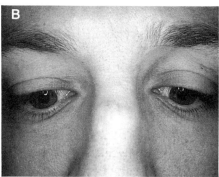

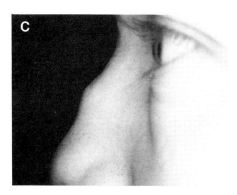

Fig. 3.10 (A) the right angle of splay is larger than the left angle; (B) the irregularity on the back of the nose shows even better as a side view (C)

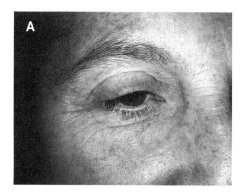

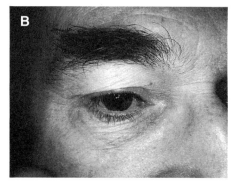

Fig. 3.11 The female's eyebrows (A) have a scantier hair growth than the male's (B). Both persons are aged 54

ner with age. In contrast, the hairs of the male brow are generally thinner in youth, and tend to grow thicker, longer and coarser with age.

Of importance is the distance between the open upper lid and the eyebrow, which measures about 10 mm. Together with the eyebrow shape it determines to a considerable extent the shape of the 'eye' of the spectacle frame that will suit a wearer best. However, wearers may have their own ideas about the position and shape of the upper rim of their frame.

3.2.6 CHEEKS

The shape of the cheeks is determined by the zygomatic (malar) and upper maxillary bones together with any adipose tissue overlying them (Fig. 3.12). This determines the vertical extent of the space between cheeks and eyebrows available to accommodate a spectacle front. It must be

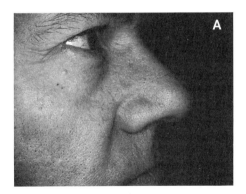

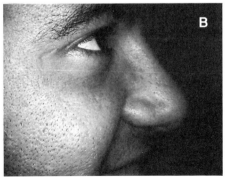

Fig. 3.12 The cheeks of person (A) are less pronounced than person (B)

admitted that spectacle frame fashion does not always take heed of this dimension. The position of the cheeks relative to the bridge of the nose determines the (maximum) inclination of the front through the angle of side.

3.2.7 EYELASHES

The length of the eyelashes of the upper eyelid (up to 8 mm), together with the thickness of that lid (about 2 mm), determine the minimum distance between the back surface of a spectacle lens and the front surface of the eye's corneal vertex (hence, vertex distance; see Chapter 20).

3.2.8 TEMPLES

The temple width of the wearer's head usually provides a good measure of the frontal width of a suitable spectacle frame.

3.2.9 EARS

The average ear has a vertical dimension of around 50 mm and a horizontal one of about 30 mm.

The position of the ears beyond the plane of the bridge of the nose determines the overall length of the sides of a frame. Their position in the vertical plane determines the angle of side. According to Fahrner (1987), the mean position of the ear point lies a little below the centre of rotation of the eye, with extreme variations of ±15 mm. A 10 mm difference is not uncommon. Fahrner also found that the mean position of the ear point beyond the centre of rotation of the eye is 70 ± 15 mm. This appears to be a reasonable finding because the centre of rotation is generally assumed to be situated 15 mm behind the anterior corneal surface (Obstfeld, 1982), to which 12–20 mm should be added as vertex distance, to arrive at a front to bend (FTB) measurement of 70–105 mm (Table 3.2).

Stimson (1951) showed two shapes of the bearing surface at the ear point (Fig. 3.13). He

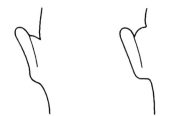

Fig. 3.13 Examples of the shape of the bearing surface at the ear point (after Stimson, 1951)

wrote that most ears are set close enough to the head to provide a definite crotch into which the side can be fitted. Some ears, however, protrude from the head, or the shape of the external ear is such that the bearing surface is perpendicular to the head.

Murrell (1976) investigated the external bearing surface of 200 spectacle wearers' ears using a

TABLE 3.3. *Classification of ear contours N = 200). (After Murrell, 1976)*

	Distribution (% of total)	
Type	Male	Female
A	20	19
B	8	3
C	11	18
D	9	9
E	3	0

moulding technique. He concluded that two further types should be added to the classification according to Stimson (1971). Murrell's classification is shown in Fig. 3.14 and the distribution is given in Table 3.3. He found that the majority of pairs of ears fell in category A.

The details contained in this section are of great importance for the design of not only the length of spectacle sides, but also the angle of side and possible adjustments thereof.

3.3 Development

Kaye (1969) carried out a detailed anthropometric examination of children between the ages of 6 and 13 years, and of children's spectacle frames (Kaye & Obstfeld, 1989). She concluded that most children's facial measurements equalled those of adults by the age of 13. The exceptions to the rule were the head width and front to bend: both increase by a further 10 mm or so after age 13.

Hantman's (1978) study of variations of facial measurements with age covers those of children. Comparing the figures from both, one finds that the values published by Kaye & Obstfeld (1989) for the 14–year-old group (mean age 13.7 years) lies between those of Hantman's (1978) age groups <15 and 15 to <61 (see Table 3.2), with the exceptions of frontal angle, apical radius,

EAR POINT

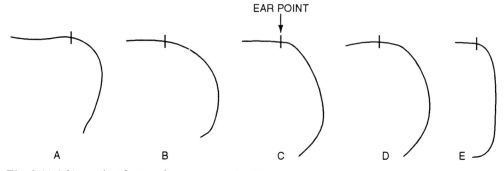

Fig. 3.14 Arbitrary classification of ear contours (after Murrell, 1976)

distance between rims (DBR) at 10 mm below crest and splay angle. These were all larger than those recorded by Hantman for each group. Note that the groupings of the two investigations are not really comparable. However, it does serve to justify placing Hantman's figures in three groups.

Murrell (1976) found for the front to bend (as head measurement) of a sample of 100 spectacle wearers (age group unspecified) a most common dimension of 95 mm with a range from >70 mm to <110 mm. This is at variance with the figures for adults in Table 3.2.

The data in Table 3.2 show also that, compared with adults, children have differently shaped faces. Figure 3.15 shows these differences diagrammatically. Note that many ranges of measurements for adjacent age groups are substantially the same, although their mean values may be significantly different. The values for the frontal angles of adults agree reasonably well with those given by Creighton (1961).

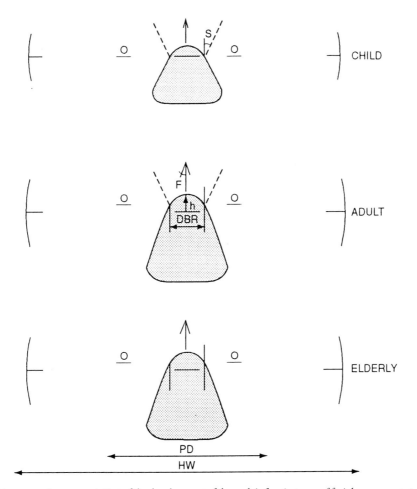

Fig. 3.15 *Diagrammatic representation of the development of the male's face in terms of facial measurements. DBR, distance between rims; F, frontal angle; h, bridge height; HW, head width; PD, interpupillary distance; S, splay angle*

There is an indication that the nose of the oldest group is subject to alteration: both frontal angle and DBR increase, assuming values close to those of the youngest group.

Kaye's (1969) and Creighton's (1961) figures also indicated that, in general, the frontal and splay angles (of the same age group) are of similar size. Although significant differences were found for some results of Hanford (1970) and Hantman (1978) (frontal angle, bridge height and front to bend), they do not materially affect the overall picture. Some of Hanford's sets of measurements were taken by various practitioners who did not always fully understand the instructions. Hant-man's measurements appear to have been less susceptible to this problem.

Woodhouse *et al.* (1994) found that the facial characteristics of children with Down's syndrome, in the age group 7–14 years, did not change with age nor did they agree with those of other children.

3.4 Racial Differences

In the following paragraphs, differences between the main racial groups will be discussed in as far as these affect spectacle frames and their fitting. See also Chapter 19: Ethnic frames.

TABLE 3.4 *Facial measurements of mongoloids aged 18 to 25. Mean values, standard deviations (between brackets) and ranges based on Symons (1979). Distances in millimetres; angles in degrees*

	N	Male	N	Female	S	C
PD	40	65.2 (12.6)	30	62.2 (1.9)	Yes	
<F	40	32.8 (5.9)	30	35.7 (5.0)		–
		20 –>45		25 –>50		
Apical radius	38	9.4 (1.0)	30	9.1 (1.4)		–
		8 –>12		7 –>12		
h.br	40	0.7 (2.1)	30	−0.7 (2.5)		–
		−3 –>+6		−5 –>+5		
DBR	30	13.3 (1.8)	13	13.1 (1.1)		–
Head width						
(HW)	40	149.9 (8.5)	30	146.4 (6.0)		
		130 –>170		130 –>155		
FTB	40	105.9 (7.1)	30	98.1 (6.6)	Yes	
		90 –>120		85 –>115		
Projection	32	−1.2 (2.7)	30	−3.9 (1.3)	Yes	NA
		−5 –>+6		−7 –>−1		
<Splay	40	41.1 (7.0)	30	46.7 (7.7)	Yes	–
		25 –>60		30 –>60		
<Crest	40	30.2 (8.4)	30	32.6 (5.6)		NA
		10 –>50		210 –>45		

C, Column indicating whether there is a significant difference between male Mongoloids and Caucasoids (compared with Hanford, 1970).
S, Column indicating whether there is a significant difference between male and female mean values.
N, Number in sample.
NA, Information not available.

The main races may be loosely described as comprising Caucasoids, Mongoloids and Negroids. (The suffix -oid means resembling or similar.) A very rough estimation indicates that of a world population approaching 5000 million individuals, 3000 million are Mongoloids, 1000 million are Caucasoids and less than 1000 million are Negroids. (The writer must stress how difficult it was to find such information which is of considerable consequence for spectacle frame design.)

Symons (1979) collected facial measurements of Mongoloids using the Facial Measurement

Gauge (Fairbanks, 1968), together with specially designed equipment to measure nasal dimensions. The results are presented in Table 3.4. Banks (1968) collected facial measurements of Negroid subjects using similar equipment. His results are summarized in Table 3.5. Note that the significant differences apply mainly to the measurements of the nose, and, therefore, have major implications for spectacle frame design. The differences are depicted in Fig. 3.17. Note the small mean DBR measurements in Tables 3.4 and 3.5. Accordingly, many Afro-Caribbean and Mongoloid patients (as well as children from

TABLE 3.5 Facial measurements of African and West-Indian male negroes aged 20 to 50. Mean values, standard deviations (between brackets) and ranges based on Banks (1968). Distances in millimetres; angles in degrees

	N	African	N	West-Indian	A	B	C	D	E
PD	30	69.7 (3.5)	26	65.3 (2.0)	S		S	S	
<F	30	42.0 (5.6) 30 –>50	26	39.2 (5.8) 25 –>50				S	S
Apical radius	30	12.4 (2.0) 8.4 –>15	26	11.1 (1.5) 8 –>14	S	S		S	S
h.br.	30	1.9 (1.9) −1 –>+7	26	1.9 (2.1) −2 –>+6				S	S
DBR	26	17.2 (1.7) 14 –>20	21	17.4 (2.2) 14 –>22	S	S			
Head width	30	151.8 (5.9) 135 –>170	26	148.7 (8.0) 135 –>165					
FTB	30	103.0 (5.3) 95 –>120	26	106.9 (6.2) 95 –>120					S
Projection	30	−0.9 (1.3) −3 –>+3	26	0.1 (1.7) −3 –>+3				NA	NA
<Splay	30	42.5 (6.1) 30 –>55	26	35.8 (7.0) 15 –>45	S	S	S	S	

A, Column showing whether there is a significant difference between Mongoloid and African males facial measurements.
B, As column A, but for Mongoloid and West-Indian males.
C, As column A, but for African and West-Indian males.
D, As column A, but for Caucasoid and African males.
E, As column A, but for Caucasoid and West-Indian nales.
N, Number in sample.
S, Significant difference present.
Columns A and B are based on Banks (1968) and Symons (1979), and columns D and E on Hanford (1970) and Banks (1968).

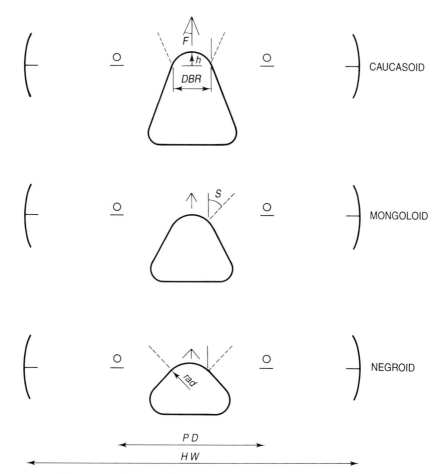

Fig. 3.17. *Facial dimensions of Caucasoids (top), Mongoloids (middle) and Negroids (bottom). DBR, distance between rims, or nasal height; F, frontal angle; h, height of bridge/crest; HW, head width; PD, interpupillary distance; rad, apical radius; S, splay angle of nose*

all races) have a negative bridge height, and the measurement must be taken below the horizontal centre line (BS3521, 1991, includes specification of bridge width of fronts at 5 mm below the horizontal centre).

Symons (1979) stressed the relationship between height of bridge and DBR, Base at 10 below crest and inset while Banks (1968) stressed the relationship between DBR, frontal angle and apical radius.

Kaye & Obstfeld (1989) provided details of the approximate differences between Caucasoid

TABLE 3.6 *Facial measurements of Afro-Caribbean children aged 14; approximations, after Kaye & Obstfeld (1989). Distances in millimetres; angles in degrees*

PD	57	<F	33
Apical radius	11	h.br.	1.5
FTB	101	<Splay	39
Projection	3		

When these measurements are compared with those for the equivalent adult group in Table 3.5, only the projection appears unsound.

and Afro-Caribbean children's facial measurements, for the age range 5–14 years. From these, Table 3.6 has been derived.

3.5 Differences Within Races

Since the aforementioned racial groups cover a large variety of ethnically different groups, it is to be expected that there will be differences within these groups. A few examples follow below.

The Front To Bend measurement of south Germans is shorter (<135 mm) than that of north Germans and British. This difference applies to central African and West-Indian males (Banks, 1968) compared with black South Africans (Turnbull, 1991).

The range of interpupillary distances (PDs) of Germans (Fleck *et al.*, 1960) is about 5 mm smaller than that of French (Darras, 1982), that of West-Indians is about 10 mm smaller than that of Africans (Banks, 1968); there is a similar difference in the Temple Width of the last two groups. The range of Temple Width of Germans (Fleck *et al.*, 1960) is 20 mm smaller than that of French (Darras, 1982).

The mean splay angle of West-Indians is 10° smaller than that of Africans (Banks, 1968).

REFERENCES

BS 3521: Part 2 (1991). *Terms Relating to Ophthalmic Optics and Spectacle Frames. Part 2: Glossary of Terms Relating to Spectacle Frames.* London: British Standards Institution.

Creighton, C.P. (1961). Spatial relationships between the eyes, the nose and the rims of the orbits. *Am. J. Optom. Arch. Am. Acad. Optom.* **38**(12), 665–680.

Fahrner, D. (1987). Brillenkunde (2): Die Ohren. *Neues Optikerj.* **29**(10), 11–15.

Hanford, R.G. (1970). An investigation of some facial measurements relevant to the design, manufacture and fitting of spectacle frames. Final Year Project. London: City University.

Hantman, D.P. (1978). A comparison of facial measurements with age. Final year project. London: City University.

Käpernick, E. (1977). Zum Leitartikel 6/1977 ein Leserbrief von Einhard Käpernick. *Neues Optikerj.* **19**(8), 657–661.

Kaye, J. (1969). Anthropometry for children's spectacles. Final year project. London: City University.

Kaye, J., & Obstfeld, H. (1989). Anthropometry for children's spectacle frames. *Ophthal. Physiol. Opt.* **9**, 293–298.

Marden, A. (1987). *Design and Realization.* Oxford: Oxford University Press.

Mercier, R. (1979). Morphologische Normen für Augenoptik und Optometrie. *Augenoptiker* **34**(11), 40–45.

Murrell, R.H. (1976). Spectacle sides – dimensions and design. Final year project. London: City University.

Obstfeld, H. (1982). *Optics in Vision*, 2nd edn, p. 278. London: Butterworths.

Spooner, J.D. (1951). The incidence of vertical centration errors. *Optician* **122**(3149), 73–74.

Stimson, R.L. (1951). *Ophthalmic Dispensing*, p. 107. St Louis: Mosby.

Stimson, R.L. (1971). *Ophthalmic Dispensing*, 2nd edn. Springfield: Thomas.

Woodhouse, J.M., Hodge, S.J., & Earlam, R.A. (1994). Facial characteristics in children with Down's syndrome and spectacle fitting. *Ophthal. Physiol. Optics* **14**(1), 25–31.

CHAPTER 4

Frame Design Criteria for Comfort and Adjustability

4.1 Introduction

When spectacle frames were small, and as a consequence, glazed frames were relatively light in weight, comfort was seldom a problem. That has changed dramatically over the years as a result of the introduction of fashion frames in the 1950s. Some of the more exaggerated examples had horizontal boxed lens sizes that approach double the size of the frames available earlier in the twentieth century. Although people may have grown taller during that same period, their facial dimensions do not appear to have changed much.

The comfortable wear of glazed frames is intimately linked with their total weight and the wearer's facial dimensions (see Chapter 3). Mechanical aspects affect the interaction of glazed spectacle frame and head (see Chapter 13). In order to make a frame fit properly and comfortably, one must be able to adjust that frame. Whether a frame is fully adjustable depends on its design and the mechanical relationships between its components.

A glazed frame should never cause its wearer more than the minimum inconvenience (Rünz, 1976). It should be wearable and bearable in addition to fulfilling its primary task: of holding the required power and type of spectacle lenses permanently in the correct position in front of the wearer's eyes. The frame should restrict the wearer's binocular field of view only minimally.

The conscientious dispenser will always advise his or her patient with these objectives in mind.

4.2 Plastics Frames

Definitions of terms used in the following sections but not defined in Chapter 1, can be found in Chapter 11.

4.2.1 THE BRIDGE AND SURROUND

The bridge of any front is of the greatest importance because it connects the two halves of the frame and plays a major role in the distribution of the weight of the spectacles on the patient's nose. In most Caucasians the bridge should curve away from the face (Fig. 4.1) to accommodate the root of the wearer's nose (a so-called 'bumped' bridge displaying a projection), and be of sturdy construction, without sharp edges. The lower the

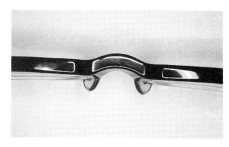

Fig. 4.1 A bumped bridge which curves away from the face thus accommodating the root of the nose

position of the crest relative to the upper rim, the greater its projection should be in order to maintain the same, or a reasonably short vertex distance (Fig. 4.2).

The bridge construction should not contain weak spots such as grooves, slots or cavities as

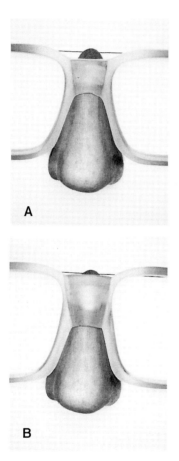

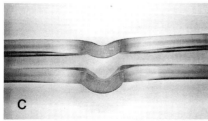

Fig. 4.2 *The lower the position of the crest (compare A and B), the greater its projection should be (C)*

these tend to have a destabilizing effect. The worst example encountered by the author was a frame where the bridge was flexible in the plane of the front so that it could fit any nasal width – but what about the stability of the axis orientation of a toric lens, or the segment top position of a multifocal lens? It is important that the mechanical forces working through the sides of a glazed front when worn do not deform the bridge. The bridge of a front is subject to the greatest stress because it is the part where the mechanical forces of a frame meet (see Chapter 13).

There are two basic bridge designs. The saddle bridge facilitates a greater continuous bearing surface and may provide less pressure per unit area for a given weight. The pad bridge features pads that increase the size of the bearing surface, thus reducing the pressure on the nasal flanks. Various modifications of each type of bridge have been manufactured.

Without experience it is difficult to determine from an empty front at the frame-selection stage whether, once glazed, a bridge will be stable on the wearer's nose as well as comfortable, particularly when the prescription is anisometropic. (Spectacle weights (see Chapter 13) can be a very useful dispensing aid.) Rünz (1976) wrote that for most glazed fronts the bearing surface should be 20 mm long. This would create a bearing surface varying between 150 and 200 mm^2, depending on the width of that surface (see Section 5.2). This does not take into account any bearing surface on the crest of the nose. The length of the bearing surface of a saddle bridge may be more than twice that of a pad bridge.

In my experience, the angle of crest in regular and saddle bridge frames can increase comfort considerably. Dispensers should adjust this angle for the individual wearer. This means, of course, that the frame must be designed and manufactured in such a way that this adjustment can be made.

The thickness of the rim in the bridge area should depend on the frontal angle (and, ideally, on the glazed front's weight): the smaller the frontal angle, the greater the pressure on the nasal bearing surfaces (Chapter 13). An important consideration is that, in the rank order of sensitivity to pressure of different body parts, the lateral surface of the nostrils is among the four most sensitive (Weinstein, 1968). From a mechanical viewpoint, therefore, the thickness (or pad width) should be increased as the frontal angle is decreased. Unfortunately, this is not a practical proposition in view of the economics of spectacle frame manufacturing.

Pads are usually placed at about the level of the horizontal centre line of the front and are usually curved in the vertical plane. Because the upper portion of the pad is normally closest to the vertical meridian, it will exert the greatest pressure on the wearer's nasal flank. To reduce the pressure, the upper portion of the pad should be wider than the lower.

4.2.2 JOINTS AND SIDES

The functions of spectacles joints (Ward, 1971) are:

- to attach the sides securely to the front,
- to facilitate stabilization of the front when the sides rest on the ears,
- to enable the sides to close parallel to the front thus making the frame compact when not in use,
- they may be used for decorative purposes,
- they are sometimes used to secure the lenses in the front.

One may add to this list:

- to hold the front at the required inclination.

With respect to the last aspect, the angle of joint is of importance. These angles vary from 0 to 15°, the majority having an angle of 10° which is in agreement with the angle of side most frequently encountered (Ward, 1971).

Joints should be adjustable. Because the position of the ear in the vertical plane may vary by ±15 mm from the average position (relative to the centre of rotation of the eye), it is necessary to be able to adjust the angle of side by some 10° either way (Fahrner, 1987a). This is three times the recommendation laid down in DIN 58 199 (1989)! One cannot usually adjust satisfactorily a joint with more than three charniers. The type of joint that has proven most suitable over the years is known as a 'mushroom' joint (Figs 4.3 and 11.17) because of its shape. The 'stalk' of the 'mushroom' must be engineered so that it can be inclined by ±10° (see above). Further details are given in DIN 58 226 (1965), 58 227 (1961), 58 228 (1961) and 58 229 (1966).

Sprung joints are defined in BS 3521 (1991) as a joint having a spring mechanism designed to exert lateral pressure on the side of the head of the spectacle wearer. Harmer (1994) identified the following additional purposes: to minimize the tension in the frame's front, especially in the

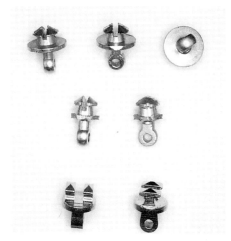

Fig. 4.3 *Examples of pinless 'mushroom' joints showing the 'anchor' above and the charnier below. The anchor is embedded in the front of the frame*

bridge, and to facilitate removal from and (re)placement of the frame on the wearer's head.

Three types of sprung joint mechanisms can be identified (Harmer, 1994), namely spring compression, spring extension and component bending sprung joints (Fig. 4.4). The latter type includes sides and joints that act as or include leafspring(s) rather than a joint assembly containing a spiral spring. Harmer (1994) found a significant increase in grip until the frame head width had been increased by 30 mm, while beyond an increase of 50 mm less force was exerted than in

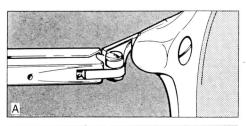

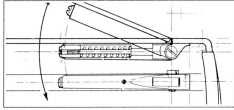

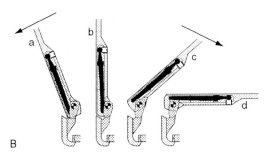

Fig. 4.4 *Diagrams of the mechanism of sprung joints. A, compression-type (courtesy of Norville Optical Co.). B, component bending type (a) side opened to its maximum and spring (shown in black) under tension; (b) side showing 0° angle of let-back, spring relaxed; (c) side in process of being closed, spring under tension; (d) side closed, spring relaxed (courtesy of Celes Optical Srl). See also Fig. 11.21*

comparable, conventionally jointed frames. Tension in the front showed a significant increase while the frame head width was increased by 30 mm but remained relatively constant beyond this point. Sprung joint design affected performance, as did poor matching with frame type. Harmer (1994) concluded that spring extension sprung joints were less effective than spring compression sprung joints.

Sprung joints cause problems for dispensers. The greatest advantage appears to be their sales potential (Rünz, 1976; Rünz *et al.*, 1977; Morel, 1981). Although most have proven to be durable and reliable, they are difficult to replace and service and in many cases the angle of side of such frames cannot (easily) be adjusted. DIN 58 199 (1989) requires the spring action of the sides to be equal. However, many heads are asymmetrical and require unequal angles of let-back. When that is the case, spectacles fitted with spring-loaded joints tend to tilt in the horizontal plane so that the vertex distances are unequal. This may affect the optical efficiency of the lenses and also the comfort of the fit on the nose, because of the unequal pressures exerted on the bearing surfaces. Hence, there are good reasons for not using such joints.

The position of the joint in the vertical plane along the front affects the fit of the frame. Low joint frames cause greater fitting and adjustment problems than high joint frames because their centre of gravity may result in a somewhat precarious balance. Moreover, low joints affect the inferior temporal field of view while high joints normally do not. A middle joint may also affect the temporal field of view. The width of the side of middle and low joint frames also affects the temporal field – it has the same effect as 'blinkers' on a horse (now outlawed in the UK) in that it prevents seeing to the temporal side. In principle, frames with wide sides are suitable only on spectacles containing a reading prescription. Such glasses should, of course, not be used when

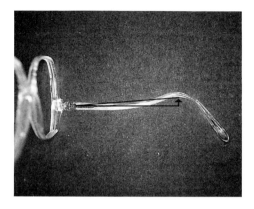

Fig. 4.5 *A low joint showing a negative angle of side*

driving (Ruffel Smith & Weale, 1966; DIN 58 216). North (1993) wrote that spectacles for motorists should have thin rims and thin sides, with as large a lens aperture as possible, bearing in mind the power of the lenses, to allow for the widest field of view.

The angle of side of a low joint frame differs noticeably from the other two types in that it usually has to have a negative value (Fig. 4.5).

The design of sides and their properties of flexibility are of major importance with respect to the removal from and also the retention of the frame on the head. Fahrner (1971–72) suggested that the vertical section through a side should be tapered, with the widest part near the joint. The pressure provided by the side at any one point along its length would then be constant. However, this applies only to a plastics side without a reinforcing core.

One should not be able to deform the core of a plastics side near the joint. It should gradually become thinner and more elastic towards the ear point, where it should be thinnest. It is then possible to adjust the downward angle of drop, and reposition the ear point in either direction. Fahrner (1987b) suggested that three lengths of side, each 8 mm longer than the previous (instead of the usual 5 mm difference), should be manufactured for each frame style. This would be

sufficient to fit practically any frame comfortably on most wearers' heads.

The core in a side should be rectangular in section between the joint and a point well before the ear point. From there onwards, it should be round. This facilitates flexibility, so that the frame may easily be removed from the head, and stability, together with adjustability in the ear-point region. The problem with cores that are rectangular in section at the ear point is that they can be adjusted only with the greatest difficulty, and usually buckle at a crucial moment – if this is not the case, the metal of which the core is made is likely to be too soft. Cores should not be made of highly flexible steel because this material has to be so over-adjusted before it will remain in the desired shape that it may affect its plastics cover.

The thickness of the drop of a plastics side should not exceed 3 mm, otherwise it may not fit comfortably in the groove between auricle and mastoid. The material should be well rounded. The drop itself need not be longer than about 35 mm. A much longer drop will seldom improve the quality of the fit in that area (but see Fig. 11.24). The overall length of side required for a proper fit varies so much that the single side length offered by so many frame manufacturers is impracticable. When the core in the drop is 10 to 15 mm shorter than the drop itself, it will be possible to reduce its length, if required, by cutting several millimetres off the drop and re-fashioning.

The larger the inner surface of the drop, the more evenly the pressure can be distributed over the skin surface covering the mastoid bone. The greater the friction between drop and skin, the better the retention of the frame on the head.

4.2.3. SCREWS

The threads of screws, taps and gauges for spectacle frames have been set out in BS 3172/EN ISO 11381 (1995). Provided that one uses the

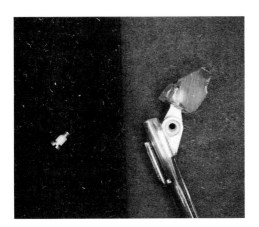

Fig. 4.6 Joint showing a plastics bush in its barrel and a plastics sleeve around its screw

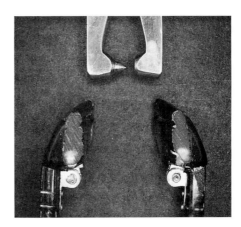

Fig. 4.7 Bottom right: the dimple in the bottom of the shaft of a screw. Above: the heads of peening pliers. Bottom left: after the application of peening pliers, the end of the screw shaft has been spread over the lower aspect of the charnier of the joint

correct size screwdriver, a single slot in the screwhead is sufficient. A few manufacturers have introduced a cross-cut slotted head which, in principle, requires a different type of screw driver. As there appear to be few advantages in the use of such screw heads, it would be advisable to discontinue their use. When ISO 11381 is implemented by manufacturers, optical dispensers will, in theory, only have to keep six types of screws in stock. At present, the number appears almost unlimited.

Screws must have gone missing ever since their invention and this problem has still not been solved. Many solutions have been introduced only to disappear after a short while (Fig. 4.6). The only way to secure a spectacle screw with certainty is to spread or peen the end of its shaft (Fig. 4.7). For this purpose, the bottom of the shaft is provided with a dimple. The spreading plier can be placed in this dimple, and applied. The disadvantage is that it then makes it difficult to remove the screw, for instance when a side needs to be replaced or the screw has been broken (see Chapter 24). Another problem is that screws tend to wear; as a result, the spectacle's side becomes loose. Efforts by screw designers to overcome this problem are to be encouraged,

provided that they can be made such that the friction is invariable and durable, and the ability to adjust the inclination of the joint is maintained.

Dowel pins (see Fig. 11.15) have sometimes been used instead of screws. When handling such frames, sides tend to open and close freely. However, some new designs include a device similar to a disc break, which restrains the free movement of sides.

Lock nuts (see Fig. 11.18) caused too many problems and have seldom been used since the 1960s.

4.3 Metal Frames

4.3.1. REQUIREMENTS
Many of the basic requirements applicable to plastics frames can also be applied to metal frames. Hence, the requirements that apply more particularly to the latter will be discussed below.

Stability is of even greater importance with metal frames than with plastics frames because any deformation is unacceptable – it can influence the fit of the lenses, especially when it affects the rims or the lens-holding device. Therefore, the construction of the bridge is of the utmost importance. Its hardness will determine its stability. Its soldering or welding must be carried out with great care so that the frame will be able to withstand daily handling. Bridge reinforcements, such as a browbar, are valuable provided that they do not bring with them any disadvantage. It is very unlikely that they will increase the mass of the appliance significantly but they will help to prevent the bridge from breaking under stress.

4.3.2 RIMS AND CLOSING BLOCKS

The properties of the material used for the rims should be carefully evaluated; their mass and hardness must prevent distortion, but one must be able to adjust them for glazing purposes. Hence, the profile or sectional shape must be carefully considered. In general, the heavier the profile, the more difficult it will be to adjust the rim. Hence, the importance of rim forming.

The closing block design is equally of major importance. There are two successful constructions in general use. In one a portion of the closing block envelops the other (Fig. 4.8)

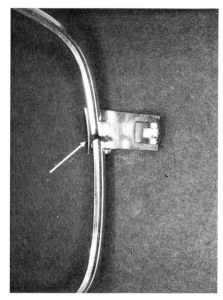

Fig. 4.9 An 'A' (above) and inverted 'V' (below) closing block

whereby the screw prevents any twisting; a modification has the two portions of the closing block fitting as a 'V' and an inverted 'A' shape (Fig. 4.9) thus preventing twisting. The closing block joint consists of two halves fixed together with two screws (Fig. 4.10), where the screws

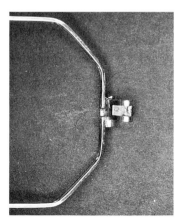

Fig. 4.8 When closed, the lower portion of this open closing block will be enveloped by the upper portion thus preventing twisting of the rims

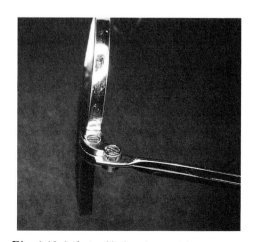

Fig. 4.10 A closing block and tenon joint

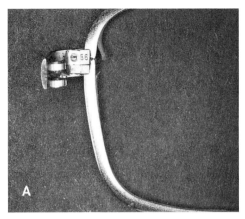
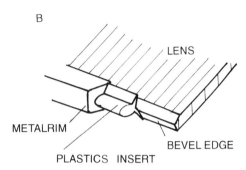

Fig. 4.11 *(A) To the left of the eye size (56) is a tiny screw which secures the closing block screw. Note the faulty plastics insert emerging from the rim above and below the closing block. (B) Diagram showing how one type of plastics insert, acting as 'shock absorber' to the spectacle lens, is secured to the metal rim*

prevent the twisting. Alternatively, the outer of the two screws is replaced by a dowel pin. A silicon inlay is sometimes fitted in the groove of the rim (Fig. 4.11), to prevent (glass) lenses from breaking under strain from the metal rim.

4.3.3 THE BRIDGE AND SURROUND
Plastics pads available for use with metal frames have surfaces varying in size from 90 to 160 mm^2 (Neill, 1978; Eber, 1987). This is considerably smaller than those of plastics pad bridges (see Section 4.2.1), and should be taken into consider-

ation when dealing with heavier spectacle lenses and frame combinations.

Pad arms must be adjustable. Ideally, one should be able to make adjustments in three dimensions. This should facilitate alterations in the distance between pad centres, vertical angle of pad and splay angle. There does not seem to be a single pad arm construction that is suitable for all metal frame designs and constructions (Fig. 4.12). Some experts (Rünz, 1976; Rünz et al., 1977) hold the opinion that a design where a pad could either be made to rock, or be fixed, is best.

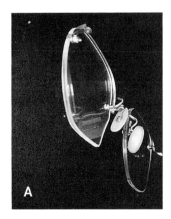
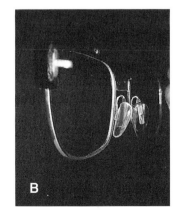
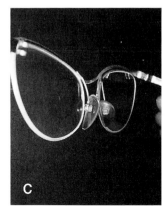

Fig. 4.12 *Three types of pad arm constructions. (A) This type of pad may be fixed, however, when the stud is not sufficiently compressed, it may rock a little. (B) A pad fixed to the pad arm. (C) A pad designed to rock*

This does not quite agree with the ideas set out by Biessels (1954). He argued against the use of rocking pads because the rocking motion tends to make pad top or bottom bury itself in the skin of the nasal flank, depending on the prevailing mechanical forces.

The hardness of the pad arms is another important factor. The dispenser should be able to adjust them with the correct tools, but they should not give way to other mechanical forces exerted on them. If they do, the rims may come to rest on the wearer's cheeks, which is undesirable.

I have come to the conclusion that the saddle bridge is the best type of bridge for any type of mass-produced frame. The plastics saddle insert bridge (see Fig. 11.28) fitted on a number of metal frames, provides a good solution provided it has the correct dimensions for the particular wearer's nose. A credible alternative is the twinned pad construction (see Fig. 11.13). This combines the relatively free adjustability of two pads with the nasal crest 'hugging' effect of the regular bridge. A further advantage is that the twinned pad design can be used as a replacement on a metal pad frame originally fitted with two pads.

Note that any part in the bridge area of the front must be designed in such a way that it will allow any power or type of lens to be properly fitted in that front, without affecting its adjustability.

4.3.4 LUG AND JOINT

The lug should be made of hard metal that is difficult to deform by the forces exerted on it by the side. If the lugs are insufficiently stable, the frame will soon lose its fit. The dimensions and construction of the lug will greatly depend on the frame's design. However, it is desirable that the dispenser, using appropriate tools, is able to make adjustments to both the angles of let-back and of the side if this cannot, or cannot sufficiently, be done at the joints.

At the joint, metal sides should be hard and relatively wide. However, the metal sides of both plastics and metal frames must be flexible. Beyond the joint, the flexibility should increase as the side becomes thinner. In the area of the ear point the profile of the side should be round, which allows adjustments to be made. The plastics tip covering the metal portion should show a gradual increase in thickness starting from well before the ear point.

4.4 Concluding Notes

The vital importance of the bridge has been touched upon. Two ear, nose and throat specialists (Dishoeck & Wal, 1985) drew attention to a problem caused by spectacles affecting breathing through the nose. They pointed out that the bridge of the spectacle frame should rest exclusively on the nasal bone. However, spectacles have a tendency to slide down the nose whereby they come to rest on the cartilage of the nose. A heavy pair of glasses may compress this so that proper breathing through the nose is affected. The patient gets the feeling that his nose is blocked up and that the mucous membranes are irritated. This is often accompanied by a headache resulting from pressure on the nerves. The patient will then start sniffling and may poke fingers in their nose. This will cause greater irritation of the nasal mucosa, which may lead to catarrh and infections such as sinusitis. Having pointed out the responsibility of the dispenser in this context, they stated that the frame manufacturer should provide a greater range of splay angles. They added that frames with large lens apertures are often undesirable because such frames have to be worn lower down the nose as a result of the position with respect to the cheeks. In such cases fashion should give way to a properly fitting, preferably lightweight, pair of spectacles.

Rünz (1976) stipulated that the basic demands of stability, elasticity and adjustability should always take precedence over the fashionable aspects of a frame style, with respect to the above points. Designers and manufacturers do not appear to have taken much notice of these recommendations. Could it be that the constraints are too severe, or that they are ignored for the sake of fashion and for pecuniary reasons.

REFERENCES

Biessels, W.J. (1954). Betere brilaanpassing en brilconstructie. *Oculus, Amsterdam*, No. 2, 2–12.

BS 3172 (EN ISO 11381) (1995). *Specification for Screw Threads for Spectacle Frames.* London: British Standards Institution.

BS 3521 (1991). *Terms Relating to Ophthalmic Optics and Spectacle Frames. Part 2: Glossary of Terms Relating to Spectacle Frames.* London: British Standards Institution.

DIN 58 199 (1989). *Brillenfassungen: Anforderungen und Prüfung.* Berlin: Deutsches Institut für Norming.

DIN 58 216 (1974–80). *Brillen für Fahrzeuglenker; Fassungen und Anpassung.* Berlin: Deutsches Institut für Normung.

DIN 58 226 (1965). *Metallgelenke für Brillenfassungen; Profile.* Berlin: Deutsches Institut für Normung.

DIN 58 227 (1961). *Metallgelenke für Brillenfassungen aus Kunststoff, 5fach geteilt.* Berlin: Deutsches Institut für Normung.

DIN 58 228 (1961). *Metallgelenke für Brillenfassungen aus Kunststoff, 3fach geteilt.* Berlin: Deutsches Institut für Normung.

DIN 58 229 (1966). *Metallgelenke für Brillenfassungen, 5fach geteilt, Rollenanordnung 2–3.* Berlin: Deutsches Institut für Normung.

Dishoeck, E.A. van, & Wal, R.J. van der (1985). De bril op de neus. *Oculus, Amsterdam*, No. 5, 35–37.

Eber, J. (1987). *Anatomische Brillenanpassung.* Heidelberg: Verlag Optische Fachveröffentlichung.

Fahrner, D. (1972). Optyl: a new basic material. Special reprint from *Neues Optikerj.*, Sept. (vol. 13) to Jan. (vol. 14).

Fahrner, D. (1987a). Brillenkunde (2): die Ohren. *Neues Optikerj.* **29**(10), 11–15.

Fahrner, D. (1987b). Brillenkunde (3): die Bügel. *Neues Optikerj.* **29**(11), 23–29.

Harmer, M.A. (1994). Investigation of sprung-hinges in spectacle frames. Final Year Project. London: City University.

ISO 11381 (1994). *Optics and Optical Instruments – Ophthalmic Optics – Screw-Threads.* Genève: International Standards Organization.

Morel, M. (1981). Les charnières dites 'Élastiques'. *Opticien – Lunetier*, No. 338, 50.

Neill, S.T. (1978). Aspects of metal spectacle frame pads. Final Year Project. London: City University.

North, R.V. (1993). *Work and the Eye*, p. 196. Oxford: Oxford University Press.

Ruffel Smith, H.P., & Weale, R.A. (1966). Obstruction of vehicle-drivers' vision by spectacle frames. *Brit. Med. J.* **2**, 445–447.

Rünz, E. (1976). Kriterien der Anpassung und des Tragekomforts moderner Brillenfassungen. Sonderdruck der Wiss. Verein. *Augenoptiker*, **26**, 180–189.

Rünz, E., Köhler, W., Norz, H., & Selwat, K-H. (1977). Kriterien der Anpassung und des Tragekomforts moderner Brillenfassungen. *Optometrie, Mainz* **25**(1), 4–12.

Ward, M.J. (1971). Spectacle joints and assembly. Final Year Project. London: City University.

Weinstein, S. (1968). Intensive and extensive aspects of tactile sensitivity as a function of body part, sex, and laterality. In: Kenshalo, D. R. (ed.) *The Skin Senses*, p. 206. Springfield, IL: C. C. Thomas.

CHAPTER 5

Designing Spectacle Frames

5.1 Introduction

5.1.1 BACKGROUND

Spectacle frames are made in response to a general need for visual aids. This means that different frame styles must be available in different sizes. These should be adjustable so that they can be made to fit the user's head. A good frame should have a form that demonstrates properties that are perfect in use and with which the wearer can identify. One single, neutral and universal frame, even when available in many sizes, will suit only a small proportion of wearers. Fahrner (1988) expressed the opinion that one single fashion frame, available in one size only, will fit, at best, no more than 1% of spectacle wearers.

5.1.2 APPROACH

Gathmann's (1977) paper appears to be the only one that deals with spectacle frame design from the designer's viewpoint. The following, in which many aspects of Mayall's (1979) design principles may be recognized, has been adapted from Gathmann's (1977) paper.

The spectacle frame designer's continuing task is to give new forms to spectacle frames. His work covers not only the overall form of the frame, but also the design of its constituent parts. Design work begins with the evaluation of the following considerations:

(1) Marketing: relationship with consumer, retailer, competitor, etc.
(2) Costs: materials, production, marketing, glazing, purchasing price.

(3) Human aspects: acceptability, relation to its surround (face/head), current fashion.
(4) Construction: application of new technology, production processes and materials, adherence to (inter)national standards.
(5) Production: unit cost, capacity.
(6) Optical workshop aspects: instrumentation, lens materials, uncut lens sizes, glazing, etc.

These stages should be followed by an investigation of comparable frames produced by competitors for the same group of wearers. Such frames may be analysed under the following headings:

(1) Form: assortment of lens aperture shapes and sizes, the sectional shape of the rim, and its strength.
(2) Material: manufacturing process of the product, strength, surface quality, structural aspects, etc.
(3) Colour: manufacturing process, producer's range and patterns, availability, etc.
(4) Function: ease of glazing and adjustment, fit of sides, etc.

Note that an aspect of overriding importance for patient and dispenser, namely that of the fit of the bridge, is not mentioned. Unfortunately, this appears to typify the approach of many contemporary designers.

This analysis should enable the designer to formulate for a frame a form concept where:

● the new frame form should present a genuine alternative to current models and might set a trend for further designs

- it should allow minor adjustments to be made enabling the dispenser to achieve the best possible and comfortable fit without undue difficulty
- the action of the frame should be simple. This will also reflect on the production and servicing costs
- the purchasing price should not be above that of comparable models. This should also be kept in mind at the design stage.

With the help of extensive studies of models, the relationship between head and frame should be ascertained for every new model.

Such studies should present alternative models that have a good fit, are technically perfect and aesthetically pleasing. Note that this scheme provides only a basis for the creative design process because a spectacle frame is a product where the designer has a relatively small degree of freedom because of anatomical and optical constraints. Therefore, the designer must possess a great deal of knowledge in order to exploit these creative constraints and provide feasible, aesthetic solutions.

5.2 Design

5.2.1 PROCEDURE

The considerations discussed in the previous section may lead to the following design procedure:

- Find and retain possible solutions through design sketches.
- Produce selected types and shapes of models, and modify them where required.
- Create alternative models, compare these with the requirements laid down in the design concept, and make a selection from these.
- Produce samples of the selected models in appropriate sizes and colours, and build up a structured assortment.

- Produce the design and detailed production drawings.

Gathmann (1977) adds a caution – although such a scheme is likely to lead to the development of a new model, it does not necessarily follow that it will be a commercial success. Hardy (1967), a long-standing observer wrote 'Precisely what qualities ensure success for a frame design remain unknown factors'.

5.2.2 BRITISH REQUIREMENTS

The British Standard BS 6625* (1985) *Specification for Spectacle Frames* contains two relevant paragraphs in Appendix F.1. They are outlined below.

Design considerations

The frame should be designed to provide secure placement and retention of lenses† in the prescribed position relative to the eyes.

Materials

The materials used must be sufficiently stable to satisfy the design considerations, but also allow adjustment and final fitting by the retailer.

5.2.3 GERMAN REQUIREMENTS

DIN 58 199 (1989) lays down some further, minimum design requirements. These are:

- An expertly chosen and fitted frame should facilitate complaint-free wear.
- The sides must be permanently connected to the front.
- Having been properly fitted, sides should retain their shape.

---

*At the time of publication, a Draft for Public Comment of BS 6625 : Part 1 had been published. This draft corresponded to pr EN ISO 12870: *Ophthalmic Optics – Spectacle Frames – Fundamental Requirements and Test Methods*.

†See BS 7394.

- When properly adjusted, the elasticity of the front and joints, together with the elasticity of the sides, should facilitate a secure fit.
- It should be possible either to shorten sides, or exchange them. At least three side lengths, in steps of 5 mm, should be available.
- Lugs must be designed so that joints or similar parts can be fixed permanently. Together, they must be able to withstand adjustments in addition to normal wear and tear.
- The spring-action of a pair of sprung joints must be approximately equal when opened equally far. The tension should increase proportionally with the size of the angle of let-back. From the moment such sides are opened beyond their point of rest, the force along the drop of the side must act as under conditions of wear.
- The bridge and adjoining parts must be able to withstand the constant demands made upon them during adjustment and normal wear.
- The angle of side should be adjustable by ±3°.
- It must be possible to distribute the anticipated combined mass of frame and lenses over an easily adjustable bridge bearing surface. The useful total area of the bridge bearing surface must measure at least 250 mm^2 for frames with a mass of up to 25 g, and at least 300 mm^2 when the mass is greater.
- Frame parts that may be in contact with the skin must be smooth to the touch. Any corners present near the opened sides should be rounded.

5.2.4 OMISSIONS

Not mentioned in the above sections are important requirements such as:

- Best use should be made of the natural field of view.
- Facial measurements outside the 'normal' range, and other features, should be accommodated.

- The best cosmetic effect should be secured.
- The anticipated life of the spectacle frame should be taken into account.

The contents of these lists were checked against design requirements of Taylor (1907), RAL (1961), Passet (1966), Clayton (1970), Fleck *et al.* (1970) and Fahrner (1988).

5.2.5 SOVIET REQUIREMENTS

A different approach is encountered in the Soviet standard Gost 18491–79. This lays down very specific requirements of which we quote the following:

Basic sizes

- Horizontal box lens size   34–60 mm
- Vertical box lens size   >27 mm
- Distance between lenses   10–28 mm in 1 mm steps
- Length to bend   55–115 mm in 5 mm steps
- Length of drop   30–50 mm
- Length of curl (ear point to end)   60–80 mm

Technical requirements

- The rim around the lenses, shall have a radius of 90 to 160 mm (to accept curved lenses).
- The let-back shall be 90 ± 5°.
- The groove in the rim shall be 0·5–1·2 mm deep for enclosed angles of 80–100°, and 0·3 to 1·0 mm deep for angles of 90–110°.
- The frontal angle shall measure 15–40° and the splay angle 20–30°, both ±10%.
- The height of crest is fixed at 3 mm above the horizontal centre line; the pads are to be placed at an unspecified distance below this line.
- The sides are to be curved along the line of the side: measured at a point 20–30 mm from the dowel point along the sides, the radius is to be 160 to 450 mm, convex towards the head. The inside curve of the drop shall be concave towards the head, with a radius of 20–30 mm

measured from a point 5–10 mm from the end.

- Plastics sides should be elastic along their whole length, and the edges should be well-rounded.
- The joint angle shall be $10 \pm 2°$, and the downwards angle of drop $60 \pm 5°$.
- The side should be able to withstand the application of 5.0 N along the axis of the joint.
- The plastics material should show no more than three bubbles of $0·15–0·25$ mm cm^{-2}.
- The shearing strength between components should be 50 ± 5 N, and the pad arms must be able to withstand 20 ± 2 N. The impact resistance shall be 30 mc^{-2}.
- Joints should withstand a minimum of 15 000 opening/closing cycles and have an actual life span of 3 years and 30 000 opening/closing cycles.

5.2.6 US REQUIREMENTS

American National Standard ANSI Z80.5–1979 provides some performance requirements. These are to be met by the frame manufacturer. They cover the following aspects: lens retention, frame performance, providing secure placement of the lenses before the eyes, bridge function and the visual field where the frame should create minimal impairment. For plastics frames a 'bridge test for minimum performance' is given. However, this test is not concerned with the fit of the bridge on the wearer's nose.

5.2.7 MISCELLANEOUS ASPECTS

With respect to vehicle driving, Bewley (1970) pointed out that whereas the average subject's binocular field of view without a spectacle frame was 196°, a frame could reduce this by 46–68°, depending on the style of frame. This lateral obstruction is reduced when the vertex distance is short, the horizontal lens size is large, the rim is thin, the sides are thin and the frame has high joints. See also Section 4.2.2 (Ruffell Smith & Weale, 1966).

With respect to a particular type of frame material, namely rolled gold, Barker *et al.* (1932) wrote that its durability depends on the combination of carat gold and base metal, the complete covering of gold over all exposed parts, and the adequate thickness of the gold laminate in those parts that come into contact with the wearer.

Correspondence and discussions with spectacle frame designers and manufacturers, and also dispensers, provided the following additional points. One dispenser maintained that only dispensers should design spectacle frames because they are aware of the technical difficulties and requirements. One manufacturer felt that a knowledge of production techniques is necessary to ensure that the frames can be mass produced; he added that a designer needs flair and should be capable of producing hand-made frames.

5.3 Practical Approach

Spectacle frames touch the head at three points – at the ear points and in the nasal area. The latter, however, is of greatest importance because it is here that the major bearing surface and area of contact between front and face is situated. Therefore, the designer of a plastics frame should start by deciding on a bridge height, frontal angle and angle of crest. The designer of a metal or combination frame must consider the configuration of the eye rim in the nasal area, and the type of pads or bridge insert that can be used with that design. The other constraint is the frontal width, which usually corresponds with the temporal width of the head. The position and shape of the eyebrows and cheek bones are of lesser importance. However, they do matter when deciding for which facial shape (see Section 14.2.2) the design is meant. Here, the lens aperture shape of the front may be a deciding factor or take precedence over the facial features.

Sides form an integral part of a frame. It is

therefore necessary to complete the design by deciding on the type of lug, joint and shape of side to complement the front. Availability of types of joints and ready-made sides may influence the designer's and manufacturer's choice.

5.4 Refinements

Köhler (1979) suggested that designer and dispenser confer on this subject. Whereas shortcomings of a design with respect to rims, joints and sides can be rectified in good time by a skilled technician, the nasal bearing surface, the bridge and also the form and type of side and its drop are often approached with distaste rather than interest, and often with hope rather than experience. Köhler (1979) maintained that prototype frames should be discussed with dispensers who have experience with fitting and adjustment problems. The dispenser should speak his mind, express preferences, make suggestions and provide constructive criticism.

When modifications to produce an optimum fit have been made, the frame should be fitted to a number of faces belonging to the group of patients targeted by the designer. Observations of the actual fit, and the blending of face and front, may indicate further desirable modifications. Köhler (1979) stressed in particular the importance of the bridge design, which can only be judged from an actual front and not from a drawing.

Next, a revised model should be made and the process repeated. It may then transpire that, for instance, the frontal angle needs to be altered. The insight and suggested modifications thus accumulated should lead to a new round of discussions. The object of the exercise is to improve only the fit of the nasal bearing surface and does not address the lens shape of the front. Hence, the essence of the design will not have been altered.

Köhler (1979) expressed the opinion that the hallmark of fruitful cooperation between designer and dispenser is the beauty of the product. The more accomplished the design, the less attention needs to be drawn to it. The less the wearer is aware of the spectacles on their face, the better the fit of the frame and blend with facial anatomy.

After creation of the design on paper (Fig. 5.1), a hand-made prototype is produced (Fig. 5.2). If the design was created with the help of a CAD (computer-aided design) program (Fig. 5.3), its prototype can be made by CAM (computer-aided manufacture) (Fig. 5.4). Refinements can then be made to this model until the designer is satisfied with it. For plastics, or plastics parts of a frame, the material and/or the colour pattern has to be chosen. Different effects, such as facets, can be added by working the surfaces with shaped cutters. These also facilitate the production of colour effects and patterns when veneered plastics are used. Alternatively, patterns may be printed onto the surface, or etched into it and filled with enamel.

5.5 Production

Once a prototype has been approved, the so-called tooling-up process for mass production (selection, production or acquisition of machine tools, setting up of production lines, etc.) may take up to 6 weeks to complete (Goodwin, 1983).

5.6 Comments

Since the 1970s 'famous' designers and fashion creators have dabbled with spectacle frames. Dowaliby (1987) wrote: 'While the original sketching of products bearing their name is often done by talented assistants, in comparing most designer eyewear with conventionally styled

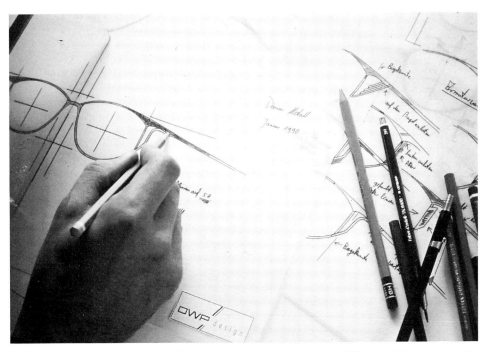

Fig. 5.1 Drawing stage of a spectacle frame design (photograph courtesy of Optische Werke Passau, Passau, Germany)

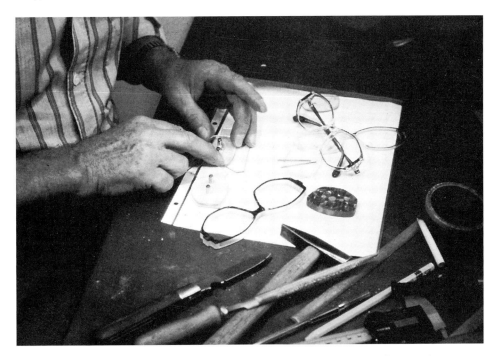

Fig. 5.2 Making of a prototype spectacle frame (photograph courtesy of Optische Werke Passau)

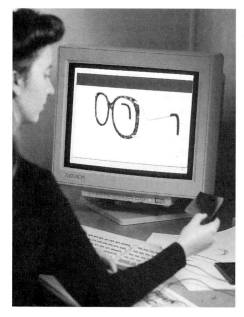

Fig. 5.3 *Computer-aided design (CAD) of a spectacle frame (photograph courtesy Cambridge Optical Company, Cambridge, UK)*

frames it is clear that a famed artist was involved in the conceptual process'; it is good to see that she adds 'Yet it must be recognized that a famed designer sometimes misjudges current taste'. Whether, and to what extent the famous designer was involved, may perhaps be judged from Brogan's (1992) investigation although note another statement by Dowaliby (1987) that 'Christian Dior died almost four decades ago, but it is common practice to continue using a famed name for fashion identification'. With respect to actual designers, perhaps Mayall (1979) hits the nail on the head: 'Designers are not well known

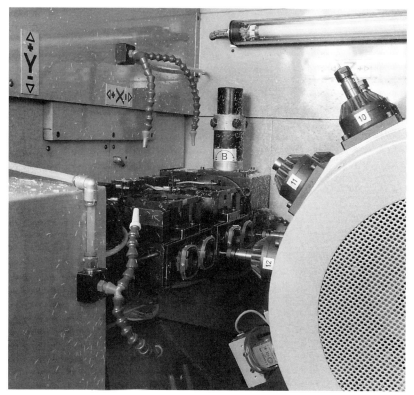

Fig. 5.4 *Computer-aided manufacturing equipment producing two spectacle fronts (photograph courtesy Cambridge Optical Company, Cambridge, UK)*

for talking about what they do; in fact they are not well known at all'. In the field of spectacle frame design in Europe, it is difficult to find even a handful of names at any one time, although there are tens of spectacle frame factories.

Since the early 1990s, some 'famed designers' have started to develop wild creations, apparently without experience in this field, whereby the actual purpose of the visual aid has been forgotten. These designers should keep an important constraint in mind, namely the function of the object. To paraphrase Read (1953) – it is interesting to note the persistence, in the modern spectacle form, of the basic design of the sixteenth century. It is unlikely that there is any conscious imitation: the forms are in each case functional; and the function being constant, there is little scope for appropriate variation. The departure from this limitation has gone so far that now one can find only a continuously reducing number of really well-assorted and adjustable frames. Even when the dispenser is familiar with the criteria for a well-fitting frame, he may be forced by fashion to make purchases against better judgement (Käpernick, 1982).

This trend has gone so far that a correspondent reviewing an optical fair, wrote that he 'was not the only man watching who found the models more alluring than the monstrous frames they wore. The emphasis was on "designer" frames and provided that the frame carried the logo of a famous fashion house the design itself seemed to be of secondary importance' (Anonymous, 1985). One can but point to the many problems that such frames can cause to wearer and dispenser alike. The dispenser may not be able to overcome these problems because the designer and/or manufacturer have left no room for reasonable adjustments to be effected. These are sad comments, echoed by a number of dispensing colleagues.

To reiterate, two points should never be overlooked: (1) the usefulness and comfortable wear of the product must be optimized so that the wearer is provided with a well-fitting spectacle frame that can be worn without any aggravation; and (2) spectacle frames are to be transformed through glazing with the required lenses into a visual aid. Some spectacle frame manufacturers do take account of these points. The firms that (still) offer to make a frame with measurements outside their normal production range are examples. Other manufacturers have carefully researched the nasal fit, and design frames around this while avoiding extreme forms (Anonymous, 1989).

Although some spectacle frame manufacturers advertise their wares to the public, one must not forget that, in the end, the patient will remember that they obtained the spectacles from Optician X or Optometrist Y. This identification of the spectacle frame with its provider demands reflection on the associated responsibilities concerned with range of measurements available, quality, and adjustability of the frames on offer. Köhler (1979) concluded that, if these obligations were taken seriously, many frames produced by many manufacturers should be excluded from one's collection.

There are exceptions on this rule: one is aware of spectacle wearers (more often, sunglass wearers) who wear their glasses only as a fashion accessory, or for psychological reasons. Such wearers may exempt themselves from these aspects, as do those who acquire a pair of 'fun' glasses (Fig. 5.5). The majority of wearers, however, indicate that fashion trends are unimportant. A German survey (reported by Kölbe, 1987) produced the averaged results shown in Table 5.1. Note that design/form/colour was given the lowest score on the importance scale and that only 29% of the participants said that it was the most important factor when deciding on a new spectacle frame. From a British survey (Pilkington, 1991), fashion trends appear unimportant, with only 1% saying they replaced their

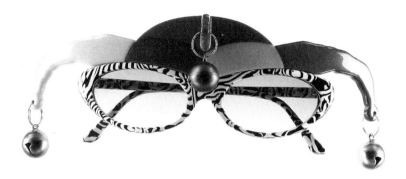

Fig. 5.5 Fun glasses: model 'Joker' (courtesy Anglo American Eyewear Co., London, UK)

TABLE 5.1 *Importance of spectacle frame aspects (after Kölbe, 1987)*

	Importance scale	Judged very important by (%)
1. **Perfect fit**	1.2	80
2. **Lightness of frame**	1.5	58
3. **Quality**	1.6	54
4. **Price**	1.7	44
5. **Design/form/colour**	2.1	29

Scale values: 1, very important; 4, unimportant.

spectacles because they wanted a more modern pair.

Alain Mikli, the optician-spectacle frame designer, is alleged to have said: 'Fashion? There is no such thing in the nineties. The notion "fashion" has become extinct, if ever it existed. Today you wear whatever takes your fancy. Every day brings another comedy: that's what it's all about in the nineties' (Andressen, 1994).

REFERENCES

Andressen, B.M. (1994). *Brillen des 20. Jahrhunderts.* München: Klinkhardt & Biermann.

Anonymous (1985). Silmo, Paris, 1985. *Optom. Today* **25**(23), 765, 766, 769.

Anonymous (1989). Stepper International: 'Wir forcieren die tragbare Brille'. *Neues Optiker.* **31**(11), 38–39.

ANSI Z80.5 1979. *American National Standard Requirements for Dress Ophthalmic Frames.* New York: American National Standards Institute, Inc.

Barker, W.B., Champness, W.H., Courlander, H., Dadd, F.W., Harwood, J., & Sutcliffe, J.H. (1932). *Enquiry into the Manufacture of Gold-filled Spectacles.* London: Joint Council of Qualified Opticians.

Bewley, L.A. (1970). Spectacle frames cause traffic hazards. *J. Maryland Optom. Assoc.* **3**(3) 8–10.

BS 6625 (1985). *Specification for Spectacle Frames.* London: British Standards Institution.

BS 7394 (1994). *Complete Spectacles. Part 2: Specification for Prescription Spectacles; Annex E: Lens retention test.* London: British Standards Institution.

Brogan, R. (1992). All in the name. *Optician* **203**(5353), 24–30.

Clayton, G.H. (1970). *Spectacle Frame Dispensing.* London: Assoc. Dispensing Opticians.

DIN 58 199 (1989). *Brillenfassungen: Anforderungen und Prüfung.* Berlin: Deutsches Institut für Normung.

Dowaliby, M. (1987). *The Art of Eyewear Dispensing.* Fullerton, CA: Southern California College of Optometry.

Fahrner, D. (1988). Brillenkunde (4): Die Köpfe. *Neues Optikerj.* **30**(10), 18.

Fleck, H., Heynig, J., Mütze, K., & Schwarz, G. (1970). *Sehhilfenanpassung.* Berlin: VEB Verlag Technik.

Goodwin, R. (1983) *Manufacture of Plastic Frames. New Insight* No. 1, p. 10. Tonbridge: Invicta Frames Ltd.

GOST 18491–79. *Spectacle Frames for Corrective Eye-glasses. General Specification.* Reprint 1985, revision no. 1. Moscow: Gosudarstvennij Komitet SSSR po Standartam.

Gathmann, L. (1977). Design der Brillenfassungen. *Neues Optikerj.* **19**(8), 662.

Hardy, W.E. (1967). Unknown factors in frame styling. *Manuf. Optics Int.* **20**(3), 130–133.

Käpernick, E. (1982). Die Brille ist eine Federwaage. *Deutsche Optikerz.* No. 11, 53–55.

Köhler, W. (1979). Zusammenarbeit zwischen Augenoptiker und Designer. *Deutsche Optikerz.* No. 2, 20–29.

Kölbe, M.J. (1987). Mode contra Technik. *Neues Optikerj.* **29**(7), 42–44.

Mayall, W.H. (1979). *Principles in Design.* London: Design Council/Heinemann Educational Books.

Passet, R. (1966). *Lunetterie.* Paris: Société Industrielle de Lunetterie.

Passet, R. (1974). Prises de mesures et adaptation en lunetterie. *Optométrie* **20**, nos. 2–5 (reprint).

Pilkington Special Glass (1991). *Spectacle Wearers Consumer Survey.* Manchester: Delphi Associates.

RAL (1961). *Güte Bestimmung im Augenoptikerhandwerk.* RAL–RG 915. Frankfurt: RAL/Beuth-Vertrieb GmbH.

Read, H. (1953). *Art and Industry,* 3rd edn. London: Faber & Faber.

Ruffel Smith, H.P., & Weale, R.A. (1966). Obstruction of vehicle-drivers' vision by spectacle frames. *Brit. Med. J.,* **2**, 445–447.

Taylor, H.L. (1907). *The Manipulation and Fitting of Ophthalmic Frames.* Birmingham: J. & H. Taylor.

CHAPTER 6

Materials: Introduction

6.1 Requirements

British Standard BS 6625, Part 1 (1992), *Specification of Spectacle Frames**, contains one paragraph in Appendix F.1 on materials. It states, in part, the following:

'*F.1.2 Materials.*

The materials used need to be sufficiently stable to satisfy the considerations in F.1.1 (see Section 5.2.2), but also need to allow adjustment and fitting by the retailer. The materials have to resist degradation sufficiently to make the frame acceptable for use over a reasonable period. Care is necessary to exclude from frame materials any that may cause skin irritation, toxic reaction or other harm during wear or during adjustment.'

It goes on to say how such reactions may occur.

A more specific list of properties and requirements for materials for spectacle frames is:

(1) Mechanical: hardness (the resistance to cutting and surface indentation)

toughness (the resistance against breaking and shock)

tensile strength (the maximum force the material can stand in tension, compression, torque and shear without breaking)

ductility (the length to which the material can be stretched without breaking)

elasticity (the length to which the material can be stretched and return to its original length when released).

---

*While going to print, a Draft for Public Comment (prEN ISO 12870), entitled '*Ophthalmic Optics – Spectacle Frames – Fundamental Requirements and Test Methods*' which is a revision of BS 6625: Part 1, had been issued.

(2) Dimensional stability, but it must be sufficiently soft to make adjustments that facilitate a comfortable fit on the wearer's head.

(3) Low density, that is, light in weight.

(4) Corrosion resistance to both atmospheric and human agents (physiological products such as skin secretions, and cosmetics).

(5) Suitability to undergo a great variety of fabrication processes.

(6) Good aesthetic properties, or to accept and retain surface treatments for this purpose.

(7) Inexpensive.

Quantification of these requirements is difficult. However, tests such as those set out in BS 6625 take care of this aspect in a practical manner.

6.2 Materials – General

Materials used for spectacle frame manufacture may be classified as follows:

- 'bio-based' materials: wood, bone, horn and tortoise shell, leather, miscellaneous
- synthesized materials: metals, alloys and laminated metals (see Chapter 8)
- 'bio-based' and synthesized materials: plastics (see Chapter 7).

Most bio-based spectacle frame materials have properties that are referred to as thermosetting and thermoplastic. Thermosetting properties are ascribed to materials that, in the final stage of production, set or harden while heated into a fixed shape. Such objects will not soften when reheated; they will burn or melt instead. An example is the spectacle lens material CR39.

Thermosetting materials are unsuitable for use in spectacle frames because the dispenser must be able to make adjustments to frames. Thermoplastics materials soften when heated and harden during cooling. When softened they can be re-shaped. When kept in their new form during cooling, they will remain in that shape. The frame material Optyl (Chapter 7) has been described variously as a thermosetting and a thermoplastic material, probably because it has a 'plastics memory' – having been deformed while heated and kept in the new form during the cooling process, it will return to its original shape when reheated.

6.2.1 BIO-BASED MATERIALS

Spectacle frame materials derived from biological substances have almost completely been superseded by artificial materials. However, spectacle frames made from such materials are available from a small number of specialist manufacturers.

6.2.1.1 Wood

The first spectacle frames (fronts; see Section 2.2: *1350*) may well have been made of wood (see Figs 2.2 and 6.5). Material from the genus *Buxus* (boxwood) of small, evergreen trees and shrubs, the beech and lime (linden) trees as well as bamboo, has been used. For further information see Appuhn (1958) and Fairbanks (1955)

Characteristics of wood:

- fibrous
- hard
- light
- yellow tinged
- swells and shrinks little, depending on variation in humidity.

Rims are closed by means of a coarse thread screw (as used in wood). Imitation 'wooden'

frames have been made in both cellulose nitrate and acetate, and may have a grained appearance.

6.2.1.2 Bone

Fish bone and bone from mammals have been used for the manufacture of spectacle frames. Use was restricted to larger, flat bones from large animals such as oxen, whale (Fig. 6.1), bear,

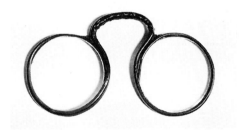

Fig. 6.1 *A frame made of whale bone*

buffalo and bull. Because the antlers of deer are solid and round in section, it is not possible to cut a flat front shape out of it. Ivory, which shows growth rings, should not be confused with bone, which does not show such rings. (For further information see: Rohr 1923–4; Fairbanks, 1955; Armitage, 1982; Rhodes, 1982; Franks, 1993; MacGregor, 1996.)

6.2.1.3 Horn and tortoiseshell

Both materials have always been expensive because they are not available in abundance and must be worked by specialist craftsmen (Hardy & Hardy, 1982). Hence, they have a certain appeal which has led to imitations, especially of the tortoiseshell pattern, in the early artificial spectacle frame materials.

Both materials are derived from the epidermis of the skin, and are composed of protein.

Horn is produced from the cavitied bones of ruminating animals (those that chew the cud). Having been kept in cold water for 2–6 weeks, the horn can be removed from its bony base.

When the solid tip has been sawn off, the tubular remainder is placed in boiling water for some hours. While being kept warm it is cut lengthwise and flattened under pressure. Chemical treatment with molten talc (magnesium silicate) improves its transparency. It is also possible to alter its appearance by dying, staining and bleaching. Cheaper horn can be made to look like tortoise shell.

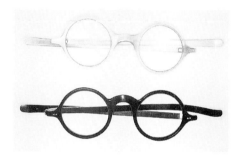

Fig. 6.2 Above: a translucent horn frame; below: a black horn frame

Characteristics of horn:

- warm, natural colours varying from creamy translucent crystal to brown and black (Fig. 6.2)
- light in weight
- does not cause allergic skin reactions
- expands a little when heated
- returns to its original dimensions when cooled
- takes a good polish
- flakes easily
- difficult to work
- cannot be joined (spliced)
- does not warp
- durable
- hard, likely to dry out and become very brittle
- unaffected by skin secretions.

Horn may be recognized by signs of flaking and the turbid appearance of crystal parts. Spec-tacle frames are likely to be fitted with so-called metal-to-metal joints (Fig. 6.3), to prevent the material from splitting.

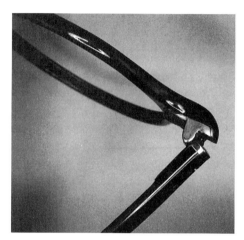

Fig. 6.3 A metal-to-metal joint on a tortoiseshell frame

Tortoiseshell is obtained from turtles. This is the name for marine species of tortoises (Rudloe & Rudloe, 1994), reptiles whose bodies are encased in a shell. This consists of curved, upper carapace (back) and flat, lower plastron (breast plate) which are joined at the sides. The species from which the semi-transparent tortoiseshell is obtained are the hawksbill, greenback and loggerhead turtles. They live in tropical seas with a minimum temperature of 25°C, as found in the East and West Indies, and around Madagascar.

The carapace consists of 13 overlapping plates; there are about 22 plastron plates and 25 V-shaped hoofs (that is, horny casings) from a rim between back and breast plate. The thin plastron plates are yellow orange while the hoofs are part yellow, part mottled. All plates have a 'skin' and a 'sand' side. Plates vary in size from about 55 × 20 to 17 × 17 cm.

Colour grading and cost (Fig. 6.4):

- blonde (amber) (most expensive)

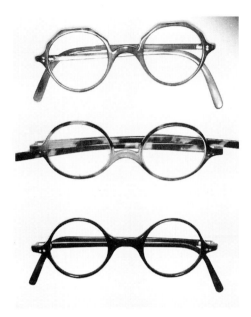

Fig. 6.4 Tortoiseshell frames. Above, demi-blonde; middle, dark mottled; below, dark. Note differences in bridge/crest height

- demi-blonde (amber with pale red splashes)
- red mottled
- even red
- dark-mottled
- dark (almost black or brown) (least expensive)

Characteristics of tortoiseshell:

- thermoplastic
- stable under normal conditions: it retains its shape perfectly
- hard
- resilient, but brittle
- takes and retains a very good polish
- mediocre strength
- good corrosion resistance
- flammability: no continuous combustion (tested according to BS 6625, 1992), and smells of burning flesh
- density: approximately 1.3 g cm^{-3}.

Turtle shell is the only natural horny material that may be joined (spliced) on the application of heat and steady pressure. It behaves like a thermoplastic material such that adjacent plates can be made to fit perfectly. This is due to its glutinous (sticky) nature and the superficial films of shell which liquify when heated. It is said that only the shell of animals that died of natural causes can be used (Hinterhofer & Fahrner, 1983; Hoffmann, 1987; Fairbanks, 1955).

Turtles are protected under The Convention on International Trade in Endangered Species of Wild Fauna and Flora (CITES) which came into force in 1975. This prohibits international commercial trade in the species listed because they are threatened with extinction; turtles are listed in Appendix I of CITES. An exception applies to parts of animals that were 'removed from nature' before 1976 (Lyster, 1985; Rudloe & Rudloe, 1994).

One German tortoiseshell spectacle frame manufacturer claimed to hold a patent which enables him to use shell remnants that had previously been unusable. It is these parts that are available in large quantities in the West Indies. They are locally treated and transformed, without the use of solvent, into shell suitable for spectacle frame manufacture (Spangemacher, 1984; MacGregor *et al.*, 1992).

Tortoiseshell fronts tend to have traditional eye shapes of relatively small diameter (<40 mm). The joints, sometimes made of gold (alloy), are metal-to-metal joints (Fig. 6.3), to prevent the material splitting. The joints are almost invariably pinned to the sides and front. They are likely to contain a dowel pin instead of a screw and may show a high degree of workmanship. The rims, bridge, lugs and sides are thin, and the drops are usually short. When the ends of the sides are made to touch, they make a distinctive ticking sound. Fronts are almost invariably made with a regular bridge which may be inset. The depth and colour of the mottled pattern is irregular.

6.2.1.4 Leather

This material was used in medieval times. Experts agree that surviving leather spectacles (see Fig. 2.6) were made using the *cuir-bouilli* technique but not much is known about this. However, Waterer (1956) quotes the following description: 'pieces of leather must be boiled in wax mixed with resin and glue. Once boiled in this manner, the leather preserves whilst it is moist, sufficient pliability to enable it to be moulded, and when it is dry it possesses a hardness and rigidity nearly equal to that of wood to which it is preferable by reason of its lightness'.

6.2.1.5 Miscellaneous

Eskimos carved snow spectacles out of walrus ivory, and used sinew, hides and grass fibre to

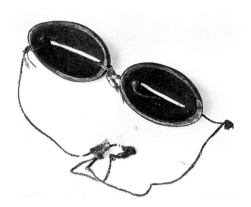

Fig. 6.5 Wooden snow goggles used by Eskimos

make bands or cords (Fig. 6.5) that kept these spectacles in position (Mandville, 1976).

Shark skin, cork and mole skin have been used to line pads (Neill, 1987).

REFERENCES

Appuhn, H. (1958). Ein gedenkwürdiger Fund. *Zeiss Werkzeitschr.,* **27**, 2–8.

Armitage, P. (1982). Note on the source of the material used in the manufacture of the spectacles. (Appendix to: Rhodes, M. (1982). A pair of fifteenth-century spectacle frames from the City of London). *Antiquaries J.* **62**, 1, 67–69.

BS 6625, Part I (1992). *Specification for Spectacle Frames.* London: British Standards Institution.

Fairbanks, P. (1955). Lecture notes. London: Northampton Polytechnic.

Franks, A. (1993). *The Seeing Eye.* Jersey (Channel Islands): Arthur Franks (private publication).

Hardy, S., & Hardy, W.E. (1982). Frame materials: a perspective; part I. *Manuf. Optics Int.* **35**, 6, 18–23.

Hinterhofer, O., & Fahrner, D. (1983). *Materialkunde für Augenoptiker.* 2nd edn. p. 9. Pforzheim: Verlag Postenrieder.

Hoffmann, J. (1987). Neue Verglasungsanleitung für Naturhorn. *Neues Optikerj.* **29**, 5, 34.

Lyster, S. (1985). *International Wildlife Law,* pp. 240, 263. Cambridge: Grotius.

MacGregor, R.J.S. (1996). Whalebone spectacles. In: MacGregor, R.J.S. (ed.) *Ophthalmic Antiques Extracts 1986–1996,* p. 34. West Kilbride, Ayrshire: Ophthal. Antiques Int. Collectors' Club.

MacGregor, R.J.S., Orr, H., Davidson, D.C. & Eadon-Allen, S. (1992). Real tortoiseshell. *Ophthalm. Antiq. Int. Collectors Newsl. (UK)* **41**, 3–8.

Mandville, R. (1976). The Eskimo and their method of eye protection. Final year project. London: City University.

Neill, S.T. (1978). Aspects of metal spectacle frame pads. Final year project. London: City University.

Rohr, M. von. (1923–4). The Thomas Young Oration. *Trans Optical Soc.* **25**(2), 41–71.

Rudloe, A., & Rudloe, J. (1994). Sea turtles in a race for survival. *Natl Geographic Mag.* **185**(2), 94–120.

Spangemacher, J. (1984). Schutzkategorie Anhang I. *Focus,* **5**, 54–58.

Waterer, J.W. (1956). *Leather in Life, Art and Industry,* p. 43. London: Faber & Faber.

Materials: Plastics

Plastic – an adjective meaning semi-solid, semi-fluid, pliable, flexible.

Plastics – a generic term for an arbitrary group of materials based on synthetic or modified natural polymers which, at some stage of manufacture, can be shaped by flow, aided in many cases by heat and pressure. This term may be used as a noun, singular or plural, and as an adjective. See BS 1755, 1982.

7.1 History

Synthetic plastic material has been in existence since the early 1860s. The subsequent development of materials relevant to spectacle frames is summarized below.

The discovery of nitrocellulose or cellulose nitrate, led to the commercial production of plastics in the 1870s. There were initial problems but by 1890 the product known as zylonite (see Hardy & Hardy, 1982) or xylonite, and colloquially abbreviated to 'zyl' in North America or celluloid (North America and elsewhere), had become established as an alternative to ivory. It was used, among other things, for knife handles. Unfortunately, cellulose nitrate is flammable and, therefore, potentially dangerous. In material for spectacle frames, a change from clear or single colour to imitation tortoiseshell took place after the First World War.

Cellulose acetate was developed around 1900, and was in commercial production at the commencement of the First World War (1914). During the war years it was applied as a dope to coat the fabric used to cover wooden aeroplane structures, thus making them waterproof. After the war there was a large surplus of production capacity which was then used to produce acetate rayon (artificial silk) for the textile industry.

Although cellulose acetate was much less flammable than cellulose nitrate, it did not have the same depth of colour and was more brittle. Notwithstanding these disadvantages, cellulose nitrate was used as a spectacle frame material until the mid-1960s.

Because of the potential fire hazard, insurance companies demanded ever-increasing premiums to cover the risks. The public also became more and more concerned, and as a result, cellulose nitrate was banned in a number of European countries.

Casein is derived from skimmed milk by the action of rennet, precipitating a solid which forms into a plastics material. It was used for a decade, from 1925. It was not a satisfactory alternative in that it was brittle, affected by even weak acids and alkalis, and could not be moulded. It deteriorates rapidly under normal conditions of patient use (see Brydson, 1975).

In the 1930s acrylic resin with trade names as Lucite, Oroglas, Perspex and Plexiglas, became commercially available. Spectacle frames made of this material were widely available in the late 1950s and early 1960s in the UK. It was also the major material from which contact lenses were made at that time.

Polyamides were developed before the Second World War and commercial production started in 1940. By 1965 spectacle frames were manufactured out of nylon, the generic name for the fibre-forming polyamides. However, it was not until the early 1980s that polyamides and co-polyamides were developed specifically for spectacle frame production. Spectacle frames made of nylon reinforced with carbon fibre appeared in the mid-1980s.

Cellulose acetate butyrate was also developed before the Second World War. It was used for injection-moulded sunglasses, contact lenses, sunglass lenses and industrial eye protectors in the 1970s (Clarke, 1978).

Cellulose propionate started to be used for spectacle frames in the early 1980s. A number of initial problems had to be overcome before it became a successful spectacle frame material used mainly for injection moulding.

The origins of the epoxy resin frame material Optyl (Obstfeld, 1988), introduced in 1964, dates back to a patent taken out in 1934.

The information in this section is summarized from Bedwell (1960), Clarke (1978), Davidson (1989), Grant (1982), Green (1963), Hardy (1982a,b), Hardy & Hardy (1982), Obstfeld (1988) and Redfarn (1951).

7.2 General Properties and Requirements for Spectacle Frames

Plastics become unserviceable at temperatures upwards of about 100°C. Their toughness (ability to absorb energy before breaking) is less than that of steel or aluminium, their surface hardness (ability to withstand scratching) is less than that of aluminium, and their abrasion resistance (ability to withstand rubbing) varies from substance to substance. All plastics can be destroyed by heat; their brittleness (breaking without much permanent distortion) varies a great deal.

In principle, the requirements for plastics materials for spectacle frames are no different from those set out in Section 6.1 for spectacle frame materials in general. However, because of their nature, a few additional notes are appropriate.

Although plastics generally do not have the same toughness as metals, polyamides are very strong indeed. Their dimensional stability is not as good as that of metals, but it is possible to work plastics to a fraction of a millimetre which is adequate for spectacle frame manufacturing purposes. They can withstand hot sunshine and also cold conditions. They have a relatively low density, which makes it possible to create frames that are light in weight. On the whole, few plastics cause skin allergies such as those experienced by sufferers from nickel sensitization. However, skin acids can cause crazing, formation of grey deposits and the embrittling of plastics (Section 9.4).

Most plastics are amenable to a variety of production processes when cold. Some processes, such as inserting metal reinforcements into sides and inserting pinless joints, require heating. The latter applies also to adjustments; if this is done using steam, plasticizer (a chemical compound added to improve its plastic properties) could leach out and affect the skin of the spectacle frame wearer. Leaching causes discoloration and brittleness of the material. Migration of large quantities of plasticizer from cellulose acetate into polycarbonate spectacle lenses may cause radial cracks within 1 year (B. Such, personal communication, 1995).

Certain pigments and dyes added to colour the transparent or translucent basic material are less stable than others. Therefore, colour stability may vary. Most modern materials are no longer subject to this problem, which was particularly troublesome with pearl and pale colours.

Plastics have very low friction, electrical and thermal conductivity characteristics, but relatively high thermal expansion. This causes a reduction of stiffness with increasing temperature. Oxidation at moderate temperatures (say, 300°C) causes 'scorching'. Most plastics are resistant to mild acids and alkalis, but vulnerable to organic solvents.

The American National Standard ANSI Z80.5 (1979) sets out requirements for plastics frame materials with respect to flammability, shrinkage, and skin irritability. British Standard BS 6625 (1985) states that it is necessary to exclude as frame materials any that cause irritation, reaction or harm during wear or adjustment.

7.3 The Nature of Plastics

7.3.1 HISTORICAL PERSPECTIVE

Plastics are mainly organic compounds. The term 'organic' is now essentially a historic one; originally, it was used to describe a group of compounds that were perceived as originating only from living organisms, that is, vegetable or animal instead of inanimate mineral sources, as described by Lemery in 1675.

Lavoisier, in the eighteenth century, showed that in some cases the same compound could be obtained from both vegetable and animal sources. These were all shown to contain carbon and hydrogen, and often oxygen. By inference, nitrogen and phosphorus were present in many compounds too. Berzelius, in the early nineteenth century, suggested that so-called organic compounds were formed from their elements by processes that differed from those by which inorganic compounds were formed. He postulated that organic compounds required a 'vital force' for their formation, and could not be prepared otherwise.

Woehler succeeded in preparing urea from ammonium cyanate in 1828. However, the synthesis was not directly from the elements. In 1845 Kolbe synthesized acetic acid (ethanoic acid) from its elements, and 11 years later Berthelot synthesized methane. With these syntheses the idea of a 'vital force' became untenable.

While the classification of compounds as organic or inorganic according to the influence of a vital force in the formation of the former was no longer accepted, the classification was retained. This was mainly because, among other reasons, all organic compounds contain carbon. These carbon-containing compounds were very numerous – more numerous than all the known compounds of the other elements put together – and almost uniquely among the elements, carbon combines with itself to form long chains. This chain formation is called catenation.

The chemistry of carbon compounds is now known as organic chemistry. Carbon forms compounds with hydrogen alone or in combination with oxygen, nitrogen, the halogens, sulphur, phosphorus and metals.

The simplest compounds involving carbon and hydrogen only, called hydrocarbons, are divided initially according to structure into two main classes – aliphatic and aromatic. Aliphatic hydrocarbons are further subdivided into families: namely alkanes, alkenes, and alkynes (and their cyclic analogues).

7.3.2. ALKANES

The alkanes, or paraffins are so named because of their comparative lack of reactivity (*para*, against; affinity, tendency to combine with others, i.e. elements or compounds). Because of the unreactive nature of their electronic structure they are said to be 'saturated'.

This can be illustrated using methane as an example. By analysis it has an empirical formula of CH_4. The element carbon is placed in group 4 of the Periodic Classification of the elements. This signifies that it has four electrons in its outer shell which take part in bond formation. The bonds formed here are covalent bonds in which a pair of electrons is shared, each atom in the bond supplying one electron to the bond pair. This can be presented diagrammatically by using dots to

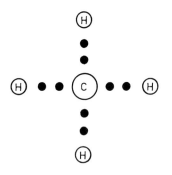

Fig. 7.1 *The black dots represent electrons shared by each atom. H – hydrogen; C – carbon*

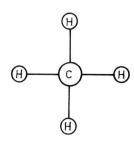

Fig. 7.2 *In this diagram the dash or line connecting the carbon C atom with each hydrogen H atom represents a pair of electrons*

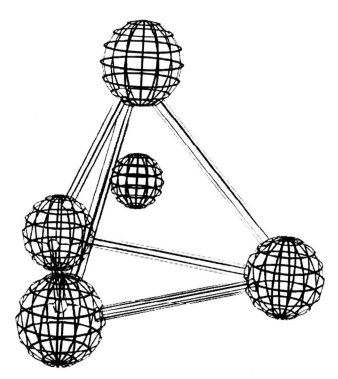

Fig. 7.3 *This spatial representation shows the hydrogen atoms at the apices of a tetrahedron with the carbon atom suspended at its centre. The 'cylinders' connecting the hydrogen atoms are used here·to emphasize the 3-dimensional effect*

represent electrons as in Fig. 7.1 or the electron pair by a dash as in Fig. 7.2. Figure 7.3 represents the spatial arrangement of the hydrogen atoms around the carbon atom at the apices of a tetrahedron with the carbon atom at its centre. This

structure has been confirmed by electron diffraction and is in agreement with the structure proposed by energy and molecular orbital theories.

The carbon atom then has a complete 'octet' (group of eight) of electrons in its outermost electronic shell. It has now acquired the stable configuration of neon, the next 'inert' or noble gas of the long Periodic Table, while each hydrogen has a complete duplet, acquiring the electron configuration of helium.

7.3.3 ALKENES

The next group or homologous series of compounds, the alkenes, historically were called olefines, then olefins and alkylenes. These hydrocarbon compounds contain a double bond and are said to be unsaturated.

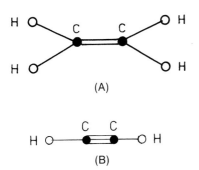

Fig. 7.4 *(A) The double bond of the simplest alkene compound, ethene or ethylene. (B) The triple bond of the simplest alkyne compound, acetylene*

We will consider the simplest member, ethene or ethylene: $H_2C=CH_2$ (Fig. 7.4A). Compared with a single bond, the double bond is (mechanically) stronger, however, it is also very reactive. This apparent contradiction results from the character of the second bond, called a π-bond. This pair of electrons forms a strong bond that adds strength to the first bond (a σ-bond) and brings the bonded atoms closer and in a more rigid embrace. However, the π-bond lies external to the σ-bond and, consequently, is more open to attack by electron-seeking species. Electrophilic attack on the π-bonding electrons leads to the formation of additional σ-bonds, with the 'predators' added to the now unsaturated molecule. This process of adding molecules by

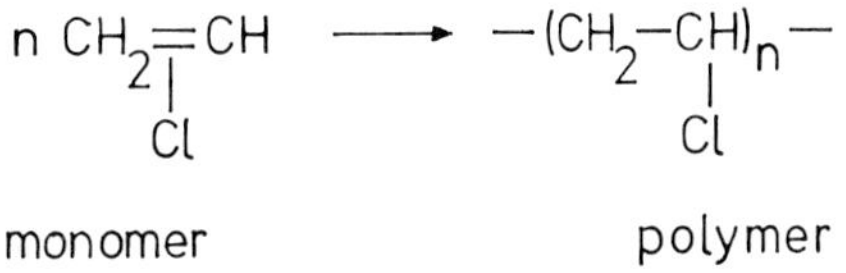

$$n\ CH_2=CH\ |_{Cl} \longrightarrow -(CH_2-CH)_n- \ |_{Cl}$$

monomer   polymer

Fig. 7.5 *A monomer is converted into a long chain molecule or polymer, through polymerization*

carbon–carbon bonding leads to long carbon chains; the single reacting molecules are referred to as monomers and the larger product molecules are called polymers; the reaction process is termed polymerization (Fig. 7.5).

The polymerization process can be effected by the application of heat, although usually catalysts (substances added in small proportion to start or accelerate a chemical reaction) are added. In this way, parts of the monomers are activated. These parts combine with other monomers to form macromolecular chains.

One can differentiate between linear polymers and crosslinked polymers. The former term refers to a polymer that consists of molecules composed of unbranched chains or of chains with very short branches. Their cohesion (sticking together) depends on the relatively weak forces of attraction between them. Crosslinked polymers have chemical bonds that form a three-dimensional, interwoven and inseparable, giant molecular network. Because of this network, the molecules cannot move or slide about. The greater the crosslinking the more difficult it is for molecules to 'move' with respect to other molecules in the network because of the great number of interconnections between the chains of molecules.

When linear polymers are heated, the intermolecular forces become weaker, and the polymer softens. On further application of heat it becomes a viscous (sticky) liquid: that is, a liquid with great internal friction between its molecules. That liquid will flow only very slowly.

When viscous liquids are cooled, solidification occurs.

A plastics material capable of being repeatedly softened by heating and hardened by cooling is called a thermoplastics. Examples are cellulose acetate and polyamide.

Heating crosslinked polymers does not significantly soften the material. They are, therefore, called thermosetting materials. Examples are polyesters and the spectacle lens material CR 39 (allyl diglycol carbonate).

7.3.4 ALKYNES

The third homologous series are the alkynes, or acetylenes as they were called after the name of the simplest homologue, acetylene. These unsaturated hydrocarbons contain a triple bond, that is, three bonds (one σ-bond and two π-bonds) between adjacent carbon atoms, usually presented as shown in Fig. 7.4B. This is even stronger and more reactive than a double bond. Alkynes are important in industrial organic synthesis.

7.4 Characteristics of Plastics

The advantages and disadvantages of rigid plastics are set out in Table 7.1, and the common characteristics of cellulose-based plastics are presented in Table 7.2. Table 7.3 gives details about handling and manufacturing properties of plastics materials.

TABLE 7.1 *Advantages and disadvantages of rigid plastics (Humphrey, 1980)*

Advantages	Disadvantages
1. Low density: 0·90 to 2·20 g cm^{-3}	1. Low coefficient of elasticity
2. Good strength/weight ratio at low strains	2. Subject to 'cold flow' if processed incorrectly
3. Good electrical and thermal insulators	3. High thermal expansion
4. Good chemical resistance	4. Majority cannot be used above 100°C
5. Permanent surface finish requiring little or no maintenance	5. Can be indented
6. Ease of fabrication and machining	6. Relatively high cost per unit of weight
7. Good impact resistance	

TABLE 7.2 *Common characteristics of cellulose-based plastics*

Can be injection moulded (exception: cellulose nitrate)
Are clear and tough
Can be formed into film and fibres
Can be given a great variety of colours, and used in lacquers
Are produced in the form of pellets, sheets and pipes.

TABLE 7.3 Handling and manufacturing properties of plastics

Material	Density (g cm^{-3})	Softening temperature (°C)	Decomposition temperature (°C)	Moulding temperature (°C)	Flammability
Cellulose acetate (CA)	1·2–1·34	50	240	130–230	Slow-SE
Cellulose acetate butyrate (CAB)	1·15–1·24	70			Slow
Cellulose propionate (CP)†	1·17–1·2	65		150	Slow
Cellulose nitrate (CN)	1·35–1·4	75	150		Rapid
Epoxide resin	1·11–1·4	110*(Optyl)	350	290	Slow-SE
Polyamide	1·09–1·15	100		230–310	SE
Polymethyl methacrylate (PMMA)	1·17–1·19	70		180–270	Slow-SE
Reinforced polyamide	1·5–1·6	80			
Silicone rubber			>250		
For comparison:					
CR 39	1·3				Slow
Crown glass	2·5				

† Ceroids: softening temperature 100–110°C. (Section 24.6.2.5).
* Can be adjusted at about 80°C.
SE, self extinguishing.
All temperatures are approximate values.
Other properties (hardness, elasticity, and flexural, impact and tensile strength) have been specified by Humphrey (1980).

7.5 Cellulose-based Plastics

7.5.1 HISTORICAL DEVELOPMENT

The first reported use of a cellulose derivative was by Schoenbein who prepared cellulose nitrate in 1845. This was used to produce films and to make collodion solutions: sticky, viscous solutions used in medicine.

Alexander Parkes, in Britain, made a mould-able thermoplastic composition of cellulose nitrate and castor oil. In 1865, he patented the use of camphor in the compositions and in 1866 the Parkesine Company was formed. However, it failed after 2 years.

The brothers I. S. and J. W. Hyatt, in America, developed mechanical production equipment and improved manufacturing techniques so that by 1870 they had successfully established the

Celluloid Manufacturing Company. Thereafter, most of the commercial cellulose nitrate materials were given the generic name of celluloid. The manufacture of celluloid was begun in France in 1875, in Germany during 1878, and in Italy and Japan by 1910.

Daniel Spill, who had earlier been associated with Parkes, continued to manufacture cellulose nitrate materials and this culminated in the establishment of the British Xylonite Company in 1877, later to become BX Plastics.

Cellulose acetate was first reported to have been prepared in 1869 and was manufactured commercially in 1894 by Lichtenberger. This was triacetate, which was soluble only in chlorinated hydrocarbons and had no satisfactory plasticizers. Around 1904, Miles patented a process for 'ripening' cellulose acetate allowing it to be readily soluble in solutions such as acetone, and also to be compatible with plasticizers. Consequently, it became a commercially viable material for injection moulding processes. The latter had been patented *c.* 1930 by Eichengruen. Cellulose acetate continued as one of the major materials for injection moulding up to the early 1950s. Cellulose acetate sheet production came to an end in Britain in the early 1990s. Pellets of this material continue to be manufactured and are now used to produce spectacle frame material by moulding into slabs, strips or spectacle fronts. Pellets are turned into sheet material by similar processes in Italy. Patterns are now more quickly produced by printing or spraying them onto the sheet material, and covering the pattern with a thin, protective layer. Various other processes, such a dip-dyeing to produce two-tone material, are also used by individual frame manufacturers.

Other cellulose-based polymeric materials are cellulose propionate and the mixed ester and copolymer cellulose acetate butyrate (CAB). Each of these materials has specific properties making it particularly useful for different sectors of the plastics industry. Cellulose propionate has

become very important in spectacle frame manufacture while cellulose acetate butyrate has been used for contact lenses.

7.5.2 CELLULOSE

Cellulose is a polymer that occurs widely in nature: it is the main constituent of the cell walls of all plants. The polymer is a complex carbohydrate (a group of complex organic compounds such as sugars, starches and cellulose, that are present in all living matter) composed of long (25 μm), open, parallel chains of glucose units; the monomeric unit (Fig. 7.6A) is D-glucose (a sugar). The polymer has the molecular formula $(C_6H_{10}O_5)n$ where *n* may be several thousands. Because of the long chains and the strong adhesion between chains, cellulose is mechanically very strong but lacks the flow properties of plastics materials.

The raw material comes in the form of cotton, flax, hemp, jute and wood. The main sources for the commercial production of cellulose are cotton linters, which look like cotton wool, and wood. Cotton linters are the short buff-coloured fuzzy fibres adhering to the cotton seed after the long staple white fibre or 'cotton' has been stripped from the seed by the process known as 'ginning'. The linters are then commercially graded into three grades. The top grade, 'first cuts', and the staple fibre are used by the textile industry; the middle grade, 'second cuts', is used by the plastics industry to produce chemical cellulose, the starting material for a wide range of cellulosic plastics.

7.5.2.1 Chemistry

The molecular formula of cellulose can be represented as shown in Fig. 7.6A. The glucose molecule, which contains three hydroxyl (OH) groups, is capable of hydrogen bonding. This is a relatively weak but important long-range bond

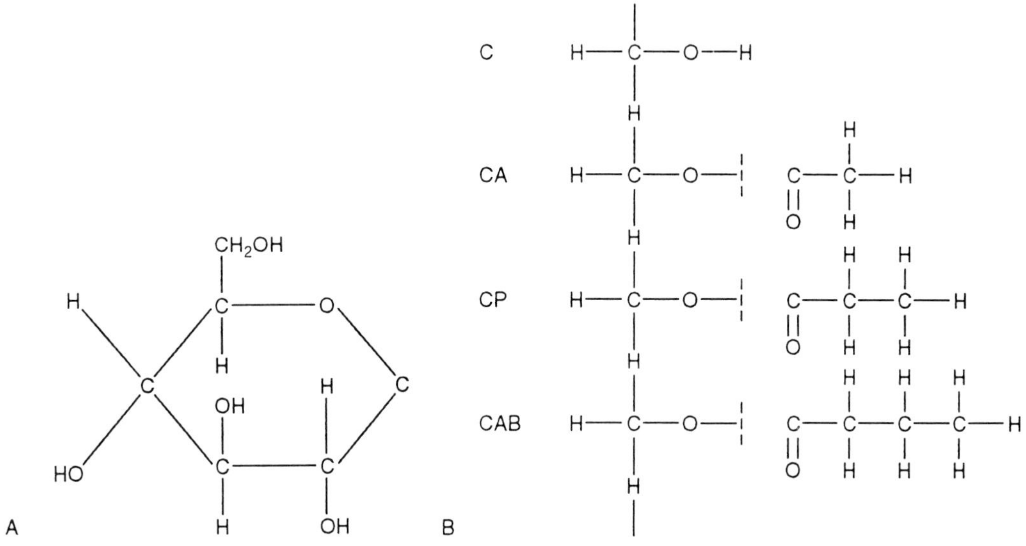

Fig. 7.6 *(A) Representation of a cellulose molecule $C_6H_{10}O_5$. (B) The molecular representations of cellulose C, cellulose acetate CA, cellulose propionate CP and cellulose acetate butyrate CAB*

formed between -OH and adjacent H-. Consequently, the great intermolecular forces, together with the regularity of the structure where there is little or no branching of the polymeric chain, give it a high degree of crystallinity. The solubility is therefore low, but the polymer does swell in hydrogen-bonding solvents, including water. Swelling takes place in the amorphous regions of the polymer. This cellulose is then converted to the cellulose ester required by esterification of the hydroxyl groups on the cellulose molecule by the corresponding acid. The esterification reaches a low product-concentration equilibrium between alcohols and acids:

$$\text{alcohol} + \text{acid} \leftrightarrow \text{ester} + \text{water}$$
$$(\text{R-OH} + \text{H-ONO}_2 \leftrightarrow \text{R-ONO}_2 + \text{H-OH})$$

To increase the yield of cellulose ester the equilibrium can be shifted to the product ester side by removal of water. This is usually carried out by the use of sulphuric acid. Because cellulose is a trihydric alcohol, the product is a mixture of mono-, di- and tri-substituted cellulose units along the polymer chain. The degree of substitution determines the physical and chemical properties of the material, and hence its end use.

Because cellulose-based plastics are derived from organic raw material, they have been described as semi-synthetic.

7.5.2.2 Manufacture

Chemical cellulose or α-cellulose, the starting material for the various cellulose esters and ethers used in the plastics industry, is produced as follows.

From cotton linters. The linters, received in bales, pass through a breaker to part and fluff the fibres. These are then separated from solid impurities (dirt) in an air separator, and saponifiable (convertable into soap) material such as fats and waxes is removed by digestion in alkaline solution, commonly sodium hydroxide (caustic soda). The digestion is carried out in large pressure vessels with continuous stirring. The reaction conditions (concentration, temperature and duration) are chosen according to the required properties, particularly the viscosity, of the end product. Digestion can take up to 6 hours for a 4500 kg batch of linters. After digestion, the linters are separated from the spent liquor and are thoroughly washed to remove saponified materials and alkali residues. The linters which, at this stage, are grey or light yellow in colour, are bleached using chlorine or hypochlorites. Careful control of time and temperature, and of the concentration and pH (the acidity or alkalinity of the solution) of the reaction mixture, is essential to avoid degradation of the cellulose and to produce the required white colour. The bleaching is carried out in two or more stages, to avoid degradation, and thorough washing follows each stage; iron is rigorously excluded. The purified, white linters are blended, and then dried to a moisture content of about 5%.

From wood. Wood contains about 50% cellulose as well as 20% hemicelluloses (water-soluble sugars) and lignin, which is an alcohol and binds the cellulose; lignin is also the binding agent in growing plants.

The wood is first reduced to wood chips and then treated with steam under pressure. This softens the lignin. When released to atmospheric pressure the wood chips, without the restraint of the lignin under high external pressure, 'explode', leaving a mass of fibres coated with lignin.

The hemicelluloses are then hydrolysed (decomposed into simpler forms by the action of water); the material can then be compressed and used as raw material, for instance, for coarse paper products.

To make it into a workable plastics the interchain adhesion has to be reduced carefully so as not to destroy desirable mechanical properties. Before the linters can be further processed, they need to be broken down and the material dried to a prescribed moisture content.

7.5.3 CELLULOSE NITRATE
7.5.3.1 Description
This is a nitric acid ester of cellulose, which produces a tough fast-burning thermoplastic material (BS 3521, 1962) typically containing 11% nitrogen (Humphrey, 1980). Its molecular formula is $CH_2N_3O_{11}$, and it is sometimes abbreviated to CN.

7.5.3.2 Production process
In earlier texts this product was described as nitrocellulose and the conversion process as nitration. However, further investigation showed that this was more correctly described as an esterification and the product as an ester, namely cellulose nitrate. This product could be cellulose mononitrate, dinitrate or trinitrate according to how many of the three hydroxyl groups were substituted on each glucose unit of the cellulose polymer chain.

The ester most commonly used for plastics is the dinitrate with a nitrogen content of 10·5–12·0%. Esters with nitrogen content between 12·5% and 13·5% are used for making explosives such as cordite.

The process of esterification is carried out (Fig. 7.7) by steeping the dried linters (see Section 7.5.2.2) in a nitrating mixture of concentrated nitric acid, sulphuric acid and water (typically, 25% HNO_3, 55% H_2SO_4, and 20% H_2O). The product is separated and conditioned in a sequence of wash, blend, stabilize, bleach and wash again. Finally, the water is removed with ethyl alcohol to give an alcohol-damp, stabilized, cellulose nitrate which can then be processed into suitable material for conversion to end product.

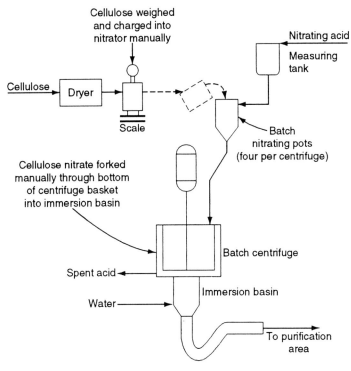

Fig. 7.7 Flow diagram of nitration (Reproduced by permission of John Wiley & Sons, Inc.)

The process is very similar to that used in the mid-1800s, but with some important modifications. A number of catastrophic explosions early in the manufacture resulted in urgent investigations into the stability of the process. Abel, in 1865, showed that the instability was caused by trace retention in the product of the nitrating acid mixture. Later investigations indicated that formation of free sulphuric acid from these residues could cause autocatalytic decomposition. Robertson, in 1906, showed that the acid was derived from sulphate groups. These could be removed almost completely by boiling in acidified water to give a much more stable product.

7.5.3.3 Production of sheet material
The production of sheet from the alcohol-damped cellulose nitrate is carried out by mixing it with a plasticizer, invariably camphor (a volatile, aromatic, organic compound containing the carbonyl (CO) group), although triphenyl phosphate and phthalates such as diethyl and dibutyl have been added but only in small quantities. The mixing is done in a dough-mixing machine which is jacketed to provide heating or cooling.

The batch is kneaded with heating and any colourants, soluble dyes or pigments are added at this stage. They are usually added as solutions or pastes to aid dispersion. Mixing is continued until the material is homogeneous and the cellulose has lost its fibrous nature. Small quantities of stabilizer such as urea, substituted urea, amines and zinc oxide are sometimes added during the mixing. The mix is then filtered under pressure and the alcohol content reduced by kneading in a gently heated vessel, under vacuum.

When the alcohol content has been reduced to about 25%, the material is discharged on to fast-running rollers heated to between 55 and 60°C. When the material is judged by the operator, from experience, to have the right 'feel', it is transferred to larger, slow-running rollers or calenders at a cooler temperature. The material is then rolled into sheets or 'hides', about half an inch (1 cm) thick. The solvent content at this stage is 12–16%.

Colour patterns and tortoiseshell patterns are trimmed to sheets measuring about 75 × 160 cm, loaded into steel boxes that are about 15 cm deep, and then three or four at a time are placed in a block press. The pressing cycle takes 4–5 h, which is the time required to turn, under the influence of heat and pressure, the separate sheets into a homogeneous solid block. The block is then cooled, still under pressure, for an even longer period. Finally, the blocks are conditioned in a cooled room for a further 24 hours until they reach ambient temperature throughout.

Cellulose nitrate is also extruded into rods and tubes, or made into film.

7.5.4 CELLULOSE ACETATE
7.5.4.1 Description
This is an acetic acid ester of cellulose, which produces a tough slow-burning thermoplastic material (BS 3521, 1962). 'Optical grade' cellulose acetate contains 38–40% acetyl (CH_3CO) (Humphrey, 1980). Its molecular formula is $C_{12}H_{16}O_8$ (Fig. 7.6B), and its name is sometimes abbreviated to CA.

7.5.4.2 Production process
Cellulose (Fig. 7.6A) is pretreated with acetic acid (Fig. 7.8) and then acetylated for about 7 h in a mixture of acetic acid (as solvent), acetic anhydride (anhydride = without water; two molecules of acetic acid with one molecule of water removed), and sulphuric acid or zinc chloride as catalyst. During acetylation the mix is continu-

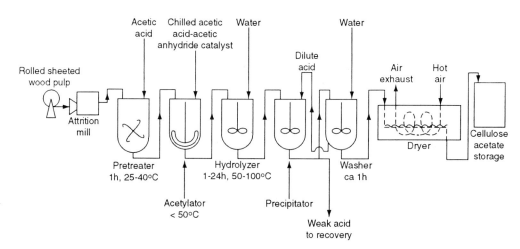

Fig. 7.8 Cellulose acetate manufacture (Reproduced by permission of John Wiley & Sons, Inc.)

ously stirred. The chemical reaction produces triacetate (after 5–6 h). At this stage the cellulose hydroxyl groups have been substituted by acetyl groups. Triacetate is a viscous, almost transparent mass. This is then 'ripened' for 72 h while water is added (hydrolysis). It stands until just over 50% of the cellulose acetate–acetic acid solution is acetate. More water is mixed with the solution to precipitate cellulose acetate, which appears as white flakes. After washing, to remove impurities, and drying it becomes a fine white powder.

To produce a plastics material, plasticizer (such as dimethyl phthalate) is mixed with the cellulose acetate in a kneader while a solvent (usually acetone C_3H_6O; Fig. 7.9) is added. The

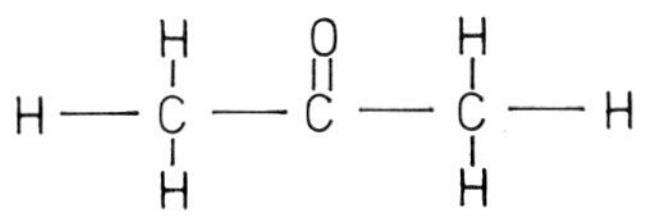

Fig. 7.9 *Acetone (C_3H_6O) molecule*

plasticizer comprises about 25% of the mix. The object of adding the plasticizer is to facilitate slippage between the cellulose chains which gives the characteristic flexibility of plastics material. The solvent also allows the mass to be worked mechanically (e.g. kneading), making it possible to add pigments and dyes.

Foreign material and ungelled particles must now be removed. To achieve this, the dough is placed in a hydraulic press to remove air pockets, which could cause an explosion. It is then passed under great pressure through a filter cloth, which is supported by fine and coarse metal gauze placed on a heavy grid. Because the solvent content is too high for the finished plastics material, it is reduced to about 15% by rolling

between pairs of cold and warm rollers, whereby fresh surfaces are continually exposed.

The hardened material is then calendered repeatedly to produce sheets (hides) 10–20 mm thick. About 10 sheets are then stacked, forming a pile about 15 cm high, on a metal plate placed in a heavy steel box. One to three boxes are placed, for several hours, between the platens of a heated hydraulic press. In this way the sheets are spliced (joined) into one unit, a block of cellulose acetate. Such a block weighs about 100 kg.

The block is slowly cooled by circulating cold water through the platens. It is then placed on the table of a planing machine which slices it into sheets. These can be made to vary in thickness between 0.1 and 20 mm, with an accuracy of 0.01 mm.

The remaining 10% or so of the solvent is finally removed during a seasoning process. Before this, each sheet destined for frame production is checked for pattern and clarity.

During the preseasoning process the sheets lie on grids; during the main process they are suspended in purpose-built chambers. Five to 12 days of seasoning at about 50°C is required per millimetre of sheet thickness. The whole process may, therefore, take well over two months.

The sheets usually become warped, and so are pressed flat between heated polished platens (like cellulose nitrate) and cooled before final inspection.

It is also possible to extrude cellulose acetate. A suitable form of the material is produced as follows. After the filtration process the material is chopped into pellets of about 3 mm diameter. These are then fed into an extrusion machine which heats the pellets to a viscous mass. It is then extruded (Section 10.2.5) under pressure through a suitable die. While cooling, the extruded material emerges from the die in the desired shape.

7.5.4.3 Production of sheet material

For sheet production the extruded material emerges as a ribbon. Two or three differently coloured ribbons from different extrusion presses may be formed into one ribbon. The continuous ribbon is cut into lengths, and flattened between a series of rollers. Finally, it may be cut into slabs of a size suitable for spectacle frame production.

Wakefield (1994) referred to a new method of manufacturing 'pressure cast' cellulose acetate material. This method is under development and allows relatively small quantities of a particular colour or pattern to be produced economically. For this purpose flakes of various colours are evenly dispersed into a mould of liquid cellulose acetate. After compression under heat, and cooling, a slab of finished material is produced.

BS 3186 (1990) gives a specification for cellulose acetate sheet for spectacle frames.

7.5.5 OTHER CELLULOSE-BASED PLASTICS

7.5.5.1 Cellulose propionate

This is prepared in much the same way as cellulose acetate. However, in addition to acetic acid (CH_3COOH) and acetic anhydride, propionic anhydride ($CH_3CH_2COOCOCH_2CH_3$) is used to treat the cellulose, and more plasticizers and stabilizers are required than in the production of cellulose acetate. Its molecular formula is $C_3H_6O_2$ (Fig. 7.6B) and its name is sometimes abbreviated to CP.

It is compatible with a number of plasticizers, and is suitable for injection moulding and extrusion. Because of its strength, spectacle frame rims can be made thinner than frames made from cellulose acetate material; this has obvious design advantages. The weight of propionate frames (Table 13.1) is less than that of cellulose acetate frames, and similar to that of Optyl frames

(Section 7.6.4), because their density is the same. Propionate frames are usually coloured by surface treatment such as dipping and lacquering.

7.5.5.2 Cellulose acetate butyrate

This material is derived from a mixed acetic acid and butyric acid reaction with cellulose, in the presence of a catalyst such as sulphuric acid (H_2SO_4).

Cellulose acetate butyrate, sometimes abbreviated to CAB, is represented by the molecular formula $C_{12}H_{18}O_7$ (Fig. 7.6B). It is available in crystal as well as in numerous colours, and requires less plasticizer and less pressure in moulding than cellulose acetate.

7.6 Other Plastics

7.6.1 POLYMETHYLMETHACRYLATE

This is a thermoplastic material composed of polymerized methylmethacrylate (BS 3521, 1962). It is frequently referred to as PMMA.

Initially, acetone ($C_3H_6O_3$) and sodium cyanide (NaCN) are made into acetone cyanohydrin. Polymerization of the latter with methanol (CH_3OH) and sulphuric acid (H_2SO_4) under the influence of heat, light and oxygen produces methylmethacrylate ($C_5H_8O_2$) (Fig. 7.10).

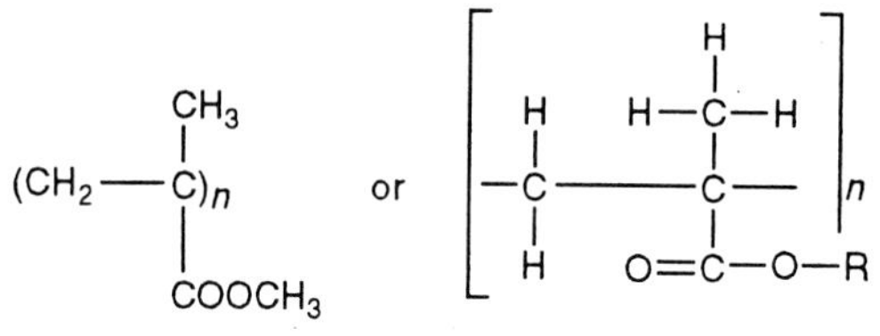

Fig. 7.10 *Two ways of representing methylmethacrylate, $C_5H_8O_2$. n, several thousands; R, rest*

Transparent sheet material may be made as follows. A monomer with a very small percentage of catalyst, such as hydrogen peroxide (H_2O_2), is allowed to thicken and harden between glass plates separated by compressible gaskets, in an oven at a moderate temperature. Allowance has to be made during polymerization for the removal of the heat caused by the reaction and for the shrinkage in volume. The sheet is then removed from between the glass plates.

To obtain optically perfect material (without bubbles, stress and irregularities), the polymerization process should be carefully controlled and progress slowly. It is possible to cast sheets that are not only larger than 1 m², but also several centimetres thick. The sheets should be cured and annealed.

Frame manufacturers have produced their own colour combinations as follows. A clear sheet is placed on a piece of plate glass and overlaid with the desired colour in liquid acrylic form. Another piece of plate glass is placed on top; they are then clipped together and left overnight to set and cure. The two-tone PMMA sheet can be used the next day. Inserts, such as lace, can be added. Pearl effects can also be achieved. Milling directionally through the layer of colours gives a three-dimensional effect.

7.6.2 POLYAMIDE

This is a polymer in which the structural units are linked by amide or thioamide groupings (BS 3521, 1962).

Nylon (Fig. 7.11) is a generic term for a long-chain polymeric amide (molecular formula $C_{12}H_{22}O_2N_2$) where the ring amide CONH-groups recur as integral part of the main polymeric chain. Polyamide compounds are formed by polymerization of amino (NH_2) acids, derived from ammonia gas (NH_3). One of the basic nylons, nylon 66, is a 1:1 combination of adipic acid ($C_6H_{10}O_4$) and hexamethylenediamine ($C_6H_{16}N_2$). They can be made in a variety of ways (see, for instance, Lever, 1966).

Nylon moulding powder can be used for injection and compression moulding and for extrusion and sintering (i.e. unite under heat without becoming a liquid). After moulding, it can be turned, milled and threaded. Although nylon was originally not available as a transparent material, this disadvantage has been overcome and it is now supplied in a range of transparent and opaque colours.

Another original problem, the propensity to snap, has not been solved completely. Polyamide frames cannot be adjusted during heating; however, reinforced polyamide sides can be adjusted. Such (B. Such, personal communication, 1995) warned that alcohol can affect polyamide spectacle frames.

The co-polyamide SPX, developed by Silhouette of Austria, has properties like the polyamides in addition to being mouldable and colourable. Frames made of SPX (and similar materials) can be designed with rims that are thinner than in conventional plastics frames. Lenses are probably best inserted 'cold'.

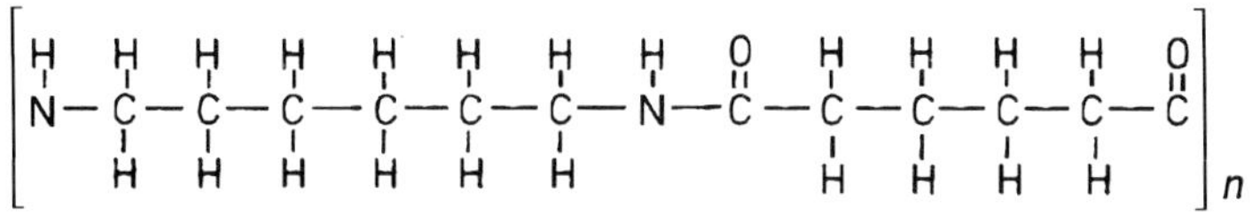

Fig. 7.11 A basic nylon structure

7.6.3 REINFORCED POLYAMIDES

In order to improve the low stiffness of polyamides, short, fibrous fillers such as glass (in its basic form, it is a mixture of sodium silicate (Na_2SiO_3) and calcium silicate ($CaSiO_3$)), carbon and silicon carbide (SiC) have been added. A typical composition of such material would be 15–20% carbon fibre, 60% nylon, the remainder consisting of other plastics. Carbon fibres are graphitic ribbons about 6 nm wide and several nanometres long.

Reinforced polyamide objects are made by moulding. They are stronger than steel and lighter than aluminium. Spectacle frames are very light (Table 13.1) and tend to have thin rims. Lenses to be inserted (Section 24.6.1) into spectacle frames not having a closing block, should be accurately edged for size and shape, and probably best inserted 'cold'.

7.6.4 EPOXIDE RESINS (*Epoxy resins*)

These are liquids or meltable solids derived from petroleum that must be mixed with hardeners or curing agents to achieve polymerization. The curing agent chosen will greatly affect the properties of the polymer.

The simplest epoxy is a three-membered ring (Fig. 7.12) consisting of an oxygen atom and two CH_2-groups; they may have more than two of the latter groups.

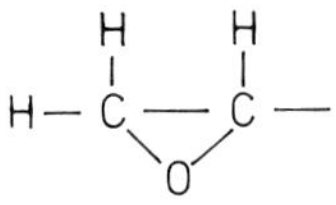

Fig. 7.12 The simplest epoxy ring

The basic resins may have modifying materials added in order to obtain a particular characteristic. When a completely rigid structure is undesirable, plasticizers, including polyamides, are added.

An epoxide resin, specially designed for spectacle frame production, was developed by Wilhelm Anger of Austria (Obstfeld, 1988); it is known as Optyl. Because of its low density, frames made from this material can be made up to 30% lighter than comparable frames made of cellulose acetate (but see Table 13.1). It has a 'plastics memory' – having been deformed at a temperature above about 85°C, when heated again above that temperature, and given the opportunity, it will return to its original shape. This process may be repeated indefinitely. Although Optyl is elastic, it is imperative to heat the material until soft, otherwise the frame part to be adjusted may snap. Optyl material can be heated to well over 200°C before permanent damage occurs. When Optyl is ignited it gives off repugnant fumes.

Reinforced epoxide resins are composites of carbon fibre (Section 7.6.3) and epoxide resin, whose properties will also depend on those of the latter.

7.6.5 SILICONE RUBBER

This type of compound is exceptional in that its basic form lacks carbon atoms. Instead, it consists of alternating silicon–oxygen (SiO_2) chains to which carbonyl (CO) groups are attached. Its molecular formula is $Si_2C_4H_{12}O_3$ (Fig. 7.13). These materials are referred to as polymeric organo-silicone compounds.

Silicone is a porous material which will absorb sweat and make-up. As a consequence, it loses its transparency, becoming milky. This

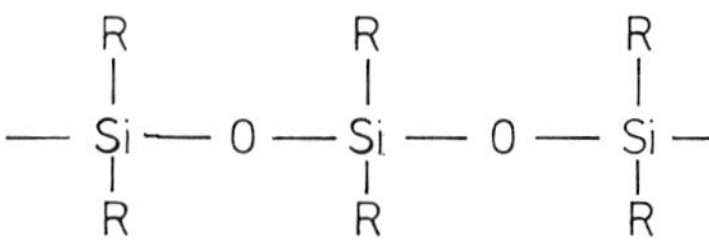

Fig. 7.13 Silicone: a silicon–oxygen chain. Si, silicon; O, oxygen; R, organic (carbon-containing) group

material has a high coefficient of friction. It is used for spectacle frame pads, and has been used as shock-absorbing lining of metal rims and as non-slip end covers of sides. It suffers from lack of rigidity and curling. To improve rigidity, silicone pads are given a hard plastics centre, which also reduces the poorer appearance of a contaminated pad.

REFERENCES

ANSI Z80.5 (1979). *American National Standard Requirements for Dress Ophthalmic Frames.* American National Standards Institute, Inc.

Bedwell, C.H. (1960). The history and production of cellulose acetate and nitrate plastic materials. *Optician* **139** (3590), 29–36.

Brydson, J.A. (1975). *Plastics Materials*, 3rd edn. London: Newnes-Butterworths.

BS 1755 (1982). *Glossary of Terms Used in the Plastics Industry. Part 1: Polymer and Plastics Technology.* London: British Standards Institution.

BS 3521 (1962). *Glossary of Terms Relating to Ophthalmic Lenses and Spectacle Frames.* London: British Standards Institution.

BS 3186 (1970). *Specification for Cellulose Acetate Sheet for Spectacle Frames.* London: British Standards Institution. (Superseded by BS 6625.)

BS 6625 (1985). *Specification for Spectacle Frames.* London: British Standards Institution.

Clarke, A.F. (1978). Cellulose acetate butyrate: an industrial plastics. *Optician* **176** (4564), 18–22.

Davidson, D.C. (1989). *Spectacles, Lorgnettes and Monocles, Album 227*, p. 31. Princes Risborough: Shire Publications.

Grant, J. (1982). The origins of plastics. *Optician* **183** (4732), 21.

Green, K.J. (1963). Plastics for the optician. *Optician* **146** (3771), 8–9.

Hardy, S. (1982a). Frame materials: plastics since 1950, part 2. *Manuf. Optics Int.* **35** (7), 34–36.

Hardy, S. (1982b). Frame materials: plastics since 1950, part 3. *Manuf. Optics Int.* **35** (8), 31–32.

Hardy, S., & Hardy, W.E. (1982). Frame materials: a perspective; part 1. *Manuf. Optics Int.* **35** (6), 18–23.

Humphrey, B. (1980). Plastics frame materials. *Manuf. Optics Int.* **33** (5), 44–45.

Hutton, K. (1966). *Chemistry: the Conquest of Materials.* Harmondsworth: Penguin Books.

Lee, H., & Neville, K. (1967). *Handbook of Epoxy Resins.* London/New York: McGraw–Hill.

Lever, A.E. (ed.) (1966). *The Plastics Manual*, 3rd edn. London: Scientific Press.

Nevell, T.P., & Zeronian, S.H. (1985). *Cellulose Chemistry and its Applications.* Chichester: Ellis Horwood.

Obstfeld, H. (1988). The Anger story, so far. *Optom. Today* **28**, 49–50.

Redfarn, C.A. (1951). *A Guide to Plastics.* London: Iliffe & Sons.

Wake, W.C., Tidd, B.K., & Loadman, M.J.R. (eds) (1983). *Analysis of Rubber and Rubber-like Polymers*, 3rd edn. London/New York: Applied Science.

Wakefield, K.G. (1994). *Bennett's Ophthalmic Prescription Work*, 3rd edn., p. 27. Oxford: Butterworth–Heinemann.

FURTHER READING

Deichmann, H. (1990). Moderne Technologien für die Produktion von Brillenfassungen im VEB Rathenower Optische Werke 'Hermann Duncker'. *Augenoptik, Berlin* **107** (1), 25–28.

Hinterhofer, O., & Fahrner, D. (1983). *Materialkunde für Augenoptiker*, 2nd edn. Pforzheim: Verlag Neues Optiker Journal/Postenrieder.

ROCEL (undated). *The Extrusion of Cellulose Acetate for Spectacle Frame Manufacture. Technical Information Bulletin no.7*, Spondon, Derby: Courtaulds.

Woodcock, F.R. (1975). Frame materials. *Manuf. Optics Int.* **28** (6), 263–275.

Woodcock, F.R. (1986). From shell to titanium. *Optician* **192** (5055), 17–25.

CHAPTER 8

Materials: Metals

8.1 The Hallmarking Act and Future Changes

The British Hallmarking Act 1973 prohibits the words gold, silver or platinum in descriptions of articles that have not been hallmarked. Hallmarking is the process of putting an authorized stamp on gold or silver articles at a place of assaying (where the proportion of a particular metal of an object is determined, and the date, maker and fineness are stamped on the object). The Act also defines the permissible descriptions of articles coated with precious metals (defined as meaning 'gold, silver or platinum, or any other metal to which by an order under this Act the provisions of the Act are applied).

Schedule 1 allows, if accurate, the word 'gold' to be qualified only by 'plated' or 'rolled', and 'silver' and 'platinum' to be qualified only by 'plated'. The American term 'gold filled' (where filled means 'to fill up a space') is, therefore, prohibited from being used in Great Britain. Terms such as 'German silver' and 'nickel silver' are also prohibited. Note that spectacle frame manufacturers based outside Britain tend to use these descriptions. Prosecutions have been brought under the Trade Descriptions Act, which makes no distinction between manufacturer, wholesaler or retailer (Bennett, 1988). However, a description is permissible if it is implicitly or in express terms confined to the colour of the article. Certain articles, such as those used for medical purposes, have been exempted and need not be hallmarked.

Articles composed of two or more precious metals may be hallmarked only if their content of precious metal fulfills criteria laid down in the Act. In general, this specifies that their precious metal content exceeds 50% of the weight of the whole article.

Note that the national legislation described above will eventually be replaced in the European Union, and elsewhere, by standards such as European Norm BS EN 29202 (1993) and International Standard ISO 9202 (1991). A European Community Draft Directive, DD 4145, deals with the fineness of articles made of gold, platinum, palladium and silver. BS EN 31426 (1994) deals with the determination of gold in gold alloys, and BS EN 31427 (1994) with the determination of silver in silver alloys.

In line with other articles traded within the Community, finished precious metal articles and articles composed of parts of precious metals and parts of base metals and other substances, will have to be marked to conform with the European Norm. A draft European Standard (prEN 1812, 1995) has been published, but one should await the definitive version.

In the USA, hallmarking requirements have been laid down in the National Stamping Act and rulings made by the Federal Trade Commission (see also ANSI Z80.5, 1979).

In order of preciousness, platinum is considered most precious, followed by gold and palladium, and silver is considered least precious (prEN 1812, 1995).

8.2 Metals

8.2.1 INTRODUCTION

As a result of their specific atomic structure, metals have relatively good conductive properties for electricity and heat, and reflect light well. Those used in spectacle frames are, in the main, easy to work, non-flammable, rigid but adjustable and durable, although some are subject to corrosion.

A number of metallic materials have been used in spectacle frame manufacture. These include iron, silver, gold, lead, copper, brass (an alloy of copper and zinc), and steel (an alloy of carbon and iron). Chinese frames were made of an alloy known as paktong; this is white, and contains copper (40–58%), nickel (8–11%) and iron (2·5%) (Davidson, 1989). Rasmussen (1950) wrote that Chinese frames and mountings were made of brass and silver, however, gold and other precious metals were apparently never used.

The following are the more common metals used in the manufacture of spectacle frames. Their characteristics are summarized in Table 8.1

8.2.2 ALUMINIUM (*aluminum*)

Pure aluminium is a soft, silver-white metal that is very light in weight, but is relatively weak. It has a soft surface, and good cold-shaping properties. It is a good electrical and heat conductor. When exposed to the air, it becomes corrosion resistant in a few seconds, during which time a thin, hard oxide develops. This layer can be made durable by compressing and 'anodizing' (an electrolytic process whereby the surface layer is converted into hard aluminium oxide, which acts as a protective coating). Anodized aluminium may be dyed to give special, highly reflective tints. Because of its heat-conducting property, aluminium spectacle sides are provided with plastics end covers (Fig. 8.1) so that they will not feel cold to the touch. At the same time, they prevent any dye from affecting the skin.

TABLE 8.1 *Characteristics of metals*

	Symbol	Density (g cm^{-3})	Melting point (°C)	Soldering properties	Type of solder
Aluminium	**Al**	2·7	660	Bad	
Beryllium	**Be**	1·86	1283		
Chromium	**Cr**	7·19	1890	Poor	
Copper	**Cu**	8·92	1083		
Gold	**Au**	19·32	1063	Good	Gold, silver
Iron	**Fe**	7·86	1530		
Lead	**Pb**	11·3	327		
Manganese	**Mn**	7·21	1250		
Nickel	**Ni**	8·9	1455	Good	Silver
Palladium	**Pd**	12	1554	Poor	
Rhodium	**Rh**	12·44	1966	Bad	
Ruthenium	**Ru**	12·3	2450	Poor	
Silver	**Ar**	10·5	960		
Silicon	**Si**	2·33	1413		
Tin	**Sn**	7·3	232		
Titanium	**Ti**	4·5	1730	Poor	
Zinc	**Zn**	7·1	420		

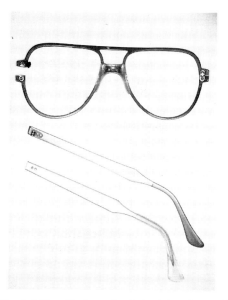

Fig. 8.1 Top: *black anodized aluminium front with riveted half joints to the front; below: silver-coloured anodized aluminium sides showing riveted half joints and plastics end covers*

Its use as a frame material is based on its strength and lightness. However, because aluminium frames become very easily ill-adjusted through normal use, it has not become popular as a frame material (Hardy & Hardy, 1982). Note that the joints are pinned to the front and/or sides. However, if they are part of the frame, they are unwieldy. The material has been used in combination frames.

8.2.3 BERYLLIUM
This is a light, silvery, hard metal that is very strong. When alloyed with copper it can be moulded and shaped while cold, into small, complicated parts. After heat treatment (hardening) it becomes highly elastic and has excellent mechanical properties.

8.2.4 CHROMIUM
This element is blueish-white and has a high melting point. It can be highly polished. In addition to being resistant to abrasion, it is very strong and withstands oxidation at very high temperatures.

On frames it is used mainly as a decorative protection against tarnish. To obtain a dull, black finish, special combinations of chromium and its oxide are used in a partly amorphous state. This finish is protected by dipping it into a special emulsion.

8.2.5 COPPER
This metal is orange-pink in colour, malleable and soft; it is tough and resistant to corrosion.

8.2.6 GOLD
This heavy, precious yellow metal is soft, durable, malleable and ductile. It is unaffected by temperature changes and is highly resistant to acids.

'Fine gold' is defined as pure gold (BS 3521, 1991). Because of its historical uniqueness, a quality designation system of its own was developed based on the 'carat' (abbreviated to 'ct' in the United Kingdom, and 'Kt' or 'K' in the USA and elsewhere). In this system 24 ct represents fine gold, that is 100% pure; hence, 12 ct refers to an alloy containing 50% fine gold.

Because of its poor wearing qualities and great cost, fine gold is not often used. Spectacle frames made of pure gold would give the best protection against corrosion and would not cause allergies but they would be very heavy, soft and expensive.

8.2.7 IRON
Iron is a shiny and relatively soft element that has no resistance to corrosion. When relatively pure (containing no more than 2·5% carbon, and up to a total of 10% of other elements), it is known as wrought iron. It was commonly used before cheap steel became available. Wrought iron is strong, tough and easy to machine. Because it

melts suddenly (between 1100 and 1200°C), it cannot be forged.

8.2.8 LEAD

Lead is a soft, blue-white metal which is used a great deal in alloys.

8.2.9 MANGANESE

This silvery-white element is used in certain types of steel and also in bronze, brass and nickel alloys.

8.2.10 NICKEL

Pure nickel is lustrous and white. It has a high melting point, low electrical and thermal conductivity, can be magnetized and is corrosion resistant. Having been hot-forged, it becomes tough, malleable and ductile on cooling. It can also be polished, welded and rolled into sheets or strung into wires.

8.2.11 PALLADIUM

This white metal of the platinum family does not tarnish in air. It is used to obtain certain surface finishes by either mechanical plating (as used for rolled gold; see Sections 8.4 and 8.5) or galvanizing.

8.2.12 RHODIUM

This silvery-white metal of the platinum group is very rare. It excels in being highly reflective (more so than chromium) after polishing. It is used for mechanical plating of base metals and galvanizing. It then takes on the finish of the surface on which it has been deposited. A rhodium-coated frame must be protected against corrosion with an appropriate intermediate layer. It is used as a colour coating and as tarnish protection only on white rolled gold material, white gold plated frames and decorations.

8.2.13 RUTHENIUM

This member of the platinum family is corrosion resistant and varies in colour from hard blue-white to silvery white to grey. It is used on frames to obtain a gun-metal effect.

8.2.14 SILICON

Most frequently encountered as its oxide (sand).

8.2.15 SILVER

This is a lustrous metal which is extremely malleable and ductile. It polishes well, but tarnishes. It conducts heat and electricity. As solder it makes good joints at 720°C.

8.2.16 TIN

Tin comes is several varieties. The most useful is a silvery white, crystalline metal which is malleable and somewhat ductile. It crumbles to a greyish powder at low temperatures. It is used as a protective coating to prevent corrosion of iron and steel.

8.2.17 TITANIUM

This lustrous, steel-like metal resembles iron and is light in weight (Table 8.1). It is expensive because of the way in which it has to be refined. It is found as oxide in rutile, a reddish-brown mineral (TiO_2), and in ilmenite, a black mineral ($FeOTiO_2$). This is chlorinated at temperatures between 800 and 1000°C to obtain titanium tetrachloride ($TiCl_4$), and then condensed and purified. After reduction with magnesium in an argon atmosphere (it burns in air) at 800°C, one is left with a spongy material. The chloride is then removed under high vacuum at temperatures between 900 and 1000°C. The titanium 'sponge' is then made into a solid in an induction furnace from which it may be poured into forms (Pajonczek, 1991).

Titanium of 90% purity containing magnesium (Titan B) is used for spectacle frame rims. It is more elastic and harder than pure titanium. Titan C is the most expensive variant. It is galvanically covered with double the usual thickness of gold, palladium, etc. and can be worked in a normal, air-containing atmosphere. Some spectacle frames have parts made from different metals including titanium. It is claimed that titanium frames can be about half the weight of conventional metal frames. The smaller the quantity of titanium, the heavier the frame.

This material does not cause allergies and its corrosion resistance is comparable to that of the precious metals. It exhibits great variations in colour and surface structure. Its oxides are used to colour spectacle frame decorations. It has been used for frame manufacture since the latter half of the 1980s. Because it requires special manufacturing processes, such as laser soldering, owing to its unusual hardness, etc., frames made of this material have remained expensive. Specialized workshops can make repairs.

8.2.18 ZINC

In its pure form zinc has a blueish colour and turns dull in air. It is used to galvanize iron.

8.3 Alloys

Alloys are mixtures of metals or of metals and non-metals. They have special properties such as corrosion resistance, great hardness and tensile strength. The following are used in spectacle frame manufacture. Their characteristics are summarized in Table 8.2.

8.3.1 ALUMINIUM ALLOYS

These alloys have great strength and were once used extensively for frames. A variety of colours can be produced by anodizing, and by etching the surface decorations are produced (Fig. 11.35).

Characteristics

The joints used with aluminium frames are either very big and clearly part of the frame part itself, or they are made of a different metal (alloy) and rivetted to front and/or sides (Fig. 8.1). Aluminium sides are provided with plastics end covers.

8.3.2 COBALT ALLOYS

A 46% cobalt, 26% nickel, 20% chromium alloy has been used (Brogan, 1994) for its strength

TABLE 8.2 *Characteristics of alloys*

Name	Components	Density $(g\,cm^{-3})$	Strength $(N\,mm^{-2})$	Melting point (°C)	Soldering properties
Aluminium	Al Cu Si Mn			650	Poor
Bronze	Cu Sn Zn (Pb)	8·9	400–1030	865–1015	Good*
Blanka Z	Cu Ni Zn Sn	8·8	400–800	1046	Good*
Copper–nickel–zinc	Cu Ni Zn	8·65	380–780	1025	Very good*
Monel	Cu Ni Fe Mn	8·9	450–930	1360	Good*
Beryllium–copper	Cu Be Co	8·3		865–980	Poor*
Gold	Cu Ar Ni Zn	14			
Nickel	Ni Mn	8·9	450–800		Good
Silver	Ar Cu Zn			625–800	Very good*
Stainless steel	Cr Ni				Good*

* Can be soldered with silver solder.

when used in thin sections, durability, corrosion resistance and low density.

8.3.3 COPPER ALLOYS
(ISO 197/1, 1983 (E))
8.3.3.1 Copper–tin alloys

Bronze. This alloy must contain at least 60% copper, from 4 to 25% tin as well as zinc and lead. Its colour is yellow or brown. It is harder than pure copper and better suited for casting. It has a low to good corrosion resistance. Bronze is used as a base metal for rolled gold material and for parts that are cold-shaped.

Feather bronze is an alloy of copper and tin. It is exceedingly flexible, but must be protected against corrosion.

8.3.3.2 Copper–nickel–zinc alloys

It should be noted that nickel-containing articles such as costume jewellery have caused allergic reactions in many people. It is with this problem in mind that draft European Union legislation and a European Norm are being prepared to restrict the use of articles containing nickel, that come into contact with the body.

The limit for nickel leaching from such articles is likely to be set at $0.5\,\mu g\,cm^{-2}\,week^{-1}$ (prEN 1811, 1995). This would mean that articles, possibly including spectacle frames, would have to be essentially free from nickel.*

Blanka Z. This alloy consists of copper, nickel, zinc and tin. The higher the proportion of nickel,

the better its corrosion resistance. It cannot be cured and is not magnetic. It has good shaping properties and can be given a galvanic surface finish. Because of its remarkable elasticity, it is widely used for spectacle frame components.

'Nickel-Silver'. This alloy does not actually contain silver. It is usually made up of 60% copper and 18% nickel to which zinc and manganese are added (BS 2870/NS 106 (1980)). It can vary in colour from pale yellow to white. The copper provides its flexibility; the nickel content determines a number of other characteristics such as corrosion resistance, thermal and electrical as well as mechanical properties. Inferior quality alloys of this nature may contain no more than 5% nickel, and have been used for spectacle frames.

The alloy has been known under a variety of other names, such as 'German silver' (because of its likeness to silver when polished) and 'alpaca'. It may cause dermatitis when worn against the skin (see Section 9.3.1).

It is used for soldering and machining; it has a suitable limited corrosion resistance, therefore spectacle frames must be covered with a corrosion-resistant agent. One variety (Akutan) cannot only be formed by cold forming, as after soldering, heat treatment of the whole frame also hardens it.

8.3.3.3 Shape memory alloys

According to one report (Claessens, 1989), these are new mixed alloys. The object of these materials is to be able to repair/restore broken or damaged frames to their original shape simply by bringing them back into a certain shape at a given temperature. Those best known are the Shape Memory Effect brasses. These contain 55–80% copper, 2–8% aluminium and some zinc (Higgins, 1987).

*At the time of press, the British Ministry of Health had withdrawn spectacle frames from the EC Nickel Directive since they fall within the General Medical Devices Directive 93/42/EEC. Discussion is ongoing at European and International Standards Level as to how the question of nickel sensitivity may best be addressed.

8.3.3.4 Copper–nickel alloys
See section 8.3.3.2.

Monel. This alloy is usually made up of 29% copper, 68% nickel, 1·25% iron and 1·25% manganese (BS 3072/3076/NA 13, 1989). It has a dull white appearance and is corrosion resistant. Manganese makes it tarnish resistant, the nickel protects against corrosion, and the copper provides its flexibility. Other elements, such as aluminium, iron and silicon, can be added to improve particular properties.

8.3.3.5 Special copper alloys
Beryllium copper. This is a shiny silver-white, very strong alloy consisting mainly of copper with 1·75% beryllium and 0·2% cobalt (Higgins, 1987). It has a very high electrical conductivity and a low coefficient of elasticity. It is very flexible and malleable, while tensile strength, yield strength and hardness increase considerably during rehardening (Kremmler, 1980). It requires special manufacturing techniques because it is too hard to be worked without annealing, after which it can be cold-shaped. However, it must be rehardened, which involves extra cost. It is suitable for moulding and can be used in very thin spectacle sides or complicated small parts without losing its resilience.

8.3.4 NICKEL ALLOYS (ISO 6372 Part 1)
See section 8.3.3.2.

8.3.4.1 Nickel manganese
Addition of 1·5–2·5% manganese to pure nickel produces an alloy which has been used for eye rims.

8.3.5 SILVER ALLOYS
Because of its softness, silver is usually alloyed

with copper. 'Sterling silver' is an alloy of 92·5% silver and 7·5% copper.

Hard solder, which is also known as silver solder, contains from 50 to 80% silver, along with quantities of copper and zinc.

Frames have been manufactured from silver alloy in past centuries. These were embossed with a hallmark and letter combinations identifying the maker (Fig. 8.2).

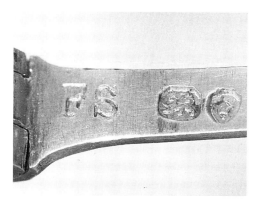

Fig. 8.2 *Silver alloy side showing hallmarks. The letter combination facilitates identification of the maker*

8.3.6 STAINLESS STEEL (BS 970)
This is an alloy of iron, chromium (18%) and nickel (8%) which is only occasionally used for spectacle frame production (Hardy & Hardy, 1982) because it is neither sufficiently malleable nor ductile, and is difficult to work. However, it is frequently used for small components such as screws. Its properties include corrosion resistance, toughness, flexibility and a low mass. Although it is extremely hard, it is reasonably pliable. It is seldom associated with skin irritation.

Because it may have been coated with silver, gold or coloured plastics materials, identification may be difficult.

8.3.7 STEEL

Steel is an alloy of iron and up to 1·7% carbon which also often contains 1% manganese (Higgins, 1987). Its properties vary with the percentage of carbon and other elements.

8.4 Laminated Metals

8.4.1 INTRODUCTION

Until the price of gold rose in the 1970s, making it become prohibitively costly for general application in the manufacture of metal ophthalmic spectacle frames, only rolled gold laminated metal was used for this purpose. Cost-cutting efforts led to the use of electrolytic depositing techniques of thin metal layers, together with surface finishes and coatings that give the impression of a gold frame.

The discovery of a method of mechanically fusing silver to copper led to the development of a method of fusing gold to copper in 1817, by John Turner (Kook, 1978).

Modern techniques have not revolutionized the manufacturing method except for the use of new base metals (BS 3521, 1991; a basic material upon which a surface of precious metal is formed). The composition of base metals was once a carefully guarded secret because it determined the quality of the frame. Currently, the alloys mentioned above are used.

8.4.2 ROLLED GOLD

BS 6625 (1985) defines rolled gold as a base metal to which an even covering of carat gold has been bonded by welding or brazing, the material subsequently being formed into gold clad wire, sheet or tube (see Section 8.5 for details). It is known in French as '*doublé*' (originally *double* or *laminé*, that is, a sheet of base metal with a carat gold laminate on both surfaces).

8.4.2.1 Quality

The nominal quality of rolled gold material may be expressed in either of two ways (BS 3462, 1962), namely as

(1) the number of parts by weight of fine gold per 1000 parts of the whole. It is usually shown as, for instance, 50/000 or the number 50 in a circle (Fig. 8.3)
(2) the proportion by weight of a specified quality of gold, such as 1/20 12 ct. This means that 1/20th of 1000 g (50 g) is 12 ct gold alloy (Fig. 8.4).

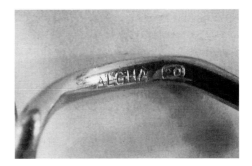

Fig. 8.3 *Rolled gold quality marking '20': 20 parts in 1000 of the whole object, are fine gold*

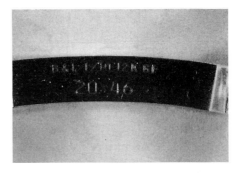

Fig. 8.4 *Rolled gold quality marking '1/10 12 K GF': 1/10th out of 1000 g is 12 carat gold. GF, gold filled (Am.) or rolled gold*

It is customary to specify the quality of rolled gold wire as the ratio of pure gold to the total weight of the wire, as in (1) above. The thickness (t) of the carat gold covering of this wire is given by the following approximate equation:

$$t = d \cdot \text{diam} \cdot ct \cdot 1000/4D(C - ct) \,\mu\text{m}$$

where
d = density of the base metal (usually 9 g cm^{-3})
diam = diameter of the wire in millimetres
ct = gold content of the wire, in thousands
D = density of the gold alloy (usually 14 g cm^{-3})
C = gold content of the alloy, in thousands
    (Essilor)

Example: for a 1 mm diameter (diam = 1) wire of 20/000 ($ct = 20$), and 14 ct = 14/24 or 583/000 ($C = 583$) gold alloy, we obtain a thickness of 5·7 μm for the rolled gold covering of the base metal of the wire.

The qualities of rolled gold that were used in spectacle frame production were 10, 12 and 14 ct (Barker *et al.*, 1932; Hardy & Hardy, 1982). Currently, 14 and 16 ct are used (Fink, 1978; UK Optical, 1988). As the proportion of gold is increased in the alloys, they become heavier, more costly and softer, but less susceptible to corrosion and atmospheric influences. A 10 ct alloy is harder than a 12 ct alloy and will resist wear and abrasion better; a 12 ct alloy is more resistant to acid skin secretions and atmospheric conditions, that is, it tarnishes less easily. A 14 ct alloy has even better properties. Higher quality gold alloy is not normally used for optical work because of its cost and lack of wearing qualities; alloy lower than 10 ct is unsuitable because it corrodes easily (Barker *et al.*, 1932; Fink, 1978).

8.4.2.2 CHARACTERISTICS

The characteristics of rolled gold are:

- expensive
- limited design (shaping) possibilities
- non-porous cladding prevents atmospheric attack (e.g. by humidity and skin secretions)
- easily repaired (soldering)
- allergic reactions are rare
- the copper in the alloy may cause black streaks when in contact with cosmetics.

8.4.3 GOLD PLATED

This is defined (BS 6625, 1985) as a base metal coated with gold or gold alloy with a minimum purity of 18 ct and a thickness not less than 1·0 μm.

8.4.4 WASHED GOLD

Washed gold refers to a base metal covered by a very thin deposit of gold by electro- or chemical deposition. This technique is unsuitable for ophthalmic frames because the thin deposit wears off very quickly. It has been used for metal sunglass frames.

8.5 Rolled Gold Production

8.5.1 INITIAL PROCESS

Carat gold is melted in an electric oven, in vacuum. It is then cast into plates from which sheets are rolled. These are cut into strips, 2–4 mm thick. From these strips, 'rounds' of 120 mm diameter are stamped. These are covered with a thin layer of solder, a nickel layer (to protect against possible corrosion and diffusion caused by a damaged carat gold layer), followed by another layer of solder. This layered round is sweated (united by partially fusing metal surfaces) in a furnace under high pressure (Fig. 8.5).

8.5.2 WIRE PRODUCTION

The round is deep-drawn in five stages and three annealing processes, into a tube 500 mm long and

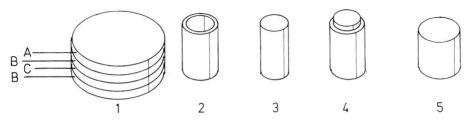

Fig. 8.5 *(1) A 'round' consisting of (A) a top layer of carat gold, and layers of solder (B) and nickel (C), which is pressed into (2) a tube with the carat gold cladding on the outside; (3) a base metal cylinder with a diameter fractionally smaller than the internal diameter of the tube; (4) the cylinder is fitted into the tube and having been heated in a furnace, becomes (5) a solid object*

45 mm diameter. Its inner surface is ground with an abrasive and thoroughly cleaned.

A base metal rod is prepared to fit exactly into the carat gold tube. The tube is then fitted around the base metal rod. Its total weight is now around 7 kg. This object is fitted into a steel mantle and placed into an annealing furnace which is then heated to 800°C. At this temperature the base metal expands more than the carat gold layer, while the steel mantle does not expand at all. Once the base and gold have been sweated in this way the layers cannot be separated mechanically.

After cooling, the steel cylinder is removed. The laminated rod is then repeatedly drawn (Fig. 8.6) through powerful wire mills. Each operation reduces its diameter and increases its length, thus producing a long wire.

The finishing process consists of several swaging and annealing processes, and passing the wire through rolling mills. Finally, the diameter is further reduced by passing the wire through dies (Fig. 8.7). These have been accurately cut to reduce the wire to the desired diameter. The result of this series of operations is a 1050 m long 1 mm diameter wire with a 20/000 carat gold layer 5·9 μm thick.

Special shapes and fancy designs are produced by feeding the wire through specially hardened

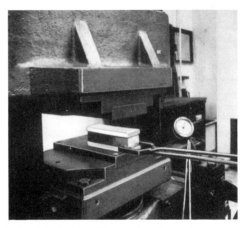

Fig. 8.6 *Rolled gold rod being drawn through wire mills (photograph courtesy Ferd. Wagner, Pforzheim)*

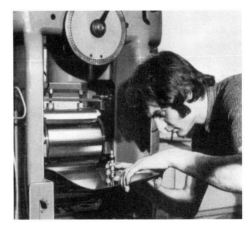

Fig. 8.7 *Reducing the diameter of rolled gold wire by drawing it through dies (photograph courtesy Ferd. Wagner, Pforzheim)*

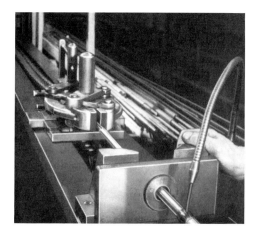

Fig. 8.8 Reshaping round rolled gold wire by passing it between rolls (photograph courtesy Ferd. Wagner, Pforzheim)

steel shaping and patterning rolls, or drawing through dies (Fig. 8.8). Throughout this process great care is taken to keep the carat gold surface spotlessly clean and free from scratches and other irregularities.

8.5.3 SHEET AND TUBE PRODUCTION

Sheet is made by welding or soldering a plate of alloyed gold to both sides of a thick block of base

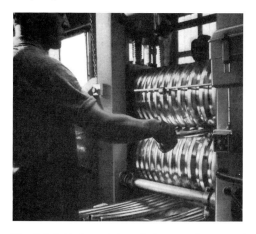

Fig. 8.9 A block consisting of a base metal centre and carat gold top and bottom, is about to be placed in a furnace (photograph courtesy Ferd. Wagner, Pforzheim)

metal (Fig. 8.9). The resulting composite block is passed repeatedly through heavy, polished steel rollers until the block has been reduced to a sheet of the required thickness (Fig. 8.10).

Tube is made out of discs that have been stamped from rolled gold sheet. The discs are then pressed into 'saucers', then into 'cups' and finally into hollow tubes (Fig. 8.11). These can be drawn to any required thickness by pulling through a series of steel drawplates, steel mandrels (conical objects) of diminishing size being

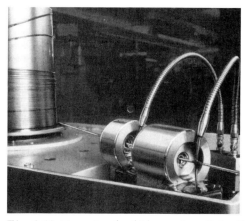

Fig. 8.10 Measuring the thickness of a rolled gold sheet with a micrometer (photograph courtesy Ferd. Wagner, Pforzheim)

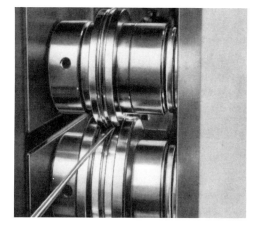

Fig. 8.11 Reducing and/or shaping a rolled gold tube by drawing it through a drawplate (photograph courtesy Ferd. Wagner, Pforzheim)

introduced to the inside to regulate the wall thickness (Barker *et al.*, 1932; Wagner, 1980).

8.5.4 COMMENT

As a result of forming profiled material from a round or flat form, the thickness of the rolled gold layer may vary in places (Fig. 8.12). This was established as long ago as 1932 (Barker *et al.*, 1932). Walsh & O'Neill (1991) pointed out that any plated frame material will act like a battery; gold will then act as a cathode and the frame's base metal as an anode while the patient's perspiration acts as electrolyte. This promotes corrosion provided there are any holes in the plating. The lacquer layer on certain metal frames acts as insulator, but we do not know how good these layers are. Because the base metal is often chosen for its mechanical rather than its chemical

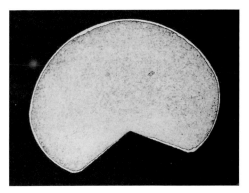

Fig. 8.12 Section through a metal rim. Note the thickness variation of the outer, rolled gold layer (from Walsh & O'Neill, 1991, by permission of Optician)

properties, the integrity of the surface coating is of paramount importance.

The application of metals and alloys in spectacle frame parts is summarized in Table 8.3 .

TABLE 8.3 Applications of metals and alloys in spectacle frame parts

	Front	Side	Rim	Bridge	Joint	Pad arms	Decor	Surface finish	Core
METALS									
Cr								*	
Cu								*	
Au	*	*					*	*	
Ni			*			*		*	*
Pd								*	
Rh							*	*	
Ru								*	
Ti	*	*	*	*	*	*			
ALLOYS									
Alum.	*	*				*	*		
Bronze		*				*			
Blanka Z	*	*	*	*		*			
Ni Cu	*	*	*	*	*				
Monel		*		*	*				
Be Cu				*	*				
Ni Mn			*						
Stainless steel	*	*	*	*	*	*	*		

FURTHER READING

Essilor (undated). *Cahiers d'Optique Oculaire, No. 8: les Montures (Ophthalmic Optics File, No. 8: Spectacle Frames).* Paris: Essilor International.

Marwitz (undated). *Brief Information Booklet on Materials.* Oberkochen: Zeiss.

Rodenstock (undated). *Information: Metal Spectacle Frames.* München: Rodenstock.

Spangemacher, J. (1977). Der Industriereport: rolled gold. (doublé) – gold too. *Augenoptiker,* p. 2–8.

Zeiss (undated) *Metallfassungen.* Stuttgart: Marwitz + Hauser.

REFERENCES

Anonymous (undated). *The Properties and Uses of Nickel Silver.* London: Henry Wiggin & Co. Ltd.

ANSI Z80.5 (1979). *American National Standard Requirements for Dress Ophthalmic Frames. Appendix: Marking and Stamping Optical Frames and Mountings Made in Whole or in Part of Gold.* New York: American National Standards Institute, Inc.

Barker, W.B., Champness, W.H., Courlander, H., Dadd, F.W., Harwood, J., & Sutcliffe, J.H. (1932). *Enquiry into the Manufacture of Gold-Filled Spectacles.* London: Joint Council of Qualified Opticians.

Bennett, F.W. (1988). Letter to the Editor: Spectacle frames and the Hallmarking Act, 1973. *Optom. Today* **28**, 181.

Brogan, R. (1994). Presenting the light fantastic. *Optician* **207**, 5448, 20–25.

BS 970 (1991). *Specification for Wrought Steel for Mechanical and Allied Engineering Purposes.* Part 1. London: British Standards Institution.

BS 2870 (1980). *Specification for Rolled Copper and Copper Alloys: Sheet, Strip and Foil.* London: British Standards Institution.

BS 3072 (1989). *Specification for Nickel and Nickel Alloys: Sheet and Plate.* London: British Standards Institution.

BS 3076 (1989). *Specification for Nickel and Nickel Alloys: Bar.* London: British Standards Institution.

BS 3462 (1962). *Specification for Metal Spectacle Frames.* London: British Standards Institution.

BS 3521: Part 1 (1991). *Terms Relating to Ophthalmic Optics and Spectacle Frames. Part 1. Glossary of Terms Relating to Ophthalmic Lenses.* London: British Standards Institution.

BS 6625 (1985). *Specification for Spectacle Frames.* London: British Standards Institution.

BS EN 29202 (1993). *Jewellery – Fineness of Precious Metal Alloys.* London: British Standards Institution.

BS EN 31426 (1994) (ISO 11426, 1993). *Determination of Gold in Gold Jewellery Alloys – Cupellation Method (Fire Assay).* London: British Standards Institution.

BS EN 31427 (1994) (ISO 11427, 1993). *Determination of Silver in Silver Jewellery Alloys – Volumetric (Potentiometric) Method Using Potassium Bromide.* London: British Standards Institution.

Claessens, B.M.L. (1989). De optische industrie in Japan: opvallende merkproducten. *Oculus, Amsterdam* **51**, 21–23.

Davidson, D.C. (1989). *Spectacles, Lorgnettes and Monocles, Album 227,* p. 31. Princes Risborough: Shire Publ.

Deichman, H. (1990). Moderne Technologien für die Produktion von Brillenfassungen im VEB Rathenower Optische Werke "Hermann Duncker". *Augenoptik, Berlin* **107** (1), 25–28.

Essilor (undated). *Cahiers d'Optique Oculaire, No. 8: les Montures (Ophthalmic Optics File, No. 8: Spectacle Frames).* Paris: Essilor International.

Fink, W. (1978). Der aktuelle Bericht: Glänzende Geschäfte. Bericht über eine Goldbrillenkollektion. *Neues Optikerjournal* No. 4, 59–61.

Hardy, S. (1983). Frame materials: metals. *Manufact. Optician Int.* **36**, 13, 17.

Hardy, S., & Hardy, W.E. (1982). Frame materials: a perspective; part 1. *Manuf. Optics Int.* **35** (6), 18–23.

Higgins, R.A. (1987). *Materials for the Engineering Technician,* 2nd edn. London: Hodder & Stoughton.

ISO 197/1 (1983) (E). *Copper and Copper Alloys – Terms and Definitions. Part 1: Materials.* Genève: International Standards Organization.

ISO 6372 (1989). *Nickel and Nickel Alloys – Terms and Definitions. Part 1: Materials.* Genève: International Standards Organization.

ISO 9202 (1991). *Jewellery – Fineness of Precious Metal Alloys.* Genève: International Standards Organization.

Kook, N.J. (1978). Metal frame materials. *Optician* **175**, 4527, 17–18.

Kremmler, J. (1980). Copper–beryllium for modern spectacle frames. *Manuf. Optics Int.* **33** (5), 49.

National Stamping Act, 15. *United States Code,* 294 et seq.

Pajonczek, R. (1991). Titan–himmlisch leicht für irdische Ansprüche. *Neues Optikerj.* **33** (7/8), 64–65.

prEn 1811 (1995). *Precious Metals – Reference Test Method for Release of Nickel.* Brussels: CEN.

prEN 1812 (1995). *Precious Metals – Marking of Precious Metal Articles.* Brussels: CEN.

Rasmussen, O.D. (1950). *Chinese Eyesight and Spectacles,* p. 27. Tonbridge: Rasmussen.

UK Optical (1988). Gold. The original classic. (advertisement). *Optician* **196** (5174), 30.

Wagner, F. (1980). Metal frame manufacturing: rolled gold. *Manuf. Optician Int.* **33** (5), 47.

Walsh, G., & O'Neill, P. (1991). All that glisters is not gold. *Optician* **202** (5317), 11–12.

CHAPTER 9

The Skin and Spectacle Frames

9.1 The Skin

The skin has a self-protecting function in that it maintains the integrity of its own structure and components; it also acts as boundary to the environment, thus protecting the inner structures of the body (Harkness, 1971) from injury and invasion by foreign organisms.

It has two layers (Fig. 9.1). The thin outer, horny layer called the epidermis, consists of squamous (scale-like) epithelial cells and provides protection. Its cells are shed constantly and are replaced by cells from deeper layers. The epidermis covers the dermis, which is a much thicker layer. The dermis is composed of fibrous and elastic tissue, richly supplied with nerve endings thus making it a huge sense organ. The fibrous tissue, collagen, has a crosslinked structure (see Chapter 7). It determines the ultimate tensile strength of the skin, which is about $1 \cdot 8\,\mathrm{kg}$ mm^{-2}; it is lower in females than in males (Wright, 1971). Despite its thinness the epidermis has appreciable tensile strength, although compared with the total strength of the skin it is negligible. The tensile strength varies with the direction in which it is measured. Its distensibility (capacity to stretch) decreases with increasing age – 50–59% at birth to 24–48% in adults (Wright, 1971).

The coefficient of friction of the skin will depend on a number of factors, such as greasiness and perspiration (see Section 13.7). In conjunction with plastics it may be taken as having a value of about $0 \cdot 4$ (Wolfram, 1989).

The skin is part of the body's temperature-regulating mechanism and helps to prevent dehydration. In addition to hairs, it contains glands. The two main types are the sebaceous and sweat glands.

Sebaceous glands open into each hair follicle through short, wide ducts. However, they can also be found independently, especially on the face. There are about 600 sebaceous glands per square centimetre on face and scalp; elsewhere, the number is about $100\ \mathrm{cm}^{-2}$. These glands excrete an oily substance, sebum, which is essential for the maintenance of the epidermis: without this oily secretion it would dry out, flake and crack thus allowing pathogenic organisms to enter the body. Sebum is a complex mixture of triglycerides, free fatty acids, waxes, sterols, squalene and paraffins. In view of the number of glands, the amount of sebum on the body surface is insignificant, with the exception of the forehead where it forms a $50\,\mu\mathrm{m}$ thick film.

Sweat glands are simple, tubular organs found all over the skin. Their secretory portion lies deep in the dermis. Their irregular distribution over the whole of the body varies from 60 to 800 glands per square centimetre.

Sweating occurs principally when the body needs to eliminate heat. On average $0 \cdot 25\,\mathrm{l}$ of sweat is produced per day. This may rise to $10\,\mathrm{l}$ in extreme conditions. When sweat evaporates it causes a loss of latent heat. This helps to maintain the body's thermal equilibrium. Sweating has special importance in hot climates where heat loss is not easily achieved by other means.

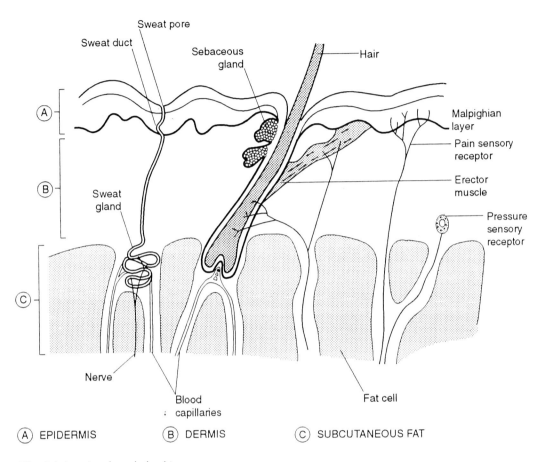

Sweat pore
Sweat duct
Sebaceous gland
Hair
Malpighian layer
Pain sensory receptor
Erector muscle
Pressure sensory receptor
(A)
(B)
Sweat gland
(C)
Nerve
Blood capillaries
Fat cell

(A) EPIDERMIS　　(B) DERMIS　　(C) SUBCUTANEOUS FAT

Fig. 9.1 *A section through the skin*

Sweat mixes with epithelial scales and sebum on the skin's surface. Its usual acidity appears to be based on the presence of lactic acid and dicarboxylic amino acids in sweat secretions mixed with sebaceous material. Its pH varies between 4 and 6 (pH of 1 is strongly acid and 11 is strongly alkali). The effect of age on the skin's pH is poorly documented (Dikstein & Zlotogorski, 1989).

After water, the next main constituent of sweat is sodium chloride. The higher the body's salt intake, the higher the concentration of sodium chloride in sweat. In people not used to sweating the sodium chloride content will be much higher than in those acclimatized to heat, unless they have a high salt intake.

According to Leveque (1989), 'dry skin' is encountered in the majority of people older than 65 years. Ageing is also associated with changes such as a lowering of the skin temperature, a reduction of the blood microcirculation, and the modification of epidermal lipids.

9.2 Allergies

An allergy may be defined as an altered or acquired state of sensitivity, or an abnormal reaction of the body to substances that are normally harmless. Such substances are called allergens and include food stuffs, pollens, animal scurf, metals (such as found in costume jewellery), house dust, chemicals (such as detergents and cosmetics), drugs, and living or dead microorganisms. Light, heat, cold and even emotional stimuli may also result in allergic reactions. They may be immediate or delayed.

An 'immediate' reaction occurs within minutes after re-exposure to an allergen. It is associated with the vascular system, and histamine plays an important part in its production. A 'delayed' reaction may occur several hours or days after exposure to the allergen. The delayed reaction is thought to involve reactions inside lymphoid cells. Histamine does not appear to play a major role.

Allergic reactions usually present themselves as an inflammation of the skin, or dermatitis. The latter term is more commonly used in the United States while in the United Kingdom it is usually referred to as eczema. The National Eczema Society (1986) classifies eczema into nine types. Each causes a similar rash of red spots, rough scaling, dryness (Fig. 9.2), and soreness of the skin, perhaps leading to the formation of blisters (Fig. 9.3) which burst and weep.

The types of eczema possibly caused by spectacle wear are presented in Table 9.1. The recognition of allergic contact eczema may be difficult as it may resemble any of the other eczematous dermatoses. Definitive diagnosis of irritant or allergic contact eczema can be made only in the context of a skillfully elicited history together with an accurate interpretation of patch tests.

Patch testing is carried out as follows. A small number of allergens are secured to the skin with a specially designed adhesive dressing. This is kept in place for 48 h. On removal the area is examined and it is noted which allergen(s) has/have caused a reaction. After a further 24–48 h, a re-examination follows. The test should be carried

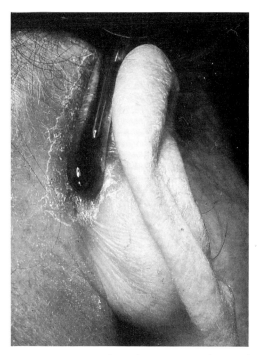

Fig. 9.2 Dry, rough, scaling eczema (photograph Central Illustration Services, United Medical and Dental Schools of Guy's and St. Thomas's Hospitals, London)

out by experienced staff. Patients with active eczema should not be subjected to a test until the rash has subsided or the test may cause the condition to flare up again.

Interpretation of the results is difficult because a positive reaction does not necessarily mean that

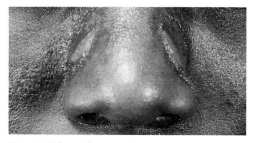

Fig. 9.3 Blisters formation due to eczema (photograph Central Illustration Services, United Medical and Dental Schools of Guy's and St. Thomas's Hospitals, London)

TABLE 9.1 *Types of eczema in spectacle wearers*

Allergic contact eczema	Sensitive skins, such as those of older people, redheads and people with fair hair as well as women post-natally, are more likely to be subject to this type of eczema. It is uncommon in children. The condition is caused by a substance actually penetrating the skin. Such substances include nickel, chromate, rubber, dyes, resins and preservatives. Sensitivity may build up over a long period and may give rise to a secondary rash at a different part of the body. It may be possible to observe seasonal variations
Atopic eczema	May appear in early childhood and is strongly associated with asthma and hayfever. It is often followed by irritant contact eczema
Irritant contact eczema	This is a delayed hypersensitivity to an external allergen as a result of a previous sensitization. It may be caused by such substances as acids, alkalis and solvents which directly damage the skin's surface cells. It tends to display seasonal variations: in winter, cold weather and low humidity it causes chapping, dryness and itching
Pompholyx	A blistering type of eczema which makes the skin very itchy. It subsequently dries out and peels. It can be aggravated by heat and sweating. Contact with rubber and plastics including polyamide could make the condition worse
Seborrhoeic eczema	Affects mainly adults and presents as an itchy, scaly scalp showing severe dandruff. It spreads over the face as a rash. The skin is then particularly sensitive to irritants

the particular allergen is responsible for the rash: it may indicate only that the patient is hypersensitive to that particular substance. The dressing might also have caused the irritation thus giving rise to a false positive result. The test is sometimes carried out with the actual suspected substance or object. Skin pigmentation may affect results (Berardesca & Maibach, 1989).

9.3 Effects of Frames on the Skin

9.3.1 NICKEL

The major sensitizer among the spectacle frame materials is nickel. It is present in many metal frames and in costume jewellery. Dowaliby (1987) wrote that approximately 6% of the US population suffers from this allergy. In Europe, about 20% of females* and 6% of males are affected. However, the recorded incidence of allergic reactions to nickel in spectacle frames is

*This percentage is also quoted by S. Carter, Senior Consultant, Health & Safety, Laboratory of the Government Chemist, London, in a letter dated 25 April 1996 addressed to the Consumer Liaison Officer of BSI Standards. However, K. Hale, Senior Executive Officer, Local Authorities Coordinating Body on Food and Trading Standards, Croydon, in a fax to the same addressee (received 7 May 1996), writes 'that at least 10% of the female population of Western Europe demonstrate a nickel allergy . . .'

proportionally quite small (Such, 1993). It may become mandatory (within the European Union) to mark as such, or prohibit the use of, nickel-containing objects that come in contact with the skin. In 1992, a nickel-free alloy for the production of eyewires became available (Bartels, 1992). This was in anticipation of the expected move to control the use of nickel in spectacle frames to items that leach no more than $0.5 \, \mu\text{g cm}^{-2} \, \text{week}^{-1}$. See prEN 1811 (1995) and Section 8.3.3.2.

Nickel is not generally kept in contact with the skin, but contact could occur when a plastics coating has been eroded, or when a metal coating not containing nickel has tarnished. There are reports of eczema caused by the nickel-containing core of plastics sides (Jirasek *et al.*, 1976; Sun, 1987). Calnan (1957) found that nickel sensitivity was more common in women but pointed out that stocking suspenders, earrings, clips and fasteners were the main sensitizing objects. Although some patients had been found to be 'nickel positive', they were often able to wear that metal in contact with their skin without showing a reaction: therefore, sweat, friction and penetration were considered to be important additional factors. Calnan noted a triad associated with the clinical pattern of nickel eczema: (1) a primary lesion at sites of direct contact, (2) a secondary symmetrical eruption of the 'sensitization' type, and (3) patches of eczema that did not appear to be directly related to the nickel sensitivity.

British Standard 3462 (1962) specifies that frames and curl sides (Fig. 9.4) made of so-called nickel silver, shall contain not less than 14% nickel by weight, and joint and pivot screws not less than 12%. This appears to be based on a statement by Duke-Elder (1954) that dermatitis is more common if the amount of nickel in the alloy is less than 15%. For greater detail see Maibach & Menné (1989).

9.3.2 OTHER METALS

Contact eczema caused by metals other than nickel, such as copper, chromium, mercury and cobalt, has been reported (Saltzer & Wilson, 1968), while Theodore & Schlossman (1958) stated that allergy to both platinum and solid gold spectacle frames can occur. Gaul (1958) reported a case where the zinc contents of a metal frame had caused a reaction.

9.3.3 PLASTICS

The problems associated with plastics materials are more complicated than with metals because there are many different manufacturing processes involved, and details of these are not always readily available. Not only the chemicals used in the making, but also those used during the processing and dyeing, together with impurities, must be considered.

Table 9.2 gives details of reports of allergies to plastics frame materials. Because cellulose nitrate is now very infrequently used as a spectacle frame material, it has not been considered.

Swinney (1951) reported on two patients who

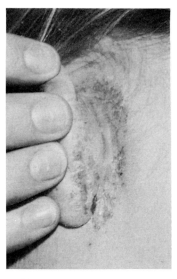

Fig. 9.4 Allergic reaction caused by a nickel curl side

TABLE 9.2 *Reported allergies to plastics frame materials*

Butyl acrylate	**Hambly & Wilkinson (1978), and Cronin (1980) reported one case each. Methyl, ethyl and butyl acrylates are all possible ingredients of acrylic (PMMA) frames. These patients did not show a reaction to the first two compounds**
Cellulose acetate	**Berkoff (1938) provided strong evidence that, before the Second World War, plasticizers were the causative factor of eczema**
Formaldehyde polymer	**Wilde (1959) reported on four women shown to have developed eczema after wearing spectacles made of phenol formaldehyde, a material not normally used for spectacle frames. Patch testing to formalin showed positive results within 24 h. This might be the result of a reaction between the skin and the polymer, formalin, having leached from the material**
Optyl	**Fisher (1976) encountered a woman who had eczema caused by an Optyl frame. She had previously been sensitized by an epoxy resin, and reacted to scrapings from such a frame, but not to polyurethane resin (with which these frames are coated). The manufacturers of Optyl emphasize the point that it is physiologically inert**

reacted to the red plastics of their frames, but not to clear plastics. Neither the type of reaction, nor the dye in question, was mentioned.

Jordan & Dahl (1971) encountered a patient who reacted to ethylene glycol monomethyl ether acetate which had been used to cement nose pads to the spectacle front. They also reported (Jordan & Dahl, 1972) on three patients who responded positively to patch testing for resorcinol monobenzoate, and on one who responded to *p*-tert-butyl phenol while three patients were found to react to colouring agents (the azo dyes, solvent yellow 3 and solvent red 26).

Bedford (1976) concluded that the likelihood of a plasticizer being responsible for an allergic reaction is small, but according to Smith & Calman (1966) it was not insignificant.

Hausen & Jung (1985) calculated that although many millions of people wear spectacles, they caused no more than 1200 to 3000 cases of contact eczema per year in the former West Germany, with a population of about 62 million

people. Of 56 cases recorded since the Second World War, 11 were caused by pigments/dyes, another 11 by chemicals in the plastics materials, and seven by plasticizers. Smith & Calman (1966) concluded that irritations are usually caused by the dyes, plasticizers and varnishes, and Jordan & Dahl (1972) added antioxidants to the list; they agreed that irritation was not caused by the actual plastics of which frames are made.

Six out of seven cases reported by Hausen & Jung (1985) were contact allergies. They hypothesized that the eczema was caused by the effect of sweat or sebum on a constituent of the plastics material, or that these had reacted with the chemical additives thus creating one or more new compounds responsible for the reaction. They were convinced that polyurethane coatings suppress the development of eczema. However, the coating must be regularly renewed because the film becomes permeable.

Walsh *et al.* (1991) cited allergies to spectacle frame materials containing triphenyl phosphate

(Carlsen *et al.*, 1986), phenyl salicylate (Sonnex & Rycroft, 1986), aliphatic isocyanate (Vilaplana *et al.*, 1987) and paraphenylenediamine (Doherty & Freeman, 1988: this article includes a review of other agents).

9.3.4 CANCEROID DEVELOPMENTS

Otto (1958) reported on four cases and concluded that 'the permanent pressure of the spectacle front (on the nasal flank) was the essential cause for the origin of their cancer. We must imagine that by this means gradually continuous epithelial lesions can appear which may lead to a pathological increase of cells'.

Miller (1971) analysed 62 cases of facial skin cancer. The study revealed that the preferential areas of development were the inner canthus and lateral nose, the cheek and pre-auricular regions, the bridge of the nose, the groove between nose and lip, and the lip and ear. Thirty-one patients were older than 60 years. Of 25 cases with cancer in the region of the eyelid and nasal flank, 15 wore spectacles permanently and 10 occasionally wore either reading or sun spectacles. Because none of the frame materials were carcinogenic, the spectacle-induced cancer could only be the result of constant pressure and skin irritation at the points of contact between face and spectacle frame.

Barnes *et al.* (1974) and Neering & Nanning (1978) describe cases variously referred to as acanthoma fissuratum, granuloma fissuratum and spectacle acanthoma. This is a benign condition often misdiagnosed, because of its clinical appearance, as a basal cell epithelioma. It appears as a raised pink nodule with a longitudinal central fissure above or behind the ear. It is thought to be the result of the continual trauma caused by the spectacle frame on the skin. It has also been observed on the bridge of the nose and above the malar area. The frame always fits into the fissure of the lesion. It can be cured by removal of the pressure through either a frame adjustment, or by fitting another frame. The nodule may be expected to resolve 3–4 weeks after removal of the cause of the trauma.

Heidenreich (1975) agreed with Otto (1958) and Miller (1972) on the cause of cancer and stressed the importance of an anatomically correct fit of the front in the wearer's nasal area. He added that as a result of fashion influences this aspect remained somewhat neglected. Because spectacle frame materials do not contain carcinogenic substances, tumours of the nasal bearing surfaces cannot be due to chemicals, but are initiated mechanically. The dispenser must avoid pressure being exerted by a spectacle frame on an area from which a carcinoma has been removed. Tumours found in the nasal area may also develop in the areas of contact with the sides (see also Section 18.2).

9.3.5 GENERAL EFFECTS

Skin irritation is usually noticed after a few hours of wearing a new pair of spectacles. The skin becomes red and tender where the frame presses into, or rubs against the skin. An adjustment usually overcomes the problem. The skin of older patients is often less resistant to trauma induced by spectacle frames (see Section 18.2).

Bedford (1976) investigated the effect of weight and quality of fit of 99 glazed spectacles with respect to mechanical irritation. He divided the spectacles into three groups according to mass, namely those < 30 g (34%), > 30 and < 60 g (56%), and those > 60 g (9%). The findings of the largest group are statistically summarized in Table 9.3. Bedford (1976) concluded that the incidence of inflammation and physical indentation of those areas of the skin in contact with the bearing surface of a pair of spectacles, varies directly with the type of bridge incorporated in, and the mass of a pair of glazed spectacles. However, the amount of inflammation and indentation produced by cellulose acetate frames with a pad bridge appeared to be independent of mass. In each case where the spectacles were said to be uncomfortable there was an increased inci-

TABLE 9.3 *Mechanical irritation due to weight and quality of fit, caused by glazed spectacles*

	%
Constantly worn	66
Having a pad bridge	86
Having a saddle bridge	14
Subjectively judged to be fitting comfortably	78
Observed to cause redness on nasal bridge	57
Observed to cause a groove on the nose	43
Fit of bridge:	
Good	65
Passable	32
Indifferent	3
Bearing surface of frame:	
Clean	30
Greasy	68
Bloomed	14
Frame material decomposing:	
Stage 0	41
Stage 1	32
Stage 2	16
Wearer washed frames	59

(After Bedford, 1976.)
Mass > 30 and < 60 g; *N* = 56.

dence of redness and indentation. Rolled gold frames with a pad bridge, when constantly worn, tended to result in an increase in discomfort with a greater incidence of redness and indentation of the skin, irrespective of the frame's mass. Almost half of the light-weight frames said to be comfortable, and all that were not, caused redness and indentation, notwithstanding a good bridge fit in most cases. Similar results were obtained for the other two groups of frames. Light-weight, saddle bridge frames, when worn constantly, did not produced any redness or indentation of the bearing surface and all felt comfortable and fitted well. Half of the medium-weight frames produced redness and indentation while most fitted well.

Bedford (1976) concluded that a saddle bridge gives the wearer greater comfort, together with a smaller incidence of indentation, but greater redness than a pad bridge on a rolled gold frame. There was a greater incidence of mechanical irritation in wearers of rolled gold frames with small plastics pads.

9.3.6 CONCLUSION

Skin irritation can be caused by a spectacle frame. If frames are not cleaned regularly the surface can become rough as a result of a build-up of foreign material (Fig. 9.5), such as dust, hair spray, perfumes, after-shave, soap, smoke, dead cells and sebum. It can form into an abrasive layer which will rub against the skin thus causing irritation. Certain chemicals and perfumes, on the other hand, erode the frame material and cause a rough surface (Fig. 9.6 and see Fig. 9.8).

Allergic eczema may be the result of spectacle frame wear, or a manifestation of a sensitivity acquired from other sources. Hence, one can only speak of true allergic eczema if the frame is found to fit perfectly, not to have abrasive surfaces and is not too heavy. Perspiration is an important factor in allergic reaction.

The most common site of irritation is behind the ear, followed by the nasal flanks. It is also

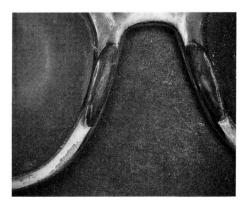

Fig. 9.5 *Foreign material build-up on back plane of the front*

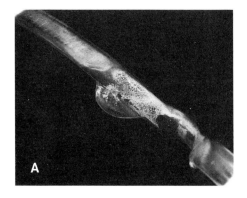

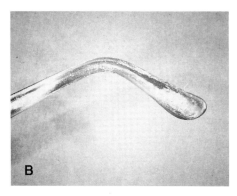

Fig. 9.6 *Rough surfaces on bridge bearing surface and inner aspect of drop cause by erosion*

found at the temples, under the sides of the frame. This, however, is also a matter of incorrect frame fitting. The eczema may be acute and of the weeping variety. However, it is often drier and more lichenified. If very severe it may spread to adjacent areas and can cause swelling of the eyelids and cheeks. The conjunctiva may become involved.

9.4 Effects of Skin on Frames

9.4.1 CORROSION OF FRAMES

This may be defined as the disturbance of materials by chemical or electrochemical reaction with their surround. Corrosion in both metals and plastics may originate on their surface and have a similar appearance. One may observe surface roughness, hairline cracks and small cavities.

The corrosion of metals is caused mainly by humidity and by electrolytic action, where ions migrate as a result of electric current that may be set up between frame and skin. The effect of ultra-violet radiation, together with atmospheric oxygen on plastics materials, not only weakens them, but it also gives rise to discoloration. This occurs to a greater extent on its surface (Hinterhofer & Fahrner, 1983).

In this context one must not overlook that spectacle frames are worn from 2–4 years, and often much longer. During this period they may be in contact with a specific part of the head for a major part of the day. Experience shows that general wear and tear and also slow corrosion takes its toll. However, the reaction is sometimes very rapid, causing extensive damage within a few months. Frequently (see Bedford, 1976, above), a layer of grease, dirt and possibly make-up will build up, especially around the bridge and on the inner aspect of the sides, if a frame is not regularly cleaned (Fig. 9.5). However, this does not constitute corrosion.

Older frames made of cellulose acetate may show corrosion, particularly in the ear point area (Fig. 9.6). Here, the upper aspect is stretched while the lower aspect is compressed, resulting in cracks, discoloration, brittleness and loss of polish. An Optyl surface may occasionally become rough to the touch and show bubbles on that surface.

Laminated metal frames may display varying degrees of corrosion, which may appear as a slightly affected surface (Fig. 9.7) to a deeply pitted, rough surface where the base metal is exposed (Fig. 9.8).

Some laminated metal frames are decorated with paint (Fig. 9.9) while others are given a clear, protective coating (Fig. 9.10). Either can become damaged. Reinforced carbon fibre

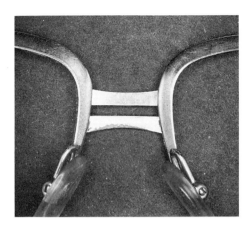

Fig. 9.7 Corrosion of surface layer of metal bridge

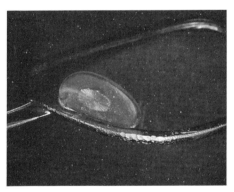

Fig. 9.8 Severe corrosion of 'gold' frame caused pitting into the base metal of the rim

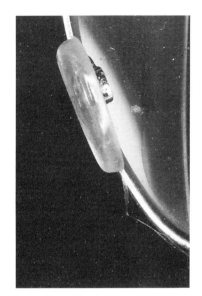

Fig. 9.10 Clear plastics coating peeling off nasal surface of right metal rim, after 1 year's wear

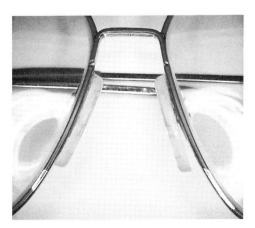

Fig. 9.9 Paint layer of a metal frame chipped within 6 months of wear

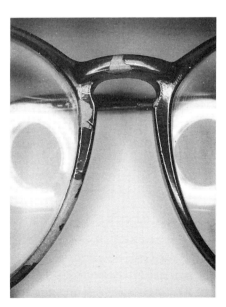

Fig. 9.11 Paint flaking off a carbon fibre reinforced plastics frame

frames have a grey tint. They are usually coated to give them a more appealing colour and shine. However, the coating can become damaged, whereupon the plastics material becomes visible (Fig. 9.11).

9.4.2 pH AS A FACTOR

Stokes (1983) investigated the effects of buffer solutions (which maintain a constant pH) with different pH values on spectacle frames made of rolled gold, plated gold, cellulose acetate and Optyl. The most susceptible material was plated gold. The greatest degree of corrosion occurred in the pH range of 6·4–7·4 and was not, as anticipated, caused by the more acid solutions. (Note that the latter were applied for only 40 days as opposed to 58 days for the other solutions.) Both rolled gold and plated gold caused a colour change of the pH 8·0 solution. The common factor was copper, which was present in each alloy.

Stokes (1983) also investigated the difference in skin pH of spectacle wearers with and without frame corrosion. She found no significant difference between the pH ranges of males and females, although there was sometimes a small difference between the values for the nose and the ear areas of skin. All corrosion was caused by skins with a pH < 5.3 after at least two years' spectacle wear. However, many frames that had been worn longer had not become corroded.

9.4.3 SWEAT AND FRAMES

Gaul (1958) found varying degrees of corrosion among rolled gold frames collected from opticians. The curls had been affected most. As it was unwound, the wire broke off; this appeared to be due to corrosion. In the worst cases, the core had almost been obliterated by a greenish deposit. This deposit was found to consist of nickel and copper salts. It had been formed by corrosion,

caused by sweat, of the core, which contained copper, nickel and zinc.

The distribution of the corrosion corresponded with the intimacy of contact between metal and skin. The sides showed discoloration where they had touched scalp and ears; also affected were the bridge and the butt of the sides. The corrosion was not limited to any one make of spectacle frame.

Burton *et al.* (1976) stated that the corrosion depended mainly upon the chloride content of the sweat: the higher the concentration, the greater the corrosion. Other components appeared to have no effect. A reduction of the pH of sweat produced a small increase in corrosive action: acidic sweat will corrode more readily than alkaline sweat. Also, people with higher rates of sweat secretion are likely to cause more corrosion. The rate of chloride excretion of an individual is relatively constant, but there are considerable interindividual variations. The higher the skin surface temperature, the higher the chloride content of the surface film. The chloride concentration also parallels the person's salt intake.

Siew (1987) reported that, in Malaysia, metal frames discolour relatively quickly and plastics materials deteriorate because of perspiration caused by high temperatures.

Hardy (1983) wrote that beryllium copper alloy, platinum and titanium are particularly suitable where perspiration poses a problem. Fahrner (1986) compared 'cheap' and 'expensive' metal frames and concluded that the latter are more corrosion resistant.

9.5 Miscellaneous Aspects

When a piece of injection-moulded cellulose acetate is exposed to a temperature of 60°C for 30 min or more, the surface loses its original lustre.

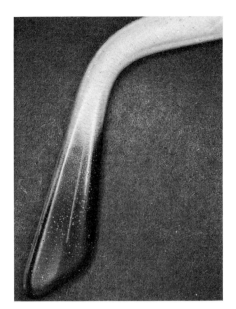

Fig. 9.12 White film deposit on cellulose acetate side. Where the deposit has been polished away a pitted surface is evident

greatest number of cosmetic allergic reactions, followed by preservatives and facial cleansers and moisturizers. Rose-coloured gold alloys, all of which contain copper, can cause black streaks when they come in contact with make-up. This has nothing to do with allergies: it is usually a chemical reaction between the copper and the make-up (Stehlin, 1986).

Medication may cause allergic dermato-conjunctivitis. Jennings (1984, personal communication) provided a list that includes many ophthalmic drugs. The major diagnostic characteristics were given as severe itching of the eyes, papillary conjunctivitis, eczema of the eyelid skin, and conjunctival eosinophilia.

MacIvor (1950) reported eight cases of allergy to plastics artificial eyes. He emphasized that poor fitting and acute or chronic infection should be excluded as causes before making a definite diagnosis.

It becomes covered with a fine white film. This deposit is the plasticizer contained in the material. This occurs less readily in extruded cellulose acetate. However, it is seen on frames that have been in use for many years (Fig. 9.12). Buffing and repolishing will usually improve the surface sheen considerably.

In referring to peri-orbital eczema, Swinney (1951) stated that nail varnish applied to either the nails or used as 'paint' on a spectacle frame, may be the causative agent. In this connection he mentions other cosmetics, namely shampoo, hair lacquer, rouges, powders, deodorants, eyelash preparations (mascara, eye shadow, eyebrow pencil, and eyecreams) and perfumes. Theodore & Schlossman (1958) discount most eyelash preparations as causing reactions; it is usually the (oil-soluble) base material, or some special additive.

Fragrances and their ingredients caused the

9.6 Remedies

Sherwin (1973) reported that he had used clear cellulose nitrate dope (as used in model and toy making) to cover cellulose acetate frames. The treatment was also suitable on metal frames, but where the metal had been affected by perspiration, it had a limited life.

A spectacle frame repair service which undertakes the coating of metal frames with a plastics layer to prevent allergic reactions has been available for some time (in Germany). For this purpose, a powder is electrostatically deposited on a metal frame (see Fig. 10.5). This becomes liquid at 180°C, and is said to cover the frame parts evenly with a tough, transparent layer of about 10 μm thus preventing contact between metal and skin. (Much of the content of this chapter is based on the work of Julia Stokes (1983), Caroline Burt (1987) and Jonathan Bedford (1976).)

REFERENCES

Barnes, H.M., Calman, C.D. & Sarkany, I. (1974). Spectacle frame acanthoma. *Trans. St. John's Hosp. Derm. Soc.* **60**, 99.

Bartels, W. (1992). Nickel- and titanium-free non-ferrous fine wires OPTOFIL(R) for the optical industry. Presseinformation nr. 060192FP. Heuchelheim, D-6301, Berkenhoff GmbH.

Bedford, J. (1976). A study of inflammation of the epithelium due to spectacle wear. 3rd Year Project. London: City University.

Berardesca, E., & Maibach, H. (1989). Allergic and irritant contact dermatitis. In: Leveque, J.L. (ed.) *Cutaneous Investigation in Health and Disease*, p.428. New York/Basel: Marcel Dekker.

Berkoff, H.S. (1938). Contact dermatitis from "horn-rimmed" spectacles. *Arch. Derm.* **38**, 746–751.

BS 3462 (1962). *Specification for Metal Spectacle Frames*. London: British Standards Institution.

Burt, C. (1987). The effects of ophthalmic materials and the skin on each other. 3rd Year Project. London: City University.

Burton, J.L., Pye, R.J. & Brooke, D.B. (1976). Metal corrosion of chloride in sweat. *Brit. J. Dermatol.* **95**, 417.

Calnan, C.D. (1957). Nickel sensitivity in women. *Int. Arch. Allergy* **11**, 73–86.

Carlsen, L., Andersen, K.E. & Egsgaard, H. (1986). Triphenyl phosphate allergy from spectacle frames. *Contact Derm.* **15**, 5, 274–277.

Cronin, E. (1980). *Contact Dermatitis*, p. 646. London: Churchill Livingstone.

Dikstein, S. & Zlotogorski, A. (1989). Skin surface hydrogen ion concentration (pH). In: Leveque J.L. (ed.) *Cutaneous Investigation in Health and Disease*, p. 67, 68, 72. New York/Basel: Marcel Dekker.

Doherty, E. & Freeman, S. (1988). Spectacle frame dermatitis due to paraphenylenediamine. *Australas. J. Dermatol.* **29** (2), 113–115.

Dowaliby, M. (1987). *The Art of Eyewear Dispensing*, p. 22. Fullerton (CA): Southern California College of Optometry.

Duke-Elder, S. (1954). The neurology of vision motor and optical anomalies. *Textbook of Ophthalmology*, **4**, 5412. London: Kimpton.

Fahrner, D. (1986). Fassungsqualitäten. *Neues Optikerj.* **28** (10), 8–11.

Fisher, A.A. (1976). Epoxy resin dermatitis. *Cutis* **17**, 1027, 1028, 1041.

Gaul, L.E. (1958). Dermatitis from metal spectacles. *Arch. Derm.* **77**, 475–478.

Hambly, E.M. & Wilkinson, D.S. (1978). Contact dermatitis to butyl acrylate in spectacle frames. *Contact Derm.* **4**, 115.

Hardy, S. (1983). Frame materials: metals. *Manuf. Optician Int.* **36** (2) 13,17.

Harkness, R.D. (1971). Mechanical properties of skin in relation to its biological function and its chemical components. In: Elden, H.R. (ed.) *Biophysical Properties of the Skin*. Ch. 11. New York/London: Wiley-Interscience.

Hausen, B.M. & Jung, H.D. (1985). Brillengestell-Dermatitis. *Akt. Dermatol.* **11**, 119–123.

Heidenreich, F. (1975). Tumore im Bereich der Auflagepunkte der Brille und der vorderen Augenabschnitte. *Augenoptik* **92** (3), 79–81.

Hinterhofer, O. & Fahrner, D. (1983). *Materialkunde für Augenoptiker*. Pforzheim: Verlag Neues Optikerjournal H. Postenrieder.

Jirasek, L., Obikova, M. & Jiraskova, M. (1976). (Retro-auricular eczema caused by the nickel of celluloid-rimmed spectacles.) *Csl. Derm.* **51**, 369–371.

Jordan, W.P. & Dahl, M.C. (1971). Contact dermatitis to a plastic solvent in eyeglasses. *Arch. Dermatol.* **104**, 524–528.

Jordan, W.P. & Dahl, M.C. (1972). Contact dermatitis from cellulose ester plastic. *Arch. Derm.* **105**, 880–885.

Leveque, J.-L. (1989). *Cutaneous Investigation in Health and Disease*, p. 143. New York/Basel: Marcel Dekker.

MacIvor, J. (1950). Contact allergy to plastic artificial eyes. *Can. Med. Ass. J.* **62** (2), 164–166.

Maibach, H.I. & Menné, T. (1989). *Nickel and the Skin*. Boca Raton, FL: CRC Press.

Miller, B. (1972). Cancer of the skin caused by spectacles. *Contacto, Chicago* **16**, 45–50.

National Eczema Society (1986). *Information pack: 4 Adults*. London: NES.

Neering, H. & Nanning, W.A.R. (1978). Het brilmontuur-acanthoom (acanthoma fissuratum). *Ned. T. Geneesk.* **122** (48), 1873–1875.

Otto, J. (1958). Entwicklung von Kankroiden bei Brillenträgern. *Klin. Mbl. Augenheilk.* **132**, 504–508.

prEN 1811 (1995). *Precious Metals – Reference Test Method for Release of Nickel*. Brussels: CEN.

Saltzer, E.I. & Wilson, J.W. (1968). Allergic contact dermatitis due to copper. *Arch. Dermatol., Chicago* **98**, 375–376.

Sherwin, L.D.G. (1973). Allergy to acetate. Letter to the Editor. *Ophthalm. Optician* **13** (7), 988.

Siew, Y.K. (1987). Setting a standard in Malaysia. *Dispensing Optics* **2** (2), 20.

Smith, E.L. & Calman, C.D. (1966). Studies in contact dermatitis. XVII: spectacle frames. *Trans. St. John's Hosp. Derm. Soc.* **52**, 10–34.

Sonnex, T.S. & Rycroft, R.J. (1986). Dermatitis from phenyl salicylate in safety spectacles. *Contact Derm.* **14** (5), 268–270.

Stehlin, D. (1986). Cosmetic allergies. *FDA – Consumer*, Nov. 28.

Stokes, J. E. (1983). To what extent does the pH of skin affect frame corrosion? Student project. Derby: Derby College of Further Education.

Such, B. (1993). The roads that lead from Rome. *Optician* **206** (5409), 34–35.

Sun, C.C. (1987). Allergic contact dermatitis of the face from contact with nickel and ammoniated mercury in spectacle frames and skin-lightening creams. *Contact Derm.* **17** (5), 306–309.

Swinney, B. (1951). Periorbital dermatitis. *Ann. Allergy* **9**, 774–778.

Theodore, F.M. & Schlossman, A. (1958). *Ocular Allergy.* Baltimore: Williams & Wilkins.

Vilaplana, J., Romaguera, C. & Grimalt, F. (1987). Allergic contact dermatitis from aliphatic isocyanate on spectacle frames. *Contact Derm.* **16** (2), 113.

Walsh, G., Patience, A. & Burgess, A. (1991). What the eye doesn't see. *Optician* **202** (5320), 16–19.

Wilde, H. (1959). Brillengestelldermatitis. *Derm. Wschr.* **140**, 1089–1090.

Wolfram, L.J. (1989). Frictional properties of skin. In: Leveque, J-L. (ed.) *Cutaneous Investigation in Health and Disease.* Ch. 3. New York/Basel: Marcel Dekker.

Wright, V. (1971). Elasticity and deformation of skin. In: Elden, H.R. (ed.) *Biophysical Properties of the Skin.* Ch. 12. New York/London: Wiley-Interscience.

CHAPTER 10

Spectacle Frame Manufacturing Processes

10.1 Introduction

In this chapter production processes used in the manufacture of frame parts, and of spectacle frames, will be defined and briefly described. Some of these processes are also used in optical workshops when spectacle frames are repaired (please consult the Index). Underlined words have their own entry in the lists.

10.2 Manufacturing Processes

10.2.1 GENERAL PROCESSES

- **Angling** Adjusting the angle of the side (BS 3521) (Fig. 10.1).

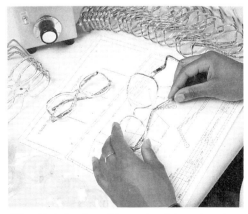

Fig. 10.1 *Angling. The angle of the side is being checked against a template (courtesy Norville Opt. Co., Gloucester)*

- **Barrelling** (*tumbling*) This is a time-consuming, but labour-saving abrasive process whereby objects are polished to a consistent and high quality. A large number of objects (for instance, 300 fronts) is placed in a multi-sided drum filled with abrasive substances (Fig. 10.2). While the drum rotates around a horizontal spindle, the objects slowly tumble about. The movement of objects over and along each other enhances the effect of the abrasive substances. Changing from coarser to finer and finer abrasives as the objects progress through the stages has the effect of removing ever smaller irregularities, and can eventually produce a finely polished surface.

  Important aspects of the barrel itself are the material of which it is made (type of wood or plastics), dimensions and speed of rotation.

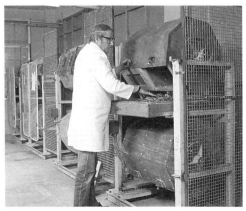

Fig. 10.2 *Barrelling. The operator removes fronts from the upper drum (courtesy Norville Opt. Co.)*

The number of operations required depends on the smoothness of the objects' surface at the start of the process and the quality of the finish required. The smoother the surfaces are (i.e. few and only small irregularities such as shallow score marks, as opposed to rough edges and routing marks) at the start of the barrelling process, the shorter the first or roughing process can be. It should not normally exceed 24 h. The abrasive materials used here include abrasive balls and granules (made of, for instance, pumice, i.e. pieces of lava), ceramic chips, hardwood and plastics pegs. The latter act as carriers for abrasive powders which are made to adhere by means of binding fluid.

The roughing stage is followed by smoothing which may take a further 24 h. It is done with an assortment of pegs impregnated with a compound (containing finer pumice than used for the first stage) designed to remove any remaining roughness. On completion, no irregularities should remain and edges should be rounded.

The third stage, honing (superficial polishing), may take less than 24 h. Small cubes and pegs impregnated with honing fluid are used to further improve the surface quality to a dull polished finish. Pointed pegs will remove abrasive material settled in groves.

In the final stage pegs impregnated with very fine polishing cream are used. It may take from 8 to 20 h. The objects finally appear from the barrel after a total of about 80 h. They will display a hard, brilliant gloss which is difficult to achieve by other polishing processes. Hand polishing a single frame to the same standard would take one person about 30 min.

Between stages the objects are separated by sieving. To prevent coarser abrasive material from entering the next barrelling stage, where it would produce scratches, objects are carefully cleaned after each stage (Fairbanks, 1955,

personal communication; Emslie, 1980; Goodwin, 1983).

Instead of tumbling, vibrating equipment is used as well.

- **Buffing (buff or mop polishing; Fig. 10.3)** Originally, polishing was carried out with a buff (buffalo-hide) and later with leather. Mops used in frame manufacture are made of flat or conically shaped felt, calico and swansdown.

Calico and swansdown mops are specified according to diameter and number of 'leaves' per mop. Felt and calico mops are used with a wax polishing compound or soap containing an abrasive (e.g. sand). The wax acts as a coolant and adheres to the mop. Polishing with swansdown 'loaded' with a glossing compound gives a highly lustrous surface.

The diameter of the mop is related to the speed of the spindle. The peripheral speed of the mop should be about 20 m s^{-1}. It is better to use large-diameter mops and low spindle speeds because such mops do not heat up so

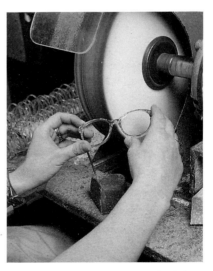

Fig. 10.3 *Buffing. Note the block of polishing compound on the shelf below the front (courtesy Norville Opt. Co.)*

quickly. Hence, the (plastics) object is less likely to get burned (Fairbanks, 1955, personal

- **Bumping**   Forming the bridge projection of a plastics front by heat and pressure (Fig. 10.4). See also Fig. 4.2.
- **Casting**   To pour liquid metal, or press soft material, into a mould (hollow form) or die (see moulding).
- **Cementing**   Bonding objects firmly by means of an adhesive substance.

    Plastics surfaces to be cemented should be cleaned (e.g. with benzene). The contact areas should then be sanded with fine abrasive paper and cleaned again. Once the appropriate solvent has been applied to both surfaces, they are held together with light pressure. The join should not be polished until the solvent has evaporated.

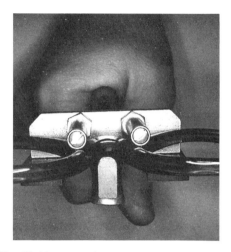

Fig. 10.4 *Bumping pliers are a workshop tool and are not used in the mass manufacture of frames*

- **Coating**   Applying a membrane or layer. On metal, it is often used as a sealant against chemical attack (Fig. 10.5A). Plastics layers are

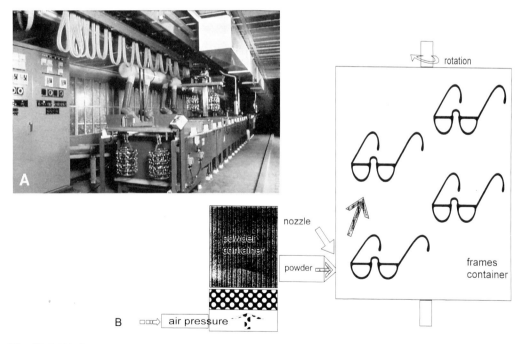

Fig. 10.5 *(A) Coating; automated electrolytic coating plant. Note the two racks with metal frames in the foreground (courtesy Essilor Ltd., Thornbury, UK). (B) Diagrammatic representation of plastics coating process for metal frames (see text)*

usually hypo-allergic, can be given varying colourings, can be bent so that the frame may be adjusted, but alcohol and other cleaning fluids may affect the coating and/or colouring. Soldering destroys plastics coatings and special techniques are required to recoat and recolour the affected part.

After production of the metal parts, they are chemically cleaned and hung on racks in a chamber (Fig. 10.5B). A negative electric charge is applied to these racks. While the racks are rotated they are sprayed with positively charged acrylic or polyester resin powder. The racks, with parts, are then heated for 15 min to 200°C. An adhesive and absorptive plastics coating is thus created that can be 30 to 70 μm thick (Crundall, 1984). Other processes, such as electrophoretic plastics coating, have also been used.

Such transparent coatings may be coloured in various combinations by passing the coated parts through dip-dyeing baths. Finally, the parts are heat treated in a low-temperature oven. The process is computer controlled, and demands great technical expertise (Sattler, 1984).

Frames made of stainless steel, titanium or rolled gold do not require coating. However, metal frames are sometimes given a partial plastics coating for decorative purposes.

- **Cresting** Shaping the arch of a plastics bridge to provide an angle of crest (BS 3521).
- **Cutting** Fashioning an object by cleaving it with a sharp edge.
- **Deburring** Removing more or less sharp edges (Fig. 10.6).
- **Die casting** See casting.
- **Drilling** Making a hole.
- **Embossing** To cover the surface of an object with raised (sometimes sunken) ornaments (Fig. 10.7). This may include alphanumerical descriptions referring to frame measurements and other identification marks,

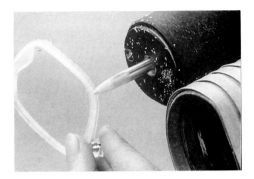

Fig. 10.6 Deburring of an Optyl frame (courtesy Carrera Eyewear Ltd)

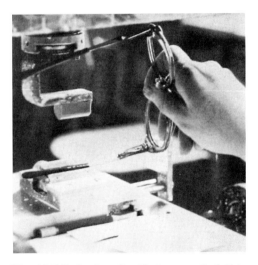

Fig. 10.7 Embossing of a side (courtesy Carl Zeiss Ltd)

the quality of rolled gold and brand marks (see pressing).

- **Engraving** Cutting or incising designs in metal, plastics, etc. A frame part may be engraved with the name of its owner, or with that of its manufacturer (Figs 10.8 and 23.7).
- **Milling** Removing material from an object by means of a rotating cutter (Fig. 10.9).
- **Polishing** Making a surface smooth and

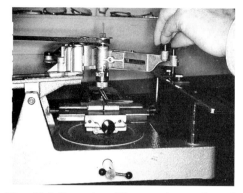

Fig. 10.8 Engraving. The text (arranged on the 'bridge', right) is transferred by means of a pantograph reducing device, and engraved on the side (centre)

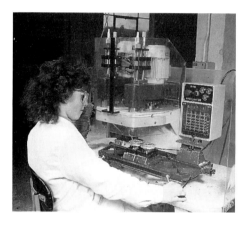

Fig. 10.9 Milling. A front being milled; the template is not visible (courtesy Norville Opt. Co.)

glossy by removing particles through rubbing (see buffing).

Acetone polishing involves the immersion of a (plastics) object in a solvent bath of acetone, ethylacetate or acetic acid. This must be carried out quickly or the solvent will soften and dissolve the material. Acetone vapour polishing involves the heating (over steam or water bath) of acetone. The article to be polished is then suspended in the vapour for a few seconds (Fairbanks, 1955, personal communication). In this way the back of pads and the grooves are given a polished appearance before barrelling.

Frames that have been polished by barrelling are usually given a final polish by hand (Fig. 10.3). This provides a lustrous surface quality.

- **Pinning**   Fitting of a joint to front or side of a frame (BS 3521) by means of a pin passed through aligned holes (see Fig. 11.17).
- **Recessing**   Forming a recess in a plastics part, generally to allow the joint plate to lie flush with the surface (BS 3521) (see Fig. 11.19).
- **Rivetting**   Fastening objects by means of a bolt passed through aligned holes and hammering the end of the bolt. A half-joint may be rivetted (or pinned) to the side or front of a frame (see Fig. 11.17).
- **Sawing**   Cutting with a toothed blade.
- **Setting up**   Adjusting a frame at the conclusion of manufacture (BS 3521) (Fig. 10.10), or before collection by the patient.
- **Splicing**   Joining together pieces of natural material by application of heat, moisture and pressure (BS 3521).
- ***Tumbling***   Barrelling.
- **Turning**   Cutting material on a lathe (a machine in which an object is clamped, and shaped with a stationary tool having a cutting edge while the object is being rotated).

10.2.2 METAL COLD FORMING PROCESSES

- **Burnishing**   Polishing by rubbing with a metal tool (Fig. 10.11).
- **Coiling**   Shaping metal eye rims out of grooved or sectional wire using a coil winding machine.
- **Countersinking**   Bevelling the edge of a hole so that the head of a screw will fit flush into it (Fig. 10.12).

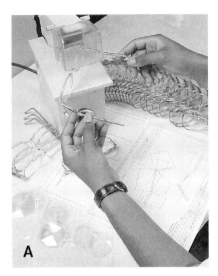

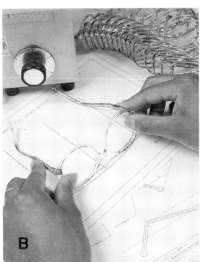

Fig. 10.10 *Setting up. A, The front is heated up so that it can be adjusted; B, checking the frame head width (courtesy Norville Opt. Co.)*

- **Crimping** Contracting or drawing together of a metal part (such as the butt end of a side so that it can take a half joint).
- **Guillotining** Cutting with a guillotine-like instrument.
- **Hammering** To beat and thus shape or fashion, with a hammer.
- **Jumping tools** Used for bending.

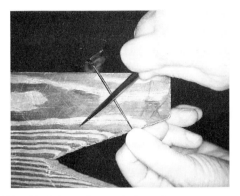

Fig. 10.11 *Burnishing. The burnishing tool is held in the operator's right hand*

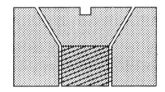

Fig. 10.12 *A countersunk screw head*

- **Piercing** To make a hole, to perforate.
- **Planishing** To flatten or polish.
- **Pressing** To imprint, stamp, flatten, shape or smooth, by weight or other squeezing force.
- **Reducing** To diminish in diameter or thickness (see wire-drawing).
- **Rim forming/rolling** Sectional shaping of metal eye rim wire between rollers.
- **Shearing** To cut, or deform in such a way that parallel planes remain parallel, but move parallel to themselves.
- **Spinning** To twist thin metal wires with a cable winder into a cable (as used for curl or cable sides).
- **Stamping** To shape with a downward blow using a die or cutter.
- **Tapping** Cutting an internal thread with a screw-like tool (Fig. 10.13).
- **Wire-drawing** To draw into wire by pull-

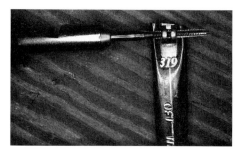

Fig. 10.13 *Tapping. The charniers of the half-joint to a side are being re-tapped*

ing through successively smaller holes in a hard steel die-block.

10.2.3 HEAT TREATMENT OF METAL

- **Annealing** To temper (to obtain the required hardness, toughness or elasticity) by heating to a high temperature and slowly cooling an object. It may also be used to remove internal stress (e.g. in glass).
- **Brazing** To join two or more metal parts by filling the capillary gaps between them with hard solder (see soldering, welding).

  Low-temperature brazing, also referred to as silver alloy soldering or brazing, silver brazing or hard soldering, is brazing between 600 and 850°C (Johnson Matthey, 1973). Heathcote (1981) drew attention to the acute toxic effects of fumes given off by cadmium bearing alloys during brazing.
- **Hardening** A process whereby a metal part is heated to a crucial temperature and then quickly cooled. This rearranges the molecular structure of the metal. As a result it becomes harder. Hardening can also be achieved through some of the cold forming processes.
- **Heat insertion** Staking.
- **Soldering** Joining metal parts by means of an alloy that, when heated, penetrates the capillary spaces between the components and

has a melting point below that of either of the parts to be joined; or joining plastics by means of heat. See: brazing, welding.

There are two types of solder used: soft and hard. Soft solders contain mainly tin and lead, and melt at relatively low temperatures (less than 450°C). Hard solders contain mainly silver and copper, melt at a much higher temperature (600–1100°C) and produce a stronger bond (Hintermeister, 1984).

A more recent development is the introduction of soft solders that are claimed to join all metals.

Sources of heat are the flame (burning on a mixture of oxygen and natural gas or butane), by passing an electric current through the parts to be joined (where the heat is created as a result of the resistance encountered by the current in the metals; Fig. 10.14A), electrically heated soldering irons, and the application of high frequency electromagnetic radiation (where an electromagnetic field is made to penetrate into the objects and spread its power thus reducing the strength of its field; Fig. 10.14B).

Chemicals, known as 'flux' (to melt or flow) are used to clean the parts to be joined. Most fluxes are solids that liquefy on heating. They degrease the surfaces, facilitate capillary flow of the solder, prevent oxidation (blackening) and leave non-corrosive residues. They usually include a rare earth such as fluor or boron. Rods of solder may have a core of resin that melts, surrounding the parts as it is applied.

- **Staking** A process whereby metal is attached to plastics. Also referred to as heat insertion.

A hole, slightly smaller than the metal component, is made in the plastics part. This helps to guide the metal part into position. Application of ultrasonic energy generates

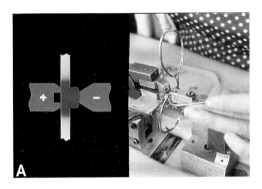 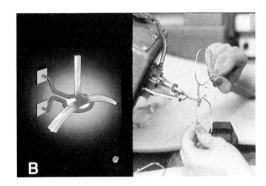

Fig. 10.14 Soldering. (A) Left: diagram of electrical resistance soldering; right: the left pad arm being soldered to the rim. (B) Left: diagram of high-frequency soldering; right: bridge and rim being soldered (courtesy Essilor)

heat at the plastics–metal interface. The heat melts the plastics which then flows around the metal part while it is pressed into the plastics. On cooling the plastics solidifies around the metal part (Lucas Dawe Ltd, London).

- **Swaging** Hammering metal, at a temperature below the melting point, whereby the diameter is reduced (Fig. 10.15).
- **Tempering** Warming metal parts so that they assume a desired degree of hardness and elasticity. See annealing.
- **Welding** Joining metal or plastics parts by raising the temperature at the joint by means

of heat, and, in the case of metal parts, applying pressure (Fig. 10.16). See: brazing, soldering, staking.

Plastics may be 'welded' by means of high frequency heating. For this purpose ultrasonic vibrations are made to pass through one component. On reaching the interface with a second component the vibratory energy will cause the parts to rub. This produces localized heating. The plastics material at the joint melts almost instantly and forms a bond after cooling (Lucas Daw).

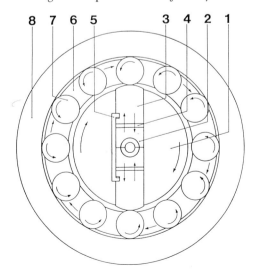 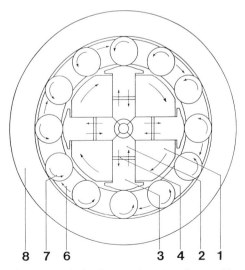

Fig. 10.15 Diagram of swaging equipment (courtesy Gebr. Felss, Koenigsbach, Germany). 1, Spindle assembly; 2, swaging dies; 3, swaging hammers; 4, shims; 5, stroke limiter; 6, roller cage; 7, rollers; 8, head ring

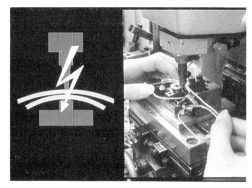

Fig. 10.16 *Welding. Left: diagram of electric spot welding; right: the right browbar being welded to the rim (courtesy Essilor)*

10.2.4 MISCELLANEOUS PROCESSES FOR METAL

- **Electrodeposition**   Deposition of a layer of metal by passing an electric current from one pole (electrode) through a bath containing a watery solution of metal salts, to the other (Fig. 10.5A). The metal ions will migrate and form a layer on the electrode such as a metal spectacle frame part. The quality and structure of the layer will depend on the chemical composition of the solution and the operating temperature. The thickness of the layer depends on the duration of the process.

    The object of these galvanic treatments is to achieve an optimum joining of the base metal and the metal layer deposited on it, where the outer layer is of sufficient strength and durability to withstand wear and tear and also adjustments to the frame. This ensures complete protection against corrosion (Bosch *et al.*, 1990).

    After barrelling and/or hand buffing of the metal frames (or parts), they undergo several chemical cleaning processes and are treated to achieve good adhesion of the layers to be deposited. High-quality frames may be subjected to some 30 separate operations, many of these being chemical cleaning and drying

operations to deposit three layers of gold: a foundation of 24 ct about 0.4 μm thick, a protective layer of 18 ct 2.5 μm thick, and a colouring layer of 22 ct 2.5 μm thick (Silhouette, 1980).

Different manufacturers use variants of this process, using various metals (chromium, paladium, rhodium and ruthenium), to obtain various surface colours and textures. To protect the metal layers, they are frequently covered with a plastics coating. (Rodenstock, 1981; Crundall, 1984; Sattler, 1984; L'Amy, 1988; Marwitz; Zeiss).

- **Plating**   Applying a thin coating of gold, silver, or other metal.

10.2.5 PLASTICS FRAME MANUFACTURING PROCESSES

- **Casting**   Manufacture of a frame from plastics material by a thermoforming process (BS 3521) whereby soft material is pressed (or metal is poured) into a shape or mould (see moulding).
- **De-gating**   Removal of the residual plastics material from the access point(s) to the mould or cast (BS 3521).
- **Extruding**   A process whereby continuous lengths of material with a constant sectional shape, such as a tube or sheet, are produced.
- **Mitring**   Making a joint (between the lug of a front and the side of a frame). For instance, when each piece is cut at (about) 45°, an angle of (about) 90° is produced when the side is fitted to the front (Fig. 10.17).
- **Moulding**   Manufacture of a frame from plastics material by a thermoforming process (BS 3521) whereby a soft material (or molten metal) is poured into a mould and assumes its shape after cooling (or drying). See casting.
- **Moulding (injection)**   A high-speed process whereby powdered or granulated thermoplastics material is heated, melted and

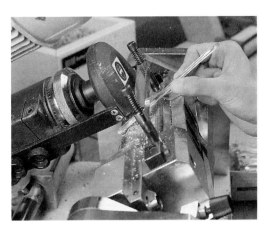

Fig. 10.17 A 45° mitre being cut onto a side

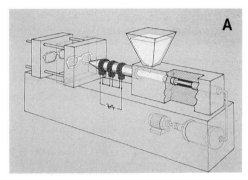

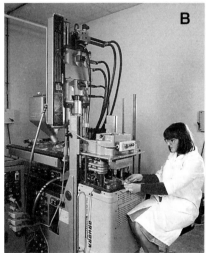

forced under pressure into a mould (Fig. 10.18). After cooling, the material takes on the form of the mould (Fig. 10.19).

- **Routing**   A <u>milling</u> process whereby the tool scoops out the lens aperture of the front and may simultaneously <u>cut</u> the groove. It is also used to cut the outer shape of a front or side (Fig. 10.20).
- **Side shooting**   Insertion of the side wire into a plastics side (BS 3521) (Fig. 10.21).

    A side blank of desired thickness (normally 3.5 or 4 mm) is softened by heat and then placed between the two cold platens of a water-cooled mould. After a few seconds the outer layers of the blank cool and harden, but the core remains soft. A side wire, preheated to about 200°C, is then pneumatically driven into the blank and will travel along the soft core. When this process has been completed, the blank can be milled to give it its final form.

Fig. 10.18 Moulding. (A) Diagram of injection moulding (courtesy Essilor) and (B) a spectacle front being removed from an injection-moulding machine (courtesy Norville Opt. Co.)

10.3 Plastics Frames: Machining and Moulding Compared

When the design stage (see Section 5.2) has been completed with the selection of the frame styles,

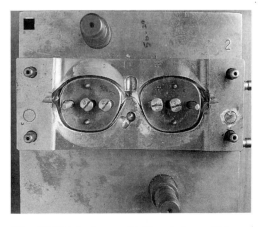

Fig. 10.19 Injection-moulded front in its mould (courtesy Norville Opt. Co.)

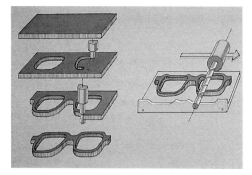

Fig. 10.20 *Diagrammatic representation of successive stages in the routing of a front (courtesy Essilor)*

the manufacturing stage is reached. Depending on the method of manufacture, different techniques will be employed.

One differentiates between two basic techniques, namely machining and moulding. The former can be used for cellulose acetate and cellulose propionate. The latter may be subdivided into injection moulding and (vacuum) casting through polymerization. They have in common that the spectacle frame(s) is/are formed in a mould(s), under the application of heat and pressure. Injection-moulded frames

(Fig. 10.18) are made out of granules of cellulose acetate, cellulose propionate or polyamides. During casting (Fig. 10.22) a liquid monomer, which is polymerized by a liquid catalyst, turns into a solid object such as a front (see Section 10.4).

Table 10.1 shows similarities and differences between the two basic techniques employed in conventional spectacle frame manufacture.

During machining operations 60–80% of the original material may be removed (Bosch *et al.*, 1990; Botton & Packford, 1994). Some manufacturers have developed more efficient techniques that combine one or more operations, thus departing from more conventional patterns (Anonymous, 1992) of frame manufacture.

Reinforced plastic spectacle sides are made in either of two ways. The older, lamination method, starts with two blanks (roughly shaped pieces to be fashioned into manufactured articles) representing vertical sections through a side. On a surface which is to become a median surface of the side, a groove is milled. This surface, and that of its counterpart, are placed in a shallow tray for a short while containing a chemical solvent. On

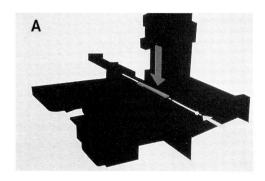

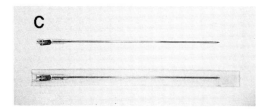

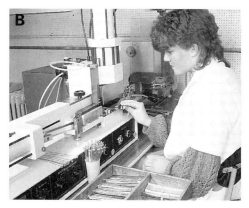

Fig. 10.21 *Side shooting. (A) Diagram of side shooting: the heated blank is secured by pressure from above while the side wire enters from the right (courtesy Essilor). (B) A side shooting machine (courtesy Norville Opt. Co.). (C) Above: a side core; below: a side blank with side core*

TABLE 10.1 *Machining and moulding compared*

Machining	Moulding
From a large stock of sheet material that has been bought in different patterns, and different colours or colour combinations	From a stock of colourless granules or liquids (together with a stock of dyes/ pigments) that occupy little space
Production of templates	Production of the two parts of the mould (Fig. 10.24).
Guillotining slabs (Fig. 10.23A) from the sheet material to a size slightly larger than that of the front required	
Slicing to the correct thickness (if necessary)	
Rough shaping by hot stamping or milling	
A pantographic routing machine cuts the aperture of one (or more) front(s) including the groove in the rims (Fig. 10.23B)	Moulding equipment forms front (Fig. 10.25) (and sides), simultaneously inserting half-joints (Fig. 10.27) (and can shape the groove in the rims)
	Routing of the groove in the rims (Fig. 10.28)
The outside shape of the front is machined (Fig. 10.23C)	
Facets/bevels are cut with inclined milling equipment	
After heating the bridge is 'bumped' (Fig. 10.23D) to give the required projection, the rims are given a 'meniscus' shape, and the lugs are rounded	
Nose pads may be cemented by hand	
Heat insertion of half-joint to front	
A nylon cap is fitted over the metal half-joint, as protection during barrelling (Fig. 10.23E)	
Side blanks milled into required shape and size, and side wire 'shot' in (Fig. 10.21) (or laminated)	

Deburring (Fig. 10.6)
Barrelling (Fig. 10.2)
Hand polishing (Fig. 10.3)

	Dip-dyeing (Fig. 10.29) and/or colour (pattern) printing
Embossing/printing of brand mark, model and sizes (Fig. 10.7)	Printing of brand mark, model and sizes (Fig. 10.7)

Lacquering
Assembly of front and sides
Setting up (Fig. 10.10)
Inspection
Packaging
Storing before dispatch

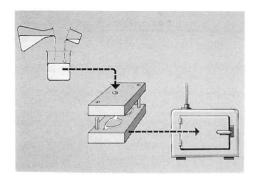

Fig. 10.22 Diagram showing the casting of a spectacle front (courtesy Essilor)

removal, a side wire is placed in the groove whereupon the two blanks, 'dipped' surfaces facing each other, are placed in a press and dried. After removal from the press, the side is given its shape by milling.

Side shooting is now the norm (Fig. 10.21; see Section 10.2.5). Whether the reinforced side has been produced through lamination or shooting, if it is to become a drop end side, it will be bent after heating.

Moulds are very expensive to make and therefore they are economic only if large production runs are made. However, computer aided design–computer aided manufacture (CAD–CAM) techniques facilitate speedy production of moulds (Figs 5.3 and 5.4). This reduces the cost considerably because it not only replaces the many days spent by an expert toolmaker, but also provides the required mould. CAD–CAM is used in similar fashion in the design and manufacture of prototypes of fronts made out of cellulose acetate and propionate. It has speeded up these processes remarkably (Goodwin, 1992).

Charlesworth (1980) described a method of injection moulding of propionate frames which did not use expensive steel moulding tools; instead, the tools were made of a special hard resin. The frame material is sucked into the mould. To produce the front takes 80 s and a further minute to cool. After de-gating, the fronts are barrelled

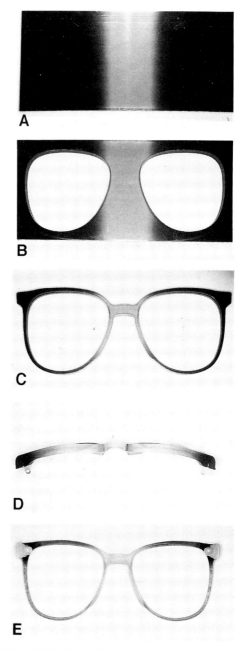

Fig. 10.23 (A) A slab, from which a front will be manufactured. (B) The lens apertures have been milled. (C) The front routed. (D) The bridge has been bumped and the rims surrounding the lens apertures have been given a meniscus shape so that the front becomes bowed. (E) Polyamide hoods are placed on the half-joints for protection during barrelling

in three stages taking 80 h. During dying the dye penetrates 0·1 mm into the surface. This process is followed by another 4 h of barrelling giving the final finish.

10.4 Optyl Frame Production

The epoxy resin Optyl behaves in a similar manner as two-component epoxy resin adhesives such as Araldite (made by Ciba–Geigy) where the resin is mixed with a hardener. The hardening process makes Optyl suitable for spectacle frame production. Appropriate doses of the resin and hardener are thoroughly mixed prior to moulding.

Prototype frames are hand-made in cellulose acetate. When the design stage has been completed, the front and sides are made in metal. From these templates, a primary set of moulds is made and duplicated such that a mass-production mould will have cavities for six to nine fronts (Fig. 10.24) and a similar number of sides. The liquid Optyl is transported into the empty mould where it is sucked into all available space. This completes the casting process. The chemical

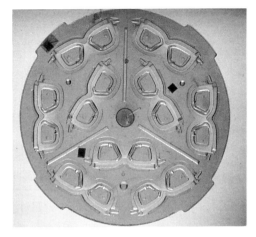

Fig. 10.24 *A mould used for the casting of Optyl fronts (courtesy Carrera Eyewear Ltd)*

reaction whereby cross-linked molecular chains are formed then takes place. This reaction consists of a series of timed and temperature-controlled cycles that are required to cure the casting. The moulds are then opened, and the moulding is removed (Fig. 10.25). It is colourless and hardens after a few seconds' exposure to air (Fig. 10.26). Next, the runners (channels through which the material runs before it reaches

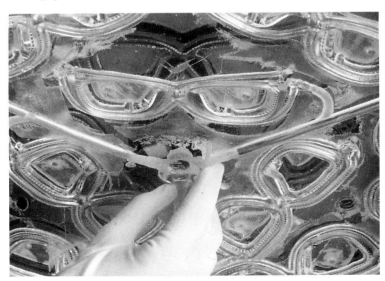

Fig. 10.25 *Removing Optyl fronts from the mould (courtesy Carrera Eyewear Ltd)*

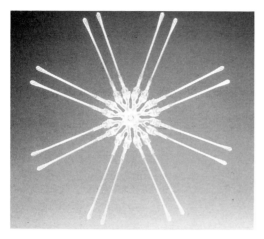

Fig. 10.26 *A set of Optyl sides. The liquid enters the mould through the centre and fills channels leading to the actual forms of the sides (courtesy Carrera Eyewear Ltd)*

that part of the mould in which the desired object is formed, and in which cured material remains) are removed so that one is left with separate fronts and sides.

All joints are moulded in during casting (Fig. 10.27). Metal trims may also be moulded in, or fitted afterwards.

The remainder of the manufacturing process is completed in much the same way as that of cellulose acetate frames: grooves are milled in the rims (Fig. 10.28), fronts and sides are barrelled to a stage where the surface quality is comparable to that after roughing, and assembled. They are then ready to receive the required colour(s).

The fronts are lowered into a dye bath (Fig. 10.29A) where the dye infiltrates the superficial layer of the object (Fig. 10.29B). A front may be dipped into more than one colour bath. Colour gradients may be introduced by angled immersion while the depth of the colour will depend on the immersion time. This time is dependent on the dye – it may require no more than a few seconds. The process is completed by totally immersing the front in a bath containing colourless, liquid polyurethane material. This hardens on removal from the bath and gives a lustrous surface. Finally, each frame is set up on a rig. (The information in this section was compiled from August, 1988; Fahrner, 1972; Hinterhofer & Fahrner, 1983; Horne, 1978; Optyl Holding, 1983; Wray, 1981.)

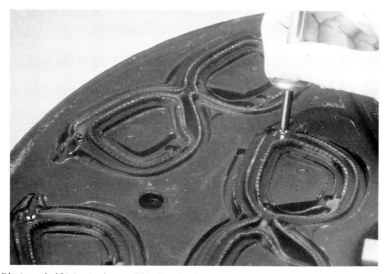

Fig. 10.27 *Placing a half-joint in the mould before the front is casted (courtesy Carrera Eyewear Ltd)*

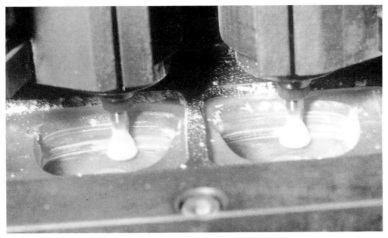

Fig. 10.28 Milling the grooves in the lens apertures of a front (courtesy Carrera Eyewear Ltd)

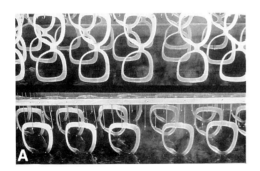
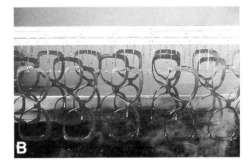

Fig. 10.29 (A) Colourless fronts suspended above a bath (above) and being dipped in a dye bath (below). (B) Dyed fronts leaving the bath (courtesy Carrera Eyewear Ltd)

10.5 Metal Frame Production

10.5.1 ROLLED GOLD FRAMES

There are now only a few metal spectacle frame manufacturers who produce frames from rolled gold material. The frame components are usually made separately or bought from component manufacturers. The front is assembled, by means of soldering operations, from two rims, a bridge and joints, and the sides are fitted to the front.

Metal spectacle frame production is a very precise process that may require well over 150 operations (including two dozen inspections), and sometimes many more.

The production stages of the different components for a conventional frame are described below.

10.5.1.1 Sides

These are made from rolled gold wire which is swaged by automated equipment fitted with tapered tungsten dies, into the required diameter. The wire is then cut into lengths suitable for a side. On one end an oval knuckle is made by pressing. This becomes the half-joint of the side. It is pierced, rounded and sheared. The butt is then formed by stamping, which simultaneously hardens it. The side is then cut to the required overall length, and the end is tapered. Finally, the plastics end cover is slid over the tapered end, and heated so that it may be bent to give a drop end side.

Curl sides are made in a similar manner. The curl itself is made with a core of base metal around which three or more strands of wire are spun. This is placed in a swaging machine which hammers the outer covering smooth and solid. The curl is then soldered to the butt and given its form by pulling it through a series of rollers. The end is sealed with a ball tip secured by soldering or hammering.

10.5.1.2 Joints

These are made from rolled gold, strip material. First the joint is preshaped by notching. During this operation the material is hardened; hence, it needs to be annealed (650°C). The individual joints are then separated. They are barrelled, cleaned and dried. This is followed by piercing, tapping and countersinking before the joint is cut into an upper and lower part.

10.5.1.3 Rims

Profile material is drawn through a number of dies to the required diameter and profile. It is simultaneously hardened and the groove, which usually has an enclosed angle of 90°, is prepared. The rim is then formed between rollers into spring-like rolls. When the material has been carefully cut into lengths suitable for individual rims, it is given the shape of the front's lens aperture by bending rollers that are controlled by a cam (a former with eccentric projections, which rotates to give the rollers the desired motion, whereby the rim is bent). Finally, the rim is cut to size.

10.5.1.4 Bridges

Metal pad bridges are made from square or round material. Having been straightened, it is cut to size. Both ends are reduced by swaging which is followed by barrelling. Each end becomes a pad arm, having been pressed flat and pierced so that it can receive a pad stud. The bridge is given its form through a small number of bending and stamping operations; the quality and trade mark is embossed during one of these. Finally, the pad arms are annealed so that adjustments can be made to it by the dispenser.

10.5.1.5 Assembly

A joint and a rim are placed in a soldering jig such that the rim fits into a small recess of the joint. They are joined by means of electric resistance soldering. Similarly, a right and a left rim is soldered to a bridge thus forming a front. This is chemically cleaned, and the nose pads are fitted to the pad arms of the bridge. The sides are then secured with screws to the joints of the front. The spectacle frame is then inspected, set up and calibrated to give the desired head width. After packaging it is stored, ready for dispatch.

10.5.2 OTHER METAL FRAMES

Metal frames not covered by a layer of rolled gold are, nevertheless, made in a similar fashion. The base metal is made into the required parts (rims, bridge, joints, sides, etc.). The rims, bridge and half-joints to the front are soldered to form the front while the other half of the joint is soldered or welded to the side. The process is completed when electrolytically, layers of gold and/or other metals have been deposited on the base metal parts. The frame is then assembled and put into stock.

10.6 Miscellaneous

It is rare for a metal frame to have no plastics parts

or covering. Rolled gold frames invariably have a plastics covering over the end of the side, the end cover (*tip*). The pads are normally made of plastics although gold pads were fitted if a patient developed an allergy to the plastics pads.

Walsh *et al.* (1991) found that the clear, rigid type of pads fitted to metal fronts are made predominantly of cellulose acetate. The polymer coatings of metal frames are largely produced from epoxy resin, with a smaller quantity being produced from polymethylmethacrylate (PMMA). End covers are made from cellulose acetate. Silicon rubber end covers are fitted on some sides and various types of pads are also made from this material.

Note that manufacturing processes may depart from the above description because of the available equipment in a given plant, or because the spectacle frame design demands a different approach.

Technical details about many processes referred to were set out by Horne (1978). They may also be obtained from articles and reviews in the technical press and from technical brochures issued by spectacle frame production machinery manufacturers.

Details of the manufacture of tortoiseshell spectacle frames are provided by Orr *et al.* (1992).

REFERENCES

Anonymous (1992). Spectacle frames cut by PCD. *Optical World* **21** (150), 13–14.

August, E.C. (1988). *Material for the Nineties* (video-tape). Optyl Eyewear Fashion Int. (USA)

Bosch, P., Kappelhof, J.P. & Kolbe, G. (1990). *Met het oog op.* The Hague: Consumentenbond / SDU.

Botton, T. & Packford, C. (1994). Material values. *Disp. Optics* **9** (9), 6–7.

BS 3521 (1991). *Terms Relating to Ophthalmic Optics and Spectacle Frames. Glossary of Terms Relating to Spectacle Frames.* Part 2. London: British Standards Institute.

Charlesworth, M. (1980). Tooling break-through at Birch. *Manufact. Optics Int.* **33** (5), 52.

Crundall, E.J. (1984). Bringing the resources to bear. *Optician* **188** (4972), 15–16.

Emslie, E.C. (1980). Barrelling: converting an enemy into a friend. *Manuf. Optics Int.* **33** (5), 51–52.

Fahrner, D. (1972). Optyl – a new basic material. Special reprint for Kunststofftechnik Wilhelm Anger KG, from *Neues Optikerjournal*, Sept. 1971 (vol. 13) to Jan. 1972 (vol. 14).

Goodwin, R. (1983). *Manufacture of Plastics Frames no. 3. New Insight, no.* **3** p. 18–19. Tonbridge: Invicta Frames Ltd.

Goodwin, R. (1992). Computed creativity. *Disp. Optics* **7**, 5, 7, June.

Heathcote, L.A. (1981). *Fumes Produced During Brazing with Silver Brazing Alloys.* Harlow: Johnson Matthey Metals Ltd. (reprint).

Hinterhofer, O. & Fahrner, D. (1983). *Materialkunde für Augenoptiker,* 2nd end. Pforzheim: Verlag Neues Optikerjournal H. Postenrieder.

Hintermeister, H. (1984). *Feinmechanische Arbeitstechniken.* Pforzheim: Verlag Bode.

Horne, D.F. (1978). *Spectacle Lens Technology.* Bristol: Adam Hilger.

Johnson Matthey (1973). *Brazing Materials and Applications.* Data sheet 1100 : 100. London: Johnson Matthey Metals.

L'Amy (1988). *Technical Handbook No. 1: Surface Treatments.* Morez: L'Amy S.A.

Lucas Dawe (undated brochure). *Ultrasonic Welding of Plastics.* London: Lucas Dawe Ultrasonics Ltd.

Marwitz (undated). *Brief Information Booklet on Materials.* Stuttgart: Marwitz + Hauser.

Optyl Holding (ed.) (1983). *Today's Frame Material for Tomorrow* (brochure). Haar/München: Optyl Holding GmbH & Co.

Orr, H., Davidson, D.C. & Eadon-Allen, S. (1992). Real tortoiseshell. *Ophthalm. Antiq. Int. Collectors Club Newsl.* (UK), No. 41, 3–8.

Rodenstock (1981). *Metal Spectacle Frames.* München: Rodenstock.

Sattler, C. (1984). The surfaces of metal spectacles. *Optician* **187**, 24–26, Feb. 17.

Silhouette (1980). *Information 3–Feb.* London: Silhouette Modellbrillen.

Walsh, G., Patience, A. & Burgess, A. (1991). What the eye

Wray, L. (1981). Plastics frame man

Zeiss (undated). *Zeiss metal frames*

CHAPTER 11

Supplementary Terminology

The general terms used for spectacles and the major parts of spectacle frames were set out in Chapter 1. In this chapter definitions, according to BS 3521 (1991), of major spectacle frame styles and a few general terms are given in Table 11.1. This is followed by terms associated with spectacle frame parts, namely bridges in Table 11.2, joints (*hinges*) in Table 11.3, sides in Table 11.4, rims in Table 11.5 and rimless mounts in Table 11.6. North American English terminology, as set out in ANSI Z80.5 (1979) and ISO 7998 (1984) as appended to BS 3521 (1991), is printed in italics.

TABLE 11.1 *Spectacle styles*

Term	Definition
Browbar spectacles (Fig. 11.1)	Rimless spectacles in which the bridge and joints are connected by bars substantially following the tops of the lenses
Combination spectacles (Figs 2.39 and 11.27–11.29)	Spectacles in which the principal parts of the front of the frame or mount are made of two distinct materials
Library spectacles (Fig. 11.2)	Spectacles of heavy weight with broad sides and usually of plastics or natural material with similar properties to plastics
Rimless spectacles (Fig. 11.3)	Spectacles without rims. The lenses are held in position by screws, keys, clamps or similar devices
Supra spectacles (Fig. 11.4)	Spectacles in which the lenses are held in position by thin bands or cords attached to the rims. Instead of polyamide cords, metal wire and bands have also been used in the past. However, these have been less successful
	The plastics lenses of a frame type that looks like a supra spectacle and is usually referred to by its brand name Polymil (Fig. 22.7), are chemically bonded to the bars
Windsor spectacles (Fig 11.5)	Comprise a metal frame and a thin channelled plastics rim covering the eyewire
General terms **Brace bar (Fig. 2.37)**	A strengthening bar joining the rims, additional to the main bridge
Bridge brace	See brace bar
Swept-back lug (Fig. 2.49)	Swept-back extension of the front to which the side is attached (lug = *endpiece*)

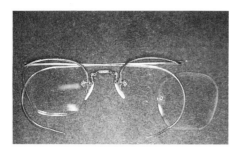

Fig. 11.1 Browbar spectacles. The left lens has been detached to show a single hole containing a small piece of plastics tubing.

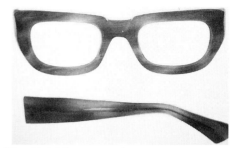

Fig. 11.2 Library spectacles

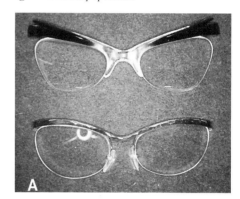

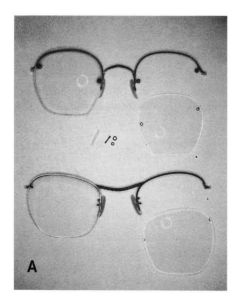

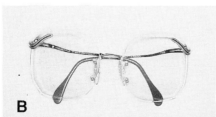

Fig. 11.3 Rimless spectacles. (A) The lenses of the upper sample are attached to the mount by means of a screw, washer, nut and plastics tubing; those of the lower sample are clamped between a pair of straps which are lodged into slots. (B) Three-piece front with four individual facets on each lens, and sinuous sides

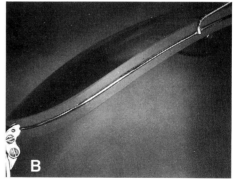

Fig. 11.4 Supra spectacles. (A) The upper mount is made of plastics. The lenses rest in V-shaped grooves in the mount. Their bevel is similarly shaped where in apposition with the mount, and flat-bevelled else-where. Below, a device which contains a polyamide cord which is hidden behind the browbar of the metal mount. This type is often refered to as a 'Nylor' frame. This cord and another, attached to either side of the device, fits tightly into the groove carved in the flat bevel of the lens. (B) The close-up photograph is of the left lens of a rather unusual supra spectacle. A metal band lies in the groove of its flat bevel. Attached to the band are a very thin brace bar (top right) and a closing block joint with side (left). In this example the bands also constitute the major part of the front

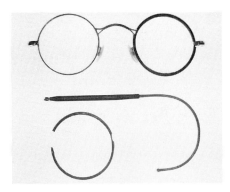

Fig. 11.5 *Windsor spectacles featuring the W-bridge. The right channelled plastics rim (below) and a curl side are shown here separately*

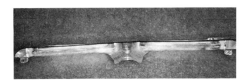

Fig. 11.6 *An inset bridge, seen from above*

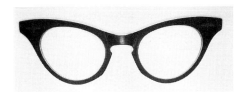

Fig. 11.7 *An 'upswept' front with a keyhole bridge*

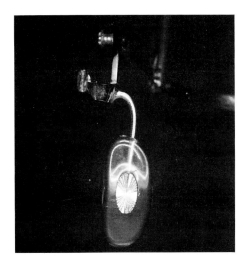

Fig. 11.8 *A plastics pad with a pad insert in the shape of a vertical oval, and a pad arm*

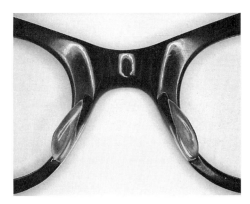

Fig. 11.9 *Rear view of the pad bridge of an opaque plastics front with transparent, rigid pads*

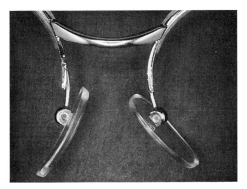

Fig. 11.10 *A pair of rocking pads. The pad stud, which is part of the pad, fits into the semicircular container at the end of the pad arm. A polyamide pin secures the stud to the container. A tiny screw is generally used instead of a pin*

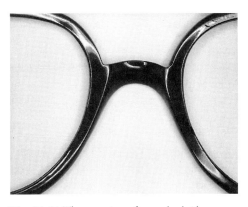

Fig. 11.11 *The rear view of a regular bridge*

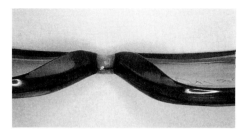

Fig. 11.12 A saddle bridge, seen from below

Fig. 11.13 Rear view of a twinned pad fitted on a ▶
metal frame

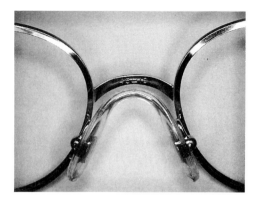

TABLE 11.2 *Bridges and their parts*

Term	Definition
Arch (see Fig. 11.11)	The main curve of a non-pad bridge forming the bearing surface
Crest (see Fig. 11.11)	The central portion of the arch of a non-pad bridge
Insert bridge (see Fig. 11.28)	A plastics bridge fitted to supplement the bridge of an otherwise metal frame
Inset bridge (Fig. 11.6)	A regular bridge shaped such that the bearing surface is wholly behind the back plane of the front
Keyhole bridge (Fig. 11.7)	A bridge with pads, shaped like the outline of the upper part of a keyhole
Pad arm (Fig. 11.8)	An extension, either integral with the bridge or as a separate attachment, to which a pad is fitted
Pad bridge (Fig. 11.9)	A bridge with two specific and limited nasal bearing areas
Pad insert (Fig. 11.8)	A piece of metal that is placed inside a plastics pad during its manufacture to give the pad rigidity in use
Pad stud (Fig. 11.10)	A protrusion from the pad, usually part of the pad insert, used to fasten the pad to the arm
Regular bridge (Fig. 11.11)	A bridge without pads designed to rest on the nose over a continuous area
Rigid pad (Fig. 11.9)	A pad formed on, or rigidly attached to, the bridge of the rim
Rocking pad (Fig. 11.10)	A pad attached by a form of hinge or toggle, allowing some self-adjustment
Saddle bridge (Fig. 11.12)	A bridge shaped such that it rests on the nose over a continuous area, but in which the ends of the bearing surface extend to lie behind the back plane of the front. (Saddle bridges include the regular bridge and inset bridge)
Twinned pad (Fig. 11.13)	A pair of rocking pads joined together to form a type of saddle bridge
Twin pad	See twinned pad

TABLE 11.3 *Joints/hinges and their parts*

Term	Definition
Barrel	See charnier
Centre joint (Fig. 11.14)	Joint positioned on or near the centre line
Charnier (Figs 11.15 and 11.18)	Tube or ring, forming part of a joint, which receives the screw or dowel pin
Closing block joint (Fig. 11.15)	Joint which also enables a metal rim to be closed and which is formed of two charniers (one threaded) and a screw
Closing block screw	A screw used to close the two parts of a closing block or a closing block joint
Concealed joint (Fig. 11.16)	Joint in which all but the charnier and pivot have been concealed within the material of front and sides
Dowel pin (Fig. 11.15)	A pivot in the form of a pin, secured in the joint by riveting
Endpiece	See closing block joint
Endpiece joint	See tenon joint
High joint (Fig. 11.14)	Joint positioned substantially above the centre line
Joint plate (Fig. 11.17)	The part of a hinge joint that provides the means of fixing it to the front and the side
Lock nut (Fig. 11.18)	A nut fitted for the sole purpose of preventing unintentional loosening of the retaining screw or dowel
Low joint (Fig. 11.14)	Joint positioned substantially below the centre line
Pinless joint (Fig. 11.17)	Joint with anchoring devices embedded in the material of front and/or side
Pinned joint (Fig. 11.17)	Joint which is attached to the front or side by means of rivets
Recessed joint (Fig. 11.19)	Joint comprising a charnier and a pivot mounted on plates which have been inset into the inside surface of front and sides
Rivet (Fig. 11.17)	A stud that is used to attach a joint plate to the front or side
Rivet plate (Fig. 11.20)	A unit comprising of two or more rivets, connected solidly together
Shield rivet	See rivet plate.
Sprung joint (Figs 4.4 and 11.21)	Joint having a spring mechanism designed to exert lateral pressure on the side of the head of the spectacle wearer
Surface joint (Fig. 11.19)	Joint comprising plates, a charnier and a pivot mounted on the inside surface of front or sides by means of which the side hinges on the front
Tenon joint (Fig. 11.15)	Joint formed by slotting either the front or side to receive a charnier formed at the end of the other component
Threaded barrel (Fig. 11.18)	One of the charniers of a closing block joint which is threaded to receive the closing block screw

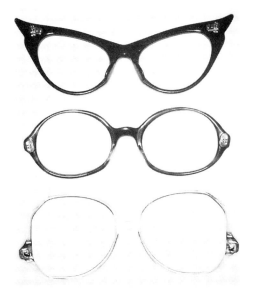

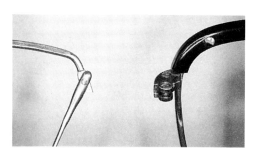

Fig. 11.15 *Left: a tenon joint with a dowel pin, seen from above; right: rear view of a metal front with a hood and a closing block joint*

Fig. 11.14 *Rear views of fronts with high joints (above), centre joints (middle) and low joints (below)*

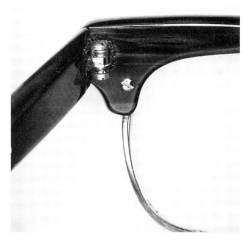

Fig. 11.16 *A concealed joint fitted into the hood of a combination frame, and its side. Compare with Fig. 1.4*

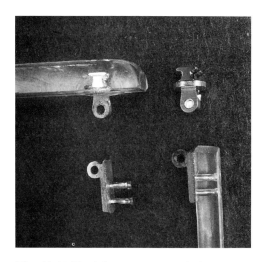

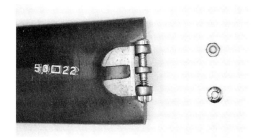

Fig. 11.17 *Top left: a transparent side fitted with a pinless joint; top right: a pinless joint; bottom left: a joint plate with a charnier and two rivets; bottom right: a transparent side fitted with a pinned joint*

Fig. 11.18 *Left: a side with a pinless joint fitted with a screw and a star-shaped lock-nut. Note that the lower portion of the screw is threaded indicating that the lowest of the three charniers is the threaded barrel. Right: a hexagonal and a round lock-nut*

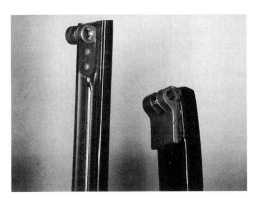

Fig. 11.19 *Sides fitted with a recessed joint (left) and a surface joint*

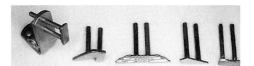

Fig. 11.20 *A joint plate fitted with a rivet plate (left) and samples of rivet plates*

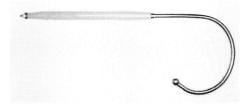

Fig. 11.22 *A curl side showing (from left to right) a butt, collet and a curl ending in a ball tip*

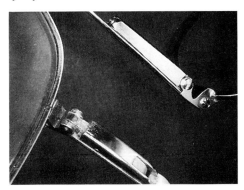

Fig. 11.21 *Sample sprung joints. Above: not under tension, top view; below: side view of a different sprung joint, fully opened. See also Fig. 4.4*

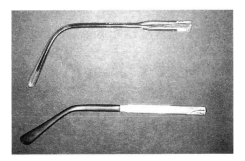

Fig. 11.23 *Above: drop-end side showing a butt (right) and the drop (left); below: a metal side fitted with an endcover*

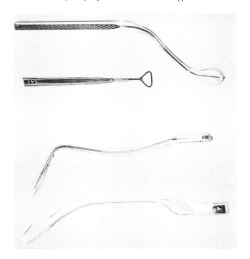

Fig. 11.24 *Top: an extended side; second from above: a loop-end side; below: two sinuous sides. The three upper sides are reinforced along the greater part of their length*

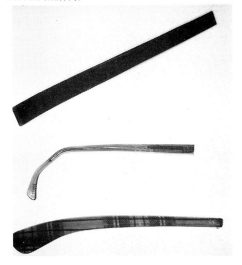

Fig. 11.25 *Above: a straight side. Middle: an 'anatomical' side with a side wire. Below: a spatula side inlaid with textile material*

TABLE 11.4 Sides/temples *and their parts*

Term	Definition
Ball tip (Fig. 11.22)	A small piece of metal in the shape of a ball, fixed to the end of a curl side
Butt (Fig. 11.23)	The part of the side nearest to the joint; it has a different form from the remainder of the side
Collet (Fig. 11.22)	A metal collar sometimes fitted at the hind end of the butt
Core	The wire on which the curl is wound
Curl (Fig. 11.22)	The flexible end of a curl side
Curl side (Fig. 11.22)	A side, the end of which is usually flexible and is designed to lie along the greater part of the groove behind the ear
Drop (Fig. 11.23)	The bent-down end of a drop-end side
Drop-end side (Fig. 11.23)	A side which is essentially straight from dowel screw to bend and the end of which is designed to lie only in the upper part of the groove behind the ear. (Various types are referred to by descriptions such as club-end and hockey-end)
Endcover (Figs 8.1 and 11.23)	A plastics covering for the end of a metal side
Extended side (Fig. 11.24)	This is not a standard term; it describes a drop-end side where the tip is designed to grip the back of the head thus providing additional anchorage
Library temple	See straight side
Loop-end side (Fig. 11.24)	A side terminating in a loop which is designed to take a tape or elastic ribbon
Reinforced side (Figs 11.24 and 11.25)	A plastics side or a side with a plastics butt with a metal insert along the greater part of the side or the whole of the butt. (When the plastics material of a side is not transparent, the metal insert may show as a small metal part embedded in the material when the side is viewed in section, nearest to the joint)
Riding bow temple	See curl side
Side wire (Figs 11.24 and 11.25)	The metal insert of a reinforced side
Sinuous side (Fig. 11.24)	A drop-end side in which the centre line describes one or more curves between the dowel screw and the bend
Skull temple	See drop-end side
Spatula side (Fig. 11.25)	A straight side but with its tip modified to give improved grip
Straight side (Fig. 11.25)	A side without a curl or drop, extending beyond, or at least to, the ear
Tip	The end of the side furthest from the front
Tip	See endcover

TABLE 11.5 *Rims and rim attachments*

Term	Definition
Closing block (Figs 11.26–11.28)	Device which enables a metal rim to be closed around the circumference of the lens. (The illustrations show a number of ways in which closing blocks have been concealed.) See also closing block screw and closing block joint (Table 11.3)
Gallery (Fig. 2.34)	A projecting wire or shelf attached to the rim, designed to exert pressure against the skin. (They have been used on monocles (Fig. 11.29) and as ptosis props)
Hood (Fig. 11.26)	A plastics covering to the upper part of the metal rim of a combination frame, to which the joint may be attached.
Top rim	See hood
Tube	See closing block.

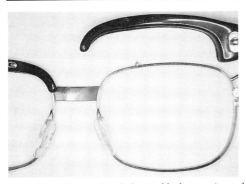

Fig. 11.26 *Conventional closing blocks are situated on the temporal side of the rim. When the hood is fitted, the closing block screw is accessible from below*

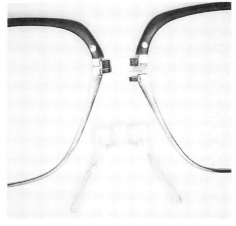

Fig. 11.28 *Occasionally, the closing blocks are situated on the nasal side of the rims. In this example, the closing blocks are covered by an insert bridge*

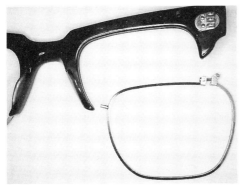

Fig. 11.27 *When the closing block is situated on the upper part of the rim access is possible only when the bar or hood has been removed*

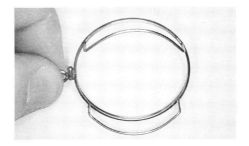

Fig. 11.29 *The galleries of a monocle seen from behind*

TABLE 11.6 *Rimless mounts*

Term	Definition
Bridge piece (Fig. 11.30)	The central component of a three-part rimless mount, comprising the bridge, pads (if any) and lens-holding devices
Claw (Figs 11.31 and 11.32)	The part of a strap extending above or below the stirrup and lying along the edge of the lens
Endpiece (Figs 11.31 and 11.32)	One of the outer components of a three-piece rimless mount, comprising the joint and lens-holding device
Strap (Figs 11.31 and 11.32)	A lens-holding device, generally in the form of a stirrup in which the lens is secured by means of a screw or a rivet
Lens-holding devices	There are a number of rimless lens-holding devices not mentioned in BS 3521 (1991). Some methods of securing the lens, are described below. Fig. 11.30: The lens is attached to the lens-holding device by means of a screw which passes through a hole in the glass or plastics lens. The lens is protected from the screw by means of a washer placed below the screw head, and plastics tubing which surrounds the screw's shaft (Fig. 11.3); Fig. 11.33 shows a lens-holding device where a rivet plate-like device is used; Fig. 11.34 shows an arrangement where two screws protrude from the back plane of the front. The screws pass through holes in the lens and a small plate, and are secured with nuts; Fig. 11.35 shows a part of a clamping device where a strap is lodged in a slot made in the flat bevel of the lens (see also Fig. 11.3). Together with a similar component placed on the nasal side, the lens is clamped in a metal arc-shaped rim. The latter is either part of the front, or suspended below a browbar. Plastics tubing may be fitted around the strap to protect a glass lens, in particular

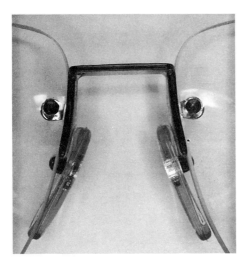

Fig. 11.30 *The bridge piece of a three-part rimless mount*

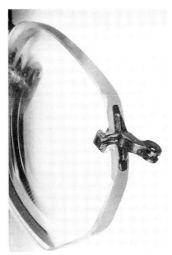

Fig. 11.31 *The claw lies in the vertical meridian, along the edge of the lens. This example consists of a thin spring nearest the lens edge, which is contained by a part fixed to the strap. The endpiece is the portion protruding to the right*

Fig. 11.32 *A strap seen from below. A screw is fitted in the stirrup-type lens-holding device. The middle portion is the claw while the endpiece is uppermost*

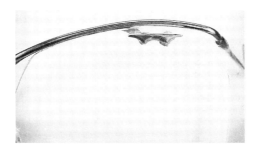

Fig. 11.33 *Frontal view of a lens-holding device resembling a rivet plate. The device is suspended from the rear aspect of the browbar*

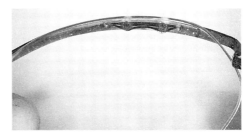

Fig. 11.34 *Rear view of a lens-holding device consisting of two screws protruding from the back plane of the front. The screws pass through holes in the lens which is secured with nuts to the screws*

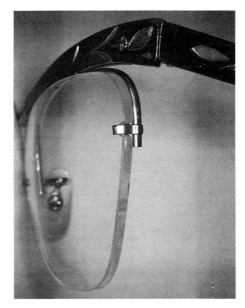

Fig. 11.35 *The temporal clamp of a two-clamp lens-holding device. Note the decorative effect obtaining by etching the anodized aluminium browbar*

REFERENCES

ANSI Z80.5 (1979). *American National Standard requirements for dress ophthalmic frames.* New York: American National Standards Institute, Inc.

BS 3521, Part 2 (1991). *Terms Relating to Ophthalmic Optics and Spectacle Frames. Part 2: Glossary of Terms Relating to Spectacle Frames.* London: British Standards Institution.

ISO 7998 (1984). *Optics and Optical Instruments – Spectacle Frames – Vocabulary and Lists of Equivalent Terms.* Genève (CH): International Standards Organisation.

CHAPTER 12

Measurement of Face and Frame

12.1 Introduction

The dimensions of a spectacle wearer's face and his spectacle frame are intimately related. This chapter features the measurement of the human face and of the frame. On the basis of the facial measurements obtained, a dispenser should be able to modify suitable spectacle frames to fit the wearer better. In addition, he should be able to design a spectacle frame for a prospective wearer, or be able to instruct a frame manufacturer to make a bespoke spectacle frame for a particular person. This frame may be based on an existing model.

12.2 Equipment for Facial Measurements

A number of authors (Sasieni, 1950; Waters, 1952; Passet, 1974; Clayton, 1977; Darras, 1982; Eber, 1987) have described equipment designed for the measurement of specific angles and distances associated with the human face. A less conventional approach was taken by Jouk (1980) who employed stereophotogrammetry.

Facial measurements are of consequence for the comfortable fit of a spectacle frame. They are indispensable when ordering a handmade spectacle frame.

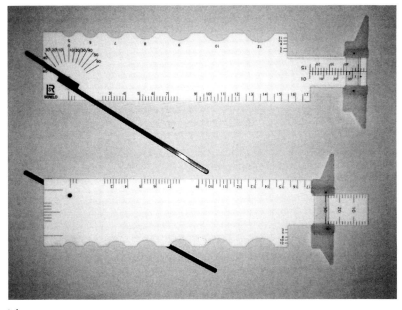

Fig. 12.1 Facial measurement gauge

The facial measurement gauge (Fairbanks, 1968; available from W. T. Rees Ltd.; see Section 12.5) is the instrument most widely used for this purpose in the UK (Fig. 12.1). The linear scales on this gauge are graduated in units that correspond to the accuracy required or attainable, varying from 2 to 5 mm. The protractor scale, which lies on the front surface of the gauge, is divided into divisions of 10°. With experience one can generally estimate to half these values.

Although the gauge can be used to measure the interpupillary distance (PD), one is referred to Chapter 21 for this measurement.

12.3 Facial Measurements

The facial measurements described in Table 12.1 are generally accompanied by a definition, illustration and sometimes remarks. Facial measurements have not been defined in a Standard. The

TABLE 12.1 Facial measurements

Term	Definition	Remarks
Angle of crest	The angle in the vertical plane between the line parallel to the nasal crest and the assumed spectacle plane (Fig. 12.2A)	
Angle of the side	The angle between the perpendicular to the assumed spectacle plane, at level with the eyebrow, and the line between eyebrow and ear point (Fig. 12.2B)	This applies to a high joint front when measured in this manner
Apical radius	The arc of the nasal crest, in the assumed spectacle plane (Fig. 12.2C)	If in doubt, record the larger radius; if necessary, the apical radius of a front may then be made steeper
Base at 10 or at 15	The width of the nose in the assumed spectacle plane, at 10 and/or at 15 mm below the nasal crest (Fig. 12.2D,E)	These two measurements give details comparable to the frontal angle
Bridge height	The sum of the crest height and 5 mm	See same entry in Table 12.2
Bridge width	The distance between the assumed areas of contact of the bearing surfaces of the front with the sides of the nose, measured at a level 5 mm below the lower limbus point in the assumed spectacle plane (Fig. 12.2F)	
Crest height	The distance in the assumed spectacle plane, between lower limbus point and nasal crest (Fig. 12.2G)	

TABLE 12.1 *Continued*

Term	Definition	Remarks
Distance between rims		Measurement taken as for bridge width, but with the edge of the rule at level with the lower limbus point. This measurement is assumed to be effective on the horizontal centre line.
Downward angle of drop	The downward inclination of the side from the assumed line of the side, measured at the ear point (Fig. 12.2H)	The line of the side of a frame rums through the dowel and ear point
Frontal angle	The angle between the vertical in the assumed spectacle plane and a parallel to the assumed bearing surface on the side of the nose (Fig. 12.2I,J)	
Front to bend	The distance from the assumed spectacle plane to the ear point (Fig. 12.2B)	
Head width	The horizontal distance between the ear points of the head (Fig. 12.2K)	The ear point is situated in the uppermost part of the groove between ear and skull
Projection	The horizontal distance between the assumed spectacle plane and the eyelashes in their most protruding position (Fig. 12.2L)	
Pupil distance		See Chapter 21
Splay angle	The angle between the assumed pad bearing area on the nose, and a normal to the assumed spectacle plane (Fig. 12.2M)	
Temple width	The horizontal distance between the temples of the head measured 25 mm behind the assumed spectacle plane (Fig. 12.2N)	
Total length of a curl side		Measure the total length required with a piece of string, from the assumed spectacle plane over the ear point to the lower aspect of the auricle. This measurement is not usually considered as a facial measurement

The nasal crest (see Section 3.2.4) may be described for the present purpose as the area of contact between the nose and the bridge of a fitted spectacle frame. The 'assumed spectacle plane' is the plane in which the spectacle front is intended to fit

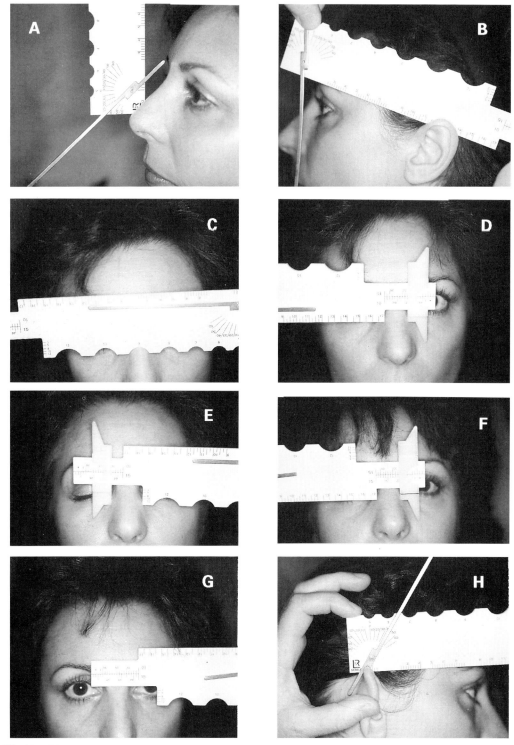

Fig 12.2 (Caption on p. 136)

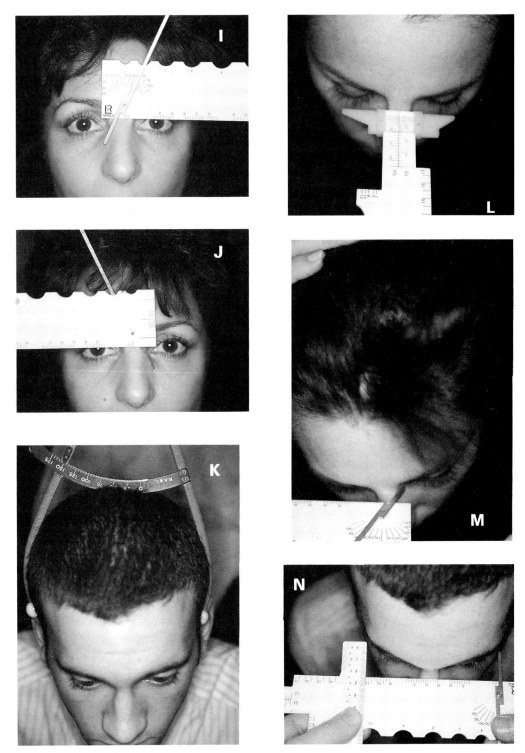

Fig. 12.2 (Continued)

definitions provided are based on the equivalent frame measurements.

Many frame measurements are based on the horizontal centre line (HCL) as reference line (see Section 12.4.2). Unfortunately, the human face has no fixed and invariable reference point or line. Conventional practice is to assume that the lower eyelid or the lowest limbus point represents the equivalent of the level of the HCL, for the purposes of taking facial measurements. In cases of gross facial asymmetry (see Section 3.2.3), one will have to specify whether the right or left eye has been used for this purpose.

12.4 Frame Measurement Systems

12.4.1 HISTORICAL BACKGROUND

In 1902, the Standards Committee of the (British) Optical Society presented a first report (Fairbanks, 1968). The completed work, which included standards for spectacle frame measurements, appeared a year later.

The Institute of Ophthalmic Opticians, together with the Association of Wholesale & Manufacturing Opticians, appointed an Ophthalmic Optical Standards Committee in 1922. Their findings did not appear until 1928 (see Emsley & Swaine, 1951). The Committee confirmed the use of the Metric System for linear measurements, but did not explicitly define the angular system to be used.

Cole & Blackburn (1935a, b) introduced the Datum Line system of frame measurements. The reference or Datum Line is situated midway between the horizontal tangents to the upper and lower edge of the lens shape. All frame measurements are given with respect to the Datum Line. The RAL 914 guidelines of 1938 showed the same system, as did RAL-RG 915 of 1961. The Datum System was enshrined in BS 3199 of 1960.

The Boxing System of Lens and Frame Measurements was 'officially' introduced by the (American) Optical Manufacturers Association in 1961 (Anonymous, 1961a–d). However, Chappell (1955) had set out his objections earlier, as had Williams (1962). Fry (1960, 1961) defended the Boxing System. Darras & Hermann (1965) described other systems, including a French proposal that borrowed concepts from both Datum and Boxing Systems, and the GOMAC System (see also Biessels, 1966a, 1966b, 1966c). Further efforts were made to resolve the dispute between the protagonists (Still, 1980; Such, 1980).

With the introduction of BS 3521 in 1991, use of the Datum System in the United Kingdom ceased. Most countries where spectacle frames are manufactured have adopted the Boxed Lens System, and it is likely that this system will soon be universal. Note that the Boxed Lens System, as set out in BS 3521 (1991), is an expanded version of the original system, as set out in 1961 (Anonymous, 1961a–d; see also Obstfeld, 1989).

Fig. 12.2 *(on preceding pages) (A) Angle of crest 40°; (B) angle of the side 20° and front to bend 112 mm; (C) apical radius 9 mm; (D) base at 10 measures 20 mm and (E) base at 15 measures 25 mm; (F) bridge width 20 mm. Because the rule was designed before the introduction of the bridge width, this measurement was not foreseen. Fortunately, an existing raised edge on the cursor lies 5 mm from another. Having blackened the raised edge, to represent the horizontal centre line, it is frequently possible to obtain the measurement; (G) bridge height 5 mm; (H) downward angle of drop 45°; frontal angles: (I) right 35°, and (J) left 25° (read on other side of rule); (K) head width 150 mm (measured with calipers); (L) projection nil; (M) splay angle (left) 27°; (N) temple width 110 mm*

TABLE 12.2 *Boxed lens system (BS 3521, 1991)*

Term	Definition
Angle of crest	The angle in a vertical plane between a line tangential to the bearing surface at its centre and the back plane of the front, of a regular bridge front. When applied to a pad bridge, it should be taken from the line approximating to the back surface of the bar in a central section (Fig. 12.7)
Back plane of the front	The surface of the frame or mount nearer to the eyes that coincides with the back surface of the rims or, in rimless mounts having a separate bridge, with the back plane of the clamps or straps
Bridge height	The vertical distance from the bridge width line to the intersection point of the vertical symmetry axis with the lower edge of the bridge (Fig. 12.3)
Bridge width	The minimum distance between the pad surfaces of the front or of the rims of regular bridge fronts measured along the bridge width line (Fig. 12.3)
Bridge width line	Line parallel to and 5 mm below the horizontal centre line (Fig. 12.3)
Boxed centre	The intersection of the horizontal and vertical centre lines of the box which circumscribes the lens and which is generally represented by a rectangle (Fig. 12.3)
Boxed lens size	The dimensions of the rectangle formed by the horizontal and vertical tangents to the lens shape (Fig. 12.3)
Centre line (horizontal)	The horizontal line drawn through the geometric centres of the rectangular boxes that just encompasses the two lenses of a front (Fig. 12.3)
Centre line of a lens	The line mid-way between, and parallel to, the horizontal tangents to the lens shape at its highest and lowest points (Fig. 12.3)
Crest height	The vertical distance from the horizontal centre line of the front to the midpoint of the lower edge of the bridge (Fig. 12.5)
Distance between centres	The distance between the geometric centres of the two lenses (Fig. 12.3)
Distance between lenses	The distance between the nearest points of the apices of the two lenses (Fig. 12.3)
Frontal width	Horizontal distance between the dowel points (Fig. 12.6; see dowel point, Table 12.5)
Horizontal lens size	The distance between the vertical sides of the rectangle which circumscribe the lens (Fig. 12.3)
Projection (or inset) of bridge	The minimum horizontal distance from the back plane of the front to the centre of the back of the bridge (Figs 12.6 and 11.6)
Vertical lens size	The distance between the horizontal sides of the rectangle which circumscribe the lens (Fig. 12.3)
Vertical symmetry axis	The central line passing vertically through the crest of the bridge (Fig. 12.3)

12.4.2 THE BOXED LENS SYSTEM (BS 3521, 1991; BS 3199, 1992/EN ISO 8624; Fig. 12.3)

The boxed lens system is defined as a system based on the rectangle formed by the horizontal and vertical lines tangential to the extremes of each lens, by which the dimensions of a front and the location of the lenses in the front may be measured. (Note: in this and following definitions this writer has replaced the word 'frame' used in BS 3521, by 'front'.) The terminology is defined in Table 12.2.

In addition to the box around the lens, or around the lens shape of a front, the centre lines are essential elements of the boxed lens system. In practice, when dealing with a (glazed) front, the horizontal centre line (HCL) is used for centration purposes and to specify the segment top position and fitting cross height.

The vertical centre line is the vertical line passing through the boxed centre (of each lens). Although it is shown in Fig. 2 of BS 3521, Part 2 (1991), it has not been defined.

The horizontal lens size is usually indicated on a frame together with the distance between lenses. The vertical lens size is seldom mentioned. However, it plays a role when deciding on the position of the horizontal centre line, and when the vertical centration of spectacle lenses is specified.

With respect to the front, a further essential measurement is the distance between the box around each lens, known as the distance between lenses (DBL). For glazing purposes, the distance between centres (DBC), needs to be noted.

Kors (1969) described modified calipers for boxing system frame measurements in the workshop. Instead of these particular calipers, a frame measurement rule (Section 12.5) may be used.

Figure 12.4 shows the greatest (horizontal) width (GW), DBL, DBC and (horizontal) lens size. The DBC may be calculated from

$$DBC = (GW + DBL)/2$$

and the (horizontal) lens size from

$$\text{lens size} = (GW - DBL)/2$$

A comparison of the likely fit of different fronts on the wearer's nose is facilitated by the bridge width.

Attention is drawn to the difference between the bridge height (Fig. 12.3) and the crest height (Fig. 12.5).

A dimension of consequence for the aesthetic relationship of the face which a front is to adorn is the frontal width, which should resemble the temple width of the wearer.

The projection (or inset) of the bridge (Fig. 12.6), and the angle of crest (Fig. 12.7) are closely

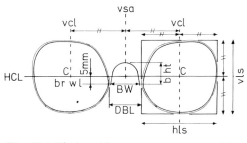

Fig. 12.3 The boxed lens measurement system: b ht, bridge height; br w l, bridge width line; BW, bridge width; C, boxed (geometric) centre; CC, distance between centres; DBL, distance between lenses; HCL, horizontal centre line; hls, horizontal lens size; vcl, vertical centre line; vls, vertical lens size; vsa, vertical symmetry axis

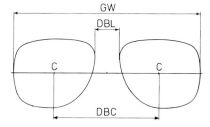

Fig. 12.4 Kors' (1969) method of ascertaining the DBC (distance between centres) and horizontal lens size from the GW (greatest horizontal width) and the DBL (distance between lenses). See Section 12.4.2

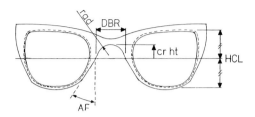

Fig. 12.5 *Measurements associated with the front: AF, frontal angle of pad; cr ht, crest height; DBR, distance between rims; HCL, horizontal centre line; rad, apical radius*

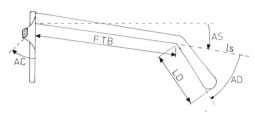

Fig. 12.7 *Measurements associated with front and side: AC, angle of crest; AD, downward angle of drop; AS, angle of the side; FTB, front to bend; LD, length of drop; ls, line of side*

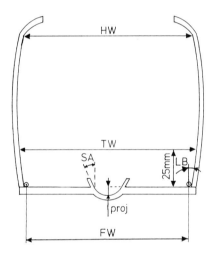

Fig. 12.6 *Measurements associated with front and sides: FW, frontal width; HW, frame head width; LB, angle of let-back; proj, projection of bridge; SA, splay angle of pad; TW, frame temple width*

associated with a well fitting front, and involve the back plane of the front. If the rims do not substantially lie in one plane, and in the case of rimless browbar and similar mounts, the back plane of the front is the one containing symmetrical small parts of both rims or both browbars immediately adjacent to the bridge.

12.4.3 MEASUREMENTS OF REGULAR BRIDGES

There are only two frame measurements specifically appertaining to regular bridges. They are given in Table 12.3. All other measurements defined in Table 12.2 also apply.

TABLE 12.3 *Measurements specific to regular bridges and in addition to those of Table 12.2 (see Section 12.5)*

Term	Definition
Apical radius	**The radius of the arc forming the lower edge of the bridge viewed perpendicularly to the back plane of the front (Fig. 12.5)**
Distance between rims	**The horizontal distance (in millimetres) between the nasal surfaces of the rims, measured at a stated level below the midpoint of the lower edge of the bridge (Fig. 12.5)** **(Usually recorded as 'DBR 20 at 10 below crest')**

12.4.4 MEASUREMENTS OF PAD BRIDGES

These are given in Table 12.4 and are in addition to those of Table 12.2.

In addition to some general terms, there are specific measurements applicable to pads mounted on arms and to pads attached directly to the rims of a front of mount.

12.4.5 MEASUREMENTS OF JOINTS AND SIDES

These are given in Table 12.5. In addition to the general terms, measurements applicable to the different types of sides are provided.

12.5 Frame Measurement Rules

Many frame measurement rules have been produced over the years. Some are also suitable for a number of facial measurements and determination of some spectacle lens details; others are no more than a modified millimetre rule. As a consequence of the introduction of the Boxed Lens System at least one measurement, the bridge width, cannot be taken with accuracy with any of these rules. To overcome this problem, the 'The City Rule' (available from W. T. Rees Ltd., Oxford Road, Wealdstone, Middx. HA3 7RG, UK) was designed (Fig. 12.18) (Campbell & Obstfeld, 1995). The rule incorporates a number of scales that can be found on its predecessor (Anonymous, 1965); however, new scales have also been introduced, while the angular scales have been rationalized. Although both old and new gauges are referred to as frame gauges, they have specific scales for multifocal lens measurement. The City Rule has two scales for this purpose: one for the measurements associated with progressive power (*progressive addition*) lenses and another which facilitates the

determination of the position of the boxed centre and all measurements based on it.

12.6 Ordering Handmade Frames

Handmade frames can be ordered from a small number of specialist workshops. The manufacture of such frames is usually limited to the common types of plastics materials for the front, and suitable types of sides. Two methods of ordering are used: one is based on an existing frame, the other on a sketch of a front or frame.

12.6.1 MODIFYING AN EXISTING FRONT

The simplest method is copying a front or frame in a colour not provided by the manufacturer. Frame workshops maintain stock of plastics sheet material or of slabs, in a great variety of colours and colour combinations of which they provide samples. Once a patient has decided on colour, only the sample frame of the correct measurements need be sent to the workshop, together with the colour reference or sample. From these details the frame can be produced. However, there may be limitations: certain effects can only be created by specialist equipment not usually found in a small frame workshop. It is therefore sometimes necessary to consult the framemaker as to the feasibility of manufacture.

When a particular facial measurement needs to be accommodated, or some other problem arises, it is also necessary to provide the frame maker with the required frame measurement(s) in addition to the sample frame. These measurements must be based on facial measurements. It may then be necessary to modify the frame style. It is sometimes wise to ask the framemaker to produce a prototype. This provides the prospective wearer with the opportunity to see what their bespoke frame is going to look like. The

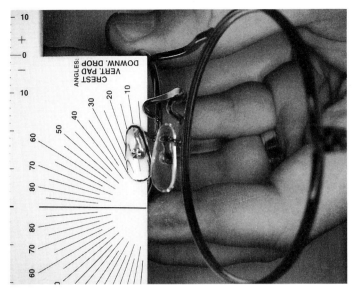

Fig. 12.8 *Vertical angle of pad (10°)*

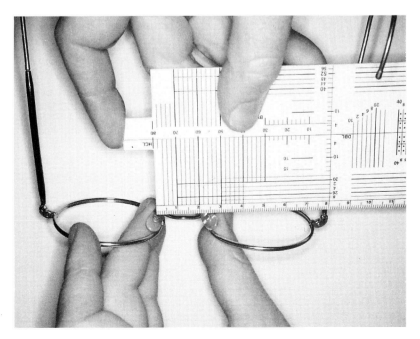

Fig. 12.9 *Distance between pad centres (24 mm)*

Spectacle frames and their dispensing

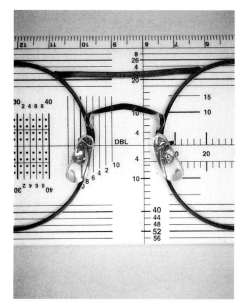

Fig. 12.10 *Height of pad centres (−4 mm)*

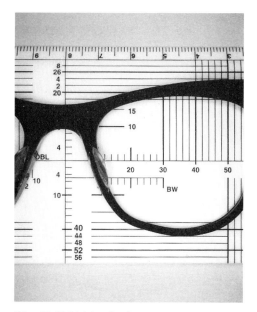

Fig. 12.12 *Height of pad tops (+4 mm)*

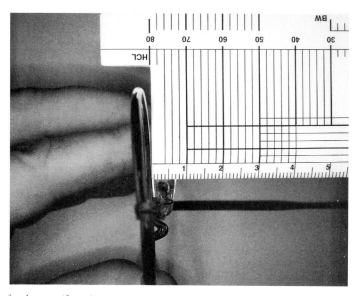

Fig. 12.11 *Inset of pad centre (3 mm)*

TABLE 12.4 *Measurements specific to pad bridges in addition to those of Table 12.2 (see Section 12.5)*

Term	Definition
General measurements	
Distance between rims	The horizontal distance between the nasal surfaces of the rims, measured either along the horizontal centre line or, if elsewhere, at a stated level above or below this centre line (Fig. 12.5)
Frontal angle of pad	The angle between the vertical and the line of intersection of the pad plane with the back plane of the front (Fig. 12.5)
Pad centre	(1) **Of fixed pads:** the point on the bearing surface equidistant from its top and bottom and front and back, edges
	(2) **Of rocking pads:** the point on the bearing surface opposite the point of attachment of the pad
Pad plane	The plane approximating to the bearing surface of the pad
Splay angle of pad	The angle between the pad plane and a normal to the back plane of the front (Fig. 12.6)
Vertical angle of pad	The angle between the back plane of the front and the long axis of the pad projected on a vertical plane at right angles to the back plane of the front (Fig. 12.8) (Unless otherwise specified, this angle will be regarded as bringing the top of the pad relatively backwards)
Pads mounted on arms	
Distance between pad centres	The horizontal distance between the two pad centres (Fig. 12.9)
Height of pad centre	The vertical distance from the horizontal centre line to the pad centre (Fig. 12.10)
Inset of pad centre	The horizontal distance from the back plane of the front to the pad centre (Fig. 12.11)
Pads attached directly to rim	
Distance between pad tops	The horizontal distance between the tops of the pads in the back plane of the front
Height of pad top	The vertical distance from the horizontal centre line to the highest point of the pad (Fig. 12.12)
Width of pad	The maximum width of the pad surface, measured from the back of the rim

TABLE 12.5 *Measurements of joints and sides (see Section 12.5)*

Term	Definition
General terms and measurements	
Angle of the side	The vertical angle between a normal to the back plane of the front and the line of the side when opened (Fig. 12.7)
Dowel point	The centre of the bottom of the dowel hole (see dowel pin, Table 11.3.)
Ear point	(1) Of a drop-end side: the midpoint of the arc of contact between the bend of the side and the circle which fits it (2) Of a curl side: the point on the lower edge of the side at the beginning of the curl (3) Of a straight side: the point on the lower edge of the side which is assumed to make contact with the top of the ear
Frame head width	The distance between the sides at the ear points (Fig. 12.6)
Frame temple width	The distance between the sides 25 mm behind the back plane of the front (Fig. 12.6)
Joint angle	The vertical angle, inherent in the construction of a joint, which contributes to the angle of the side (Fig. 12.13)
Joint height	The distance from the horizontal centre line to the horizontal plane through the centre of the joint (Fig. 12.14)
Joint size	The overall axial length of the charniers
Let-back of side	The horizontal angle between the inner surface of the fully opened side, adjacent to the joint, and a normal to the back plane of the front (Fig. 12.6)
Line of the side	A straight line through dowel and ear points (Fig. 12.7)
Lug point	The point on the back surface of the lug where it begins its backward sweep, approximately level with the dowel point (Fig. 2.49) (its position is not always clear in frames where the radius of the lug is relatively large; see Figs 2.40 and 2.41)
Drop-end sides	
Downward angle of drop	The downward inclination of the drop from the line of the side, measured near the ear point and in the vertical plane containing the line of the side (Fig. 12.7)
Front to bend	The distance between the lug point and the ear point (Fig. 12.7)
Inward angel of drop	The inward inclination of the drop near the ear point from the vertical plane containing the line of the side (Fig. 12.15)

Continued

TABLE 12.5 *Continued*

Term	Definition
Length to bend	The distance between the dowel point and the ear point
Length of drop	The distance from the ear point to the extreme end of the side (Fig. 12.7)
Overall length of side	The distance between the dowel point and the tip. (Fig. 13 of BS 3521, Part 2 (1991) shows this measurement. Manufacturers indicate it on sides as the sum of the front to bend and length of drop and it is recommended to use the latter)
Curl sides **Length to tangent**	The distance from the dowel point to the tangent to the inner surface of the curl at rest which is perpendicular to the line of the side (Fig. 12.16)
Total length	The overall length from the dowel point to the extreme end (Fig. 12.17)
Straight sides **Length**	The distance from the dowel point to the extreme end, the side being flattened

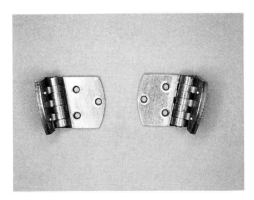

Fig. 12.13 *Joint angle: because the charniers are inclined, the line of the side will not be perpendicular to the back plane of the front*

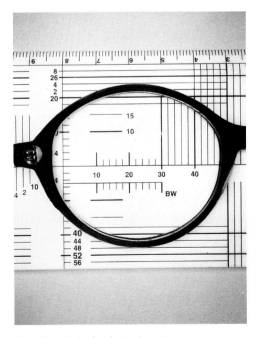

Fig. 12.14 *Joint height (+3 mm)*

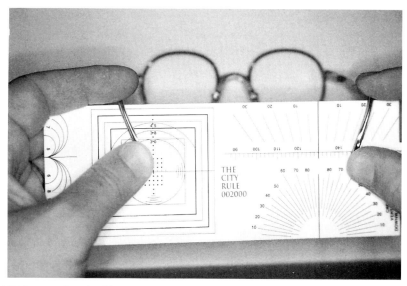

Fig. 12.15 *Right inward angle of drop (20°)*

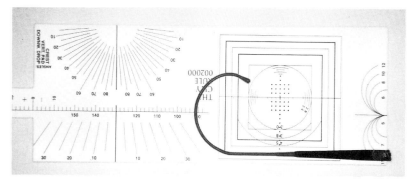

Fig. 12.16 *Length to tangent (90 mm)*

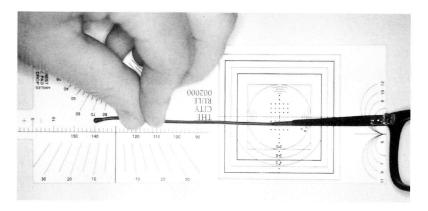

Fig. 12.17 *Total length (140 mm)*

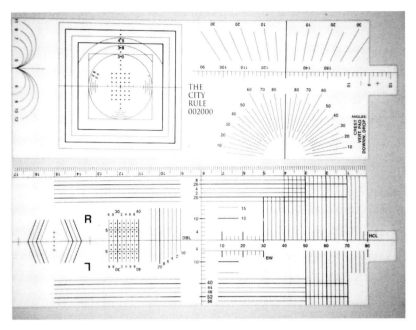

Fig. 12.18 *The City Rule*

TABLE 12.6 *Minimum frame measurements for a bespoke frame*

General front measurements	bridge height or crest height bridge width distance between lenses frontal width horizontal and vertical boxed lens sizes
For a regular bridge front	angle of crest apical radius projection or inset of bridge
For a pad bridge front	frontal angle height of pad top splay angle
Joint and sides	angle of the side joint height length of drop length to bend

dispenser can simultaneously ascertain that the frame measurements stipulated are correct so that the frame will fit once glazed. Alterations can still be made at this stage.

12.6.2 DESIGNING A 'SPECIAL' FRAME

If a patient wishes to obtain a frame that is not available from a mass manufacturer the following approach may be taken. The prospective wearer may either produce a sketch or, with the assistance of the dispenser, they may select from available samples details that they would like incorporated in their 'special'. The dispenser may then be able to produce a sketch and send this, together with the frame measurements, to the framemaker. Once a prototype has been seen by the patient further modifications may be made. When the patient's approval has been obtained, the final frame can be made and glazed.

Sketches may also be produced using an existing frame, or parts thereof, as template, and by modifying the sketch until the patient's specification has been met. It is imperative to take the necessary facial measurements carefully.

The minimum frame measurements to be provided to the framemaker are given in Table 12.6.

REFERENCES

Anonymous (1961a). The boxing system of lens and frame measurements – I. *Opt. J.-Rev.* **98** (14), 31–43.

Anonymous (1961b). The boxing system of lens and frame measurements – II: lens measurements. *Opt. J.-Rev.* **98** (15), 29–30.

Anonymous (1961c). The boxing system of lens and frame measurements – III: pattern measurements. *Opt. J.-Rev.* **98** (16), 42.

Anonymous (1961d). The boxing system of lens and frame measurements – IV. *Opt. J.-Rev.* **98**, 17, 32–38.

Anonymous (1965). New frame gauge and manual. *Optician* **150** (3892), 454.

Biessels, W.J. (1966a). The normalization of ophthalmic frame measurements – part 1. *Ophthalm. Optician* **6**, 170–172, Feb. 19.

Biessels, W.J. (1966b). The normalization of ophthalmic frame measurements – part 2. *Ophthalm. Optician* **6**, 213–215, March 5.

Biessels, W.J. (1966c). GOMAC-normalisatie. *Oculus, Amsterdam*, No. 5, 225–237.

BS 3199 (1960). *Measurement of Spectacles; Methods and Glossary*. London: British Standards Institution.

BS 3199/EN ISO 8624 (1992). *Specification for Measuring System for Spectacle Frames*. London: British Standards Institution.

BS 3521 (1991). *Terms Relating to Ophthalmic Optics and Spectacle Frames. Part 2: Glossary of Terms Relating to Spectacle Frames* (which includes ISO 7998 (1984): *Optics and Optical Instruments – Spectacle Frames – Vocabulary and lists of equivalent terms*). London: British Standards Institution.

Campbell, J. & Obstfeld, H. (1995). Made to measure. *Optician* **209** (5485), 43.

Chappell, N. (1955). My case against the boxing system. *Optician* **129** (3335), 169–170 & 172.

Clayton, G.H. (1977). *Spectacle Frame Dispensing*, 2nd edn. London: Association of Dispensing Opticians.

Cole, J. & Blackburn, A. (1935a). Bridge measurements and shaped eyes. *Optician* **89** (2301), 217, 224.

Cole, J. & Blackburn, A. (1935b). Frame measurement by Datum Line. *Optician* **89** (2302), 235–236.

Darras, C. (1982). *La Tête et ses Mesures*, 3rd edn., Chapter 3. Paris: Centre de protection oculaire.

Darras, C. & Hermann, F. (1965). The standardisation of nomenclature in spectacle-making. *Ophthalm. Optician* **5**, 63–80, Jan. 23.

Eber, J. (1987). *Anatomische Brillenanpassung*. Heidelberg: Optische Fachveröffentlichung GmbH.

Emsley, H.H. & Swaine, W. (1951). *Ophthalmic Lenses*, 6th edn., p. 305. London: Hatton Press.

Fairbanks, P. (1968). The facial measurement gauge. *Ophthalm. Optician* **8** (3), 114–116, 127–129.

Fry, G.A. (1960). Standardize: use of the boxing method. *Opt. J.-Rev.* **98** (19), 36–39.

Fry, G.A. (1961). The major issue of the datum-boxing controversy. *Optician* **141** (3643), 65–67.

Jouk, G. (1980). Méthode stéréophotogrammétrique des mesures anthropométriques pour le choix optimal des paramètres des montures. *Optométrie, France* **26** (3), 6–7.

Kors, K. (1969). Modification of inside-outside calipers to make boxing system frame measurements. *Am. J. Optom.* **46** (11), 880–881.

Obstfeld, H. (1989). DBR and other frame measurements. *Optician* **198** (5231), 26–27.

Passet, R. (1974). Prises de mesures et adaptation en lunetterie, part 2. *Optométrie, France* **20** (3).

RAL 914 (1938). *Bezeichnungsrichtlinien für Brillenteile.* Berlin: Beuth-Vertrieb GmbH.

RAL-RG 915 (1961). *Gütebestimmungen im Augenoptikerhandwerk. Individuell angepasste und handwerklich fertiggestellte Korrektionsbrillen.* Berlin: Beuth-Vertrieb GmbH.

Sasieni, L.S. (1950). *Spectacle Fitting and Optical Dispensing.* London: Hammond, Hammond & Co.

Still, D.C. (1980). The boxing system compared with the datum system. *Optician* **180** (4668), 18–20.

Such, B. (1980). Vital statistics in Paris. *Optician* **180** (4668), 14–15.

Williams, A.F. (1962). The forgotten man in the 'boxing method'. *Opt. J.-Rev.* **99** (18), 39–40.

Waters, E.H. (1952). *Ophthalmic Mechanics,* Vol. 1, 5th edn, Chapter XI. Corpus Christi (Texas): Waters.

CHAPTER 13

Equilibrium of Spectacles

13.1 Introduction

Spectacles exhibit a tendency to slide down their wearer's nose. There is rather more to this problem than meets the eye. It will be considered, at a first approximation, from the position of the centre of gravity of the complete appliance, that is, a spectacle frame fitted with spectacle lenses.

13.2 The Mass of Frame Fronts

The first aspect to consider is the mass of the front of a spectacle frame. At one time (1950s) some frame manufacturers indicated on the frame card the mass of a frame. However, all that manufacturers' information may include now is perhaps the type of material of the frame. The proliferation of new frame materials posed the question whether or not it would be useful to include the material from which a frame was manufactured and also the temperature for adjustments, presence of varnish and degrading effect of alcohol (Camau, 1985). All BS 6625 (1992) recommends is that the horizontal lens size, distance between lenses, and bridge width should be marked on the front, and the overall length on a sides. The same Standard also contains a recommendation that the mass of a frame for an identified frame size shall be provided. To date, the author has failed to find the last item.

The relationship between weight and mass is the following. The weight W, or downward force, of an object is an effect of the earth's gravitational force and is measured in newtons (N). One newton is a force of 1 kg m s^{-2} which gives a mass of 1 kg an acceleration of 1 m s^{-2}. The gravitational force g is very nearly 10 m s^{-2}. The relationship between the mass m of an object and its weight W, is given by the equation

$$W = m \cdot g$$

Hence, an object with a mass m of 1 kg, has a weight W of 10 N. Because spectacle frames have a very much smaller mass, it is reasonable to express their weight in hundredths of a newton, or centinewton (cN). However, one is more used to the gram as a measure of weight, although it is incorrect. In the tables in this chapter the mass of spectacle parts is expressed in grams.

Because no measurement of the mass of spectacle fronts appears to have been published, I have compiled Tables 13.1 and 13.2. The data were collected as follows. A number of frames of a particular type and/or material was collected, and the sides were removed from the frames (where possible). Each empty front and one of its sides were measured to the nearest gram, with an electronic scale. The boxed lens size, boxed distance between lenses (DBL) and total length of the side were also recorded. These measurements were averaged and the standard deviation calculated. Because a difference in DBL has no noticeable effect on the mass of the frame, it is not presented in the tables.

Table 13.1 shows that, on average, metal, metal combination and cellulose acetate fronts have about the same mass. Although Optyl and cellulose propionate are materials with a much lower density, because of larger lens sizes their mass is not much less than that of the first group.

TABLE 13.1 *The average mass of spectacle fronts of adults' frames (standard deviation in parentheses)*

Frame type	N	Material	Density (g cm^{-3})	Boxed lens size horizontal (mm)	vertical (mm)	Mass (g)
Metal	10		8·9	51·1(2·8)	36·1(5·9)	10·9(1·8)
	29	Cellulose acetate	1·3	48·8(4·1)	36·7(5·1)	10·2(3·7)
	8		–	46·5(5·4)	34·9(2·0)	10·0(3·5)
Metal comb.	11	Optyl	1·2	55·2(2·1)	49·2(2·9)	8·8(2·7)
	10	Cellulose propionate	1·2	53·1(3·0)	46·2(2·4)	8·1(2·0)
Half-eye	8	Various	–	48·0(4·1)	23·2(3·1)	6·7(1·7)
	5	Polyamide	1·1	54·4(4·3)	48·3(8·7)	5·8(1·7)
Supra	12	Various	–			5·8(1·5)
	3	Carbon reinforced	1·5	56·7(3·1)	49·7(1·5)	4·3(0·5)
Semi-rimless	5	Metal	8·9	42·7(2·3)		2·7(0·7)
Polymil	3		–			2·7(0·5)
*	10	Tortoiseshell	?	39·5(1·7)	38·0(1·2)	7·3(1·4)

* Front with pair of sides.

TABLE 13.2 *The average mass of fronts of children's frames (standard deviations in parentheses)*

N	Material	Density (g cm^{-3})	Boxed lens size horizontal (mm)	vertical (mm)	Mass (g)
7	Metal	8·9	46·1(2·9)	40·3(2·4)	8·1(1·0)
4	Optyl	1·2	48·0(1·4)	42·2(3·0)	6·7(0·4)
7	Cellulose acetate	1·3	38·9(3·0)	34·4(3·8)	6·6(0·7)

TABLE 13.3 *The overall size and average mass of spectacle sides*

Material	Adult N	length (mm)	mass (g)	Children N	length (mm)	mass (g)
Metal	10	137	4·5	7	121	3·6
Cellulose acetate	29	138	6·7	7	124	5·0
Metal combi	8	135	4·6			
Optyl	8	130	4·4	4	121	4·0
Cellulose propionate	9	137	5·1			
Polyamide	3	130	3·0			
Carbon reinforced	2	135	2·7			

While polyamide and carbon reinforced fronts have lens sizes similar to the second group, they have a smaller mass because of their thinner rims. The half-eye fronts have a greater mass than expected. The reason is that they are made of relatively heavy cellulose acetate and metal materials. The supra fronts are made mainly of polymethylmethacrylate (density only slightly less than that of cellulose acetate), and of metal. Hence, their relatively great mass. Semi-rimless and Polymil fronts were found to have the smallest mass. Because there were a number of tortoiseshell frames available, these were included as a curiosity.

In essence, the same comments apply to the children's fronts (Table 13.2).

The average mass of the sides is shown in Table 13.3, in the same order as in the previous tables. It is likely that the two types of sides made of cellulose-based plastics are slightly heavier than the others because of the mass of the side wire. The sides of children's frames are about 1 g lighter and about 15 mm shorter than those used with adults' fronts.

13.3 The Mass of Spectacle Lenses

Henke & Paesler (1982) considered different methods to determine the mass of edged spectacle lenses from a theoretical point of view, while Gottlob (1978) had earlier described a lens 'selector' for this purpose. Obstfeld (1990, 1991a,b) took a pragmatic approach by edging the lenses to size, before they were weighed. Table 13.4 provides a summary of the mass of edged lenses for adults' (horizontal lens size 54 mm) and children's frames (horizontal lens sizes 48 and 38 mm; see also Chapter 17). The weight of other combinations of back vertex power, uncut diameter and horizontal lens size may be estimated from the data provided. The results are in reasonable agreement with those of Maxam (1983). The author (Obstfeld, 1991b) concludes that:

(1) The shape of an edged lens has very little influence on its mass.
(2) Neighbouring horizontal lens sizes show very small differences in mass.

TABLE 13.4 The average mass of an edged meniscus spectacle lens weight in grams (after Obstfeld, 1991a,b)

Material		CR 39	Crown glass				
size:		54 mm	54	48*		38*	
BVP	diam.:	65 mm	65	65	58	65	45
+ 9 D		21	40	34	22	25	9
+ 5		14	26	21	14	15	7
+ 1		7	12	9	9	6	6
0		6	8				
− 1		6	10	7		5	6
− 5		11	15	10		6	6
− 9		13	23	15		9	6

BVP, back vertex power.
size, horizontal lens size.
diam., nominal uncut diameter.
* See also Chapter 17.

(3) Edged plastics lenses are about half the mass of their crown glass equivalent.

(4) The mass of edged, high refractive index lenses is not only dependent on their density, but also on other characteristics such as refractive index and the minimum centre thickness required for mechanical stability.

(5) Spectacle glazing shop operators should ensure that they use minimum diameter uncut lenses for positive prescriptions.

(6) Edged negative lenses weigh about half the mass of their original uncut form while edged positive lenses weigh about three-quarters of the mass of their uncut form.

Obstfeld (1992) queried the statement (Jalie, 1992) that 'aspheric lenses are lighter', on the grounds that the mean mass of six aspheric lenses of power +5·00 DS from various manufacturers, was only 0·5 g less than the mean mass of equivalent meniscus CR 39 lenses. In response, Norville (1992) pointed out that it is important that each aspheric lens be surfaced individually to obtain the thinnest lens achievable. He added that high-index resin aspheric lenses provided further improvements, and complications. This shows that there are many aspects that need to be taken into account. Table 13.5 will give an indication of the saving in mass when non-aspheric edged lenses are replaced by equivalent aspheric lenses.

With respect to bifocal lenses, Cheswick (1992) reached the following conclusions for lenses of equivalent back vertex power:

(1) With the exception of negative E-style lenses, bifocal lenses are heavier than single vision lenses.

(2) CR 39 edged negative bifocal lenses are about 70%, and positive bifocal lenses are about 40% of the weight of crown glass bifocal lenses.

(3) 25 mm diameter D-segment fused bifocal lenses are heavier than 22 mm diameter round segment fused bifocal lenses.

(4) Concerning E-style bifocal lenses, positive lenses are the heaviest, and negative are the lightest of all bifocal lenses made of the same material.

(5) The approximate weight of E-style bifocal lenses may be determined by adding half the weight of an equivalent single vision edged lens of the distance portion back vertex power, to half the weight of that of the near portion back vertex power.

TABLE 13.5 *Comparison of the mass of comparable aspheric and non-aspheric edged spectacle lenses. Nominal details: uncut diameter 65 mm, edged size 54 mm*

BVP (D)	Material	Type	Refractive index	Mass (g)
+2·50	CR 39	Non-aspheric	1·498	8
	crown	Non-aspheric	1·523	16
	CR 39	Rodenstock Cosmolit	1·498	5
	resin	Hoya HL2 Asp	1·56	5
+5·00	CR 39	Non-aspheric	1·498	14
	CR 39	Rodenstock Cosmolit	1·498	11
	resin	Nikon Lite II AS	1·56	10
	glass	Non-aspheric	1·6	20
	glass	Essilor Aspheral	1·6	17
+7·50	CR 39	Non-aspheric	1·498	18
	crown	Non-aspheric	1·523	34
	CR 39	Rodenstock Cosmolit	1·498	18

(6) The average plastics-to-glass weight ratio of edged bifocal lenses is 1:2.

To arrive at an estimated value, (2) above should be used in conjunction with the values in Table 13.4. As a rule-of-thumb, a 60 mm round flat-edged CR 39 bifocal lens of 3 D back vertex power weighs from 11 to 15 g. Gunaratnam (1991) stated that the weight of high refractive index lenses is not only dependent on their density, but also on characteristics such as refractive index and the minimum centre thickness required for mechanical stability.

13.4 The Mass of Glazed Frames

From the information provided on the mass of empty fronts, sides and lenses, it is possible to arrive at the mass of glazed spectacle frames. A front will weigh 3–10 g, a pair of sides 10–15 g, and a pair of lenses 10–80 g (or 10–80 cN). Hence, it appears reasonable to consider glazed frames having masses varying from 20 to 65 g. These figures are also in good agreement with Fischbach's (1986) findings, while Maxam (1983) wrote that the mass of a reasonably comfortable frame would be 20–30 g. He also stipulated that the mass of a glazed spectacle frame should not exceed 50 g, adding that if it were greater, pressure point(s) will usually occur on the nasal bearing surface(s) notwithstanding careful adjustment. In exceptional cases, namely for very high back vertex powers, one may encounter glazed frames weighing up to 100 g.

From the point of view of mechanics (the study of the effect of forces on objects), the nose, ears and mastoid bones have to oppose the forces resulting from the mass of the spectacle frame, so that the latter will stay in place and function as required. Figure 13.1A shows diagrammatically how the reaction force R of the nose, acts perpendicularly to the nasal bearing surface. Only the upward force U counteracts the portion of the glazed frame's weight acting through the pad. The forward force F must be counteracted by the backwards force B of the drop of the side (Fig. 13.1B). The size of the downward force D will vary with the inward angle of the drop. The latter will depend on the angle of the mastoid: the larger the angle, the greater force D will be. Finally, note that in Fig. 13.1 only the forces on the left side of the head and frame are shown, and that these are complemented by those of the right side. The forces on either side of the median plane of the head will be identical only when the head is symmetrical (see 'friction' in Section 13.7).

The force exerted in the horizontal plane by the bridge of the frame, and through the sides on the skin covering the mastoid bone, is perhaps best thought of as counteracted by the lateral component L, as shown in Fig. 13.1B (see also Section 13.9).

13.5 The Position of the Centre of Gravity

Figure 13.2 shows the variation in the position of the centre of gravity (which represents that point where an object, when supported, will balance) of glazed spectacles. The figure shows that the heavier the glazed front and the lighter the pair of sides, the nearer to the front the position of the centre of gravity will be situated. For a pair of sides with greater mass, the centre of gravity lies further away from the front.

What are the practical consequences? Based on the above figures, the point(s) of contact between front and nose may be considered to lie close to the back plane of the front of spectacles. Hence, the forces of glazed fronts together with their sides may be said to have a moment (or turning-point) around the nasal bearing sur-

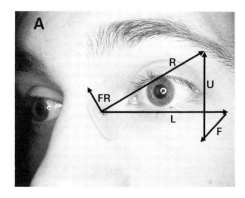

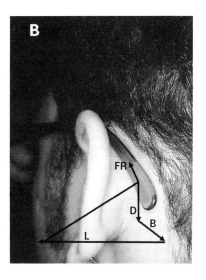

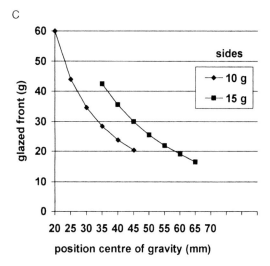

Fig. 13.1 (A) The components of the mechanical forces of the nose reacting to the force caused by the mass of the spectacle frame which acts through the pad: F, forward force; L, lateral force; R, resultant of forces F, L and U; U, upward force; FR, friction at skin–pad interface. (B) The components of the mechanical forces of the mastoid bone reacting to the force of the drop of the side: B, backward force; D, downard force; L, lateral force; R, resultant of forces B, D and L; FR, friction at skin–drop interface. (C) The position of the centre of gravity behind the glazed front depends on the mass of the pair of sides. Assumptions: sides 135 mm long and of uniform construction, weighing 10 g or 15 g per pair

face(s). The turning moment or torque of the glazed front and the pair of sides (Fig. 13.2) is calculated in Table 13.6.

To put these figures in perspective, it is useful to quote Pople (1987):

'torque required to turn a door handle: 0·3 Nm torque produced by an electric drill: 5 Nm'

This shows that the torque for glazed spectacles is very small indeed and, therefore, easily altered, causing any stable fitting pair of spectacle to become unstable. What then happens is the following.

When the anticlockwise torque is greater than the clockwise torque, the drops of the sides start to rotate anticlockwise, that is, they start to rise (Fig. 13.3). If the head's equivalent of the side's inward angle of drop is zero, the pressure exerted by the sides will not be counteracted by the mastoid bone and the front will slip down the nose. As a result, the drops will rise further, allowing the front to slide further down the nose.

Conversely, if the mastoid shows some measure of inward angle of drop, the pressure on the sides may increase as the drops rise. When this pressure on the sides, together with the

Spectacle frames and their dispensing

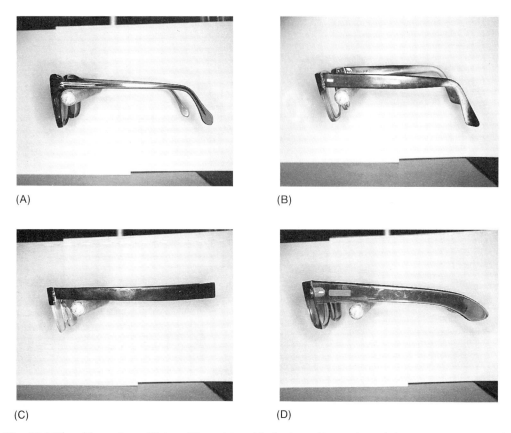

Fig. 13.2 Glazed frames in equilibrium. The position of the horizontal bar, acting as balancing point, supports the sides from 13 to 46 mm beyond the frontal plane of the front

TABLE 13.6 Torque in glazed front and sides

Glazed front			Sides		
distance (m)	weight (cN)	torque anticlockwise (cN m)	distance (m)	weight (cN)	torque clockwise (cN m)
0·005	20	0·1	0·06	5	0·3
0·005	40	0·2	0·06	10	0·6
0·005	60	0·3	0·06	15	0·9
0·005	80	0·4			

Anticlockwise torque when the centre of gravity of the front lies at 5 mm from the turning point, and clockwise torque when the centre of gravity of the side lies at 6 cm from the turning point.

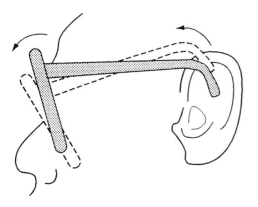

Fig. 13.3 When the anticlockwise torque is greater than the clockwise torque, the drops will rise and the front will move forward and down the wearer's nose

pressure exerted by the sides, and the forward force caused by the glazed front's weight are in equilibrium, the spectacles will become stable.

13.6 Pressure and Pain

So far 'pressure' has been used in the sense of the amount of force acting on a given area. However, there is also the physiological aspect where 'pressure' refers to the sensitivity of a part of a person's body to pressure. The following discussion is based on Geldard's (1972) work.

The stimulus for the pressure sensation is usually a mechanical deformation of the skin. In order to 'feel' pressure, a pressure gradient must be present because merely applying mechanical pressure to a part of the skin does not necessarily result in the sensation of pressure. When a steep enough pressure gradient has been formed, the required condition for pressure to be felt has been fulfilled. The significant variable is the tension, expressed in terms of force per linear extent of skin surface contacted.

Hairs are usually associated with pressure-sensitive spots on the skin. However, not all skin portions possess hairs. Measurements have

shown that the just-noticeable pressure sensation on, for instance, the ball of the thumb requires an impact of 0.026×10^{-7} J, but on various points on the underside of the forearm it varies from 0.032 to 0.113×10^{-7} J. Direct comparison of absolute intensive threshold with the eye shows that the skin absorbs 100 million to 10 billion times more energy before minimal action results. The differential pressure threshold function (the Weber fraction) of skin resembles that of other sense organs.

Adaptation to pressure depends on several variables. However, of interest is that a weight, once placed on a horizontal skin surface, does not rest there. It continues to move downward for some time. Pressure is felt as long as a supraliminal rate of movement is maintained. When tissue resistance reduces motion to an undetectable level, the sensation fades and the end point of adaptation has been reached. On removal of the weight, the pressure sensation is aroused again, as an after-sensation.

Does pressure on the skin lead to a sensation of pain? Some of the terms used to describe the various types of pain are associated with pressure (Geldard, 1972). The pain sensation, brought about by mechanical stimulation, either impairs tissue or produces radical deformations in it. The pain threshold for a given skin area is constant and proportional to the pressure exerted on the tissue. It can be shown that the common factor in pain arousal is lateral stretch of skin tissue.

At one time there was controversy about pain adaptation: did pain change into pressure when it was sufficiently weakened? It is now agreed that in the course of adaptation, pain becomes progressively less intense and disappears without passing over into pressure. Unless the adaptation stimulus is also a pressure stimulus, pain fails to leave a 'residue' of pressure.

Spectacle wearers seldom, if ever, complain of pain in the nasal region, but do mention pressure. However, they do complain about pain behind their ear(s) when continuous distortion, such as an imprint of the drop, can be observed in the groove between outer ear and mastoid, or on the outer ear itself. This is usually caused by the length to bend being too short, the downward angle of drop being too large, and/or the inward angle of drop not being large enough. Pressure on the mastoid itself seldom causes any complaint. Note that, in this area, there is only a minimal amount of subcutaneous soft tissue containing sensory receptors.

13.7 Mechanical Forces and Comfortable Spectacle Wear

Several authors (such as Sutter, 1937a,b; Spooner, 1942; Biessels, 1954, 1955; Tänzer, 1965; Käpernick, 1982) made contributions in this field, it appears that Fischbach (1986) made the definite study of the mechanical forces involved in maintaining a pair of glasses on the wearer's head. He identified the following aspects as contributing to comfortable spectacle wear (Fischbach, 1989):

- the frontal angle
- the angle of crest
- the angle of the side
- the inward angle of the mastoid bone corresponding to the side's inward angle of the drop
- the mass of the spectacles
- the force exerted by the sides on the head
- the surface area of the bridge
- the age of the wearer
- the friction of the materials of bridge and sides.

There is no need to comment on the first three angles. However, Fischbach (1986) demonstrated that the inward angle of the mastoid is one of the most important contributors to the mechanical forces that keep a pair of spectacles on the wearer's head. This confirmed the viewpoint

expressed by Sperling & Fahrner (1976) and by Käpernick (1982). (See section 13.4.)

It is surprising that the angle of let-back does not feature in the above list. In this author's opinion, it is most important. For the present purpose, the head may be considered as consisting of two triangles which, from a mechanical view, act as wedges (Fig. 3.2). Included in the anterior wedge is the temporal width and head width, where the latter is usually larger than the former. Hence, the frame temporal width should be smaller than the frame head width. However, when these head measurements are nearly the same, both frame measurements may be equal to the head width less 10 mm (see below). If the inner aspects of the sides (*temples*) are in contact with the temples of the head, the anterior wedge will be operational. As a result, the frame will be pushed forward and slide down the wearer's face.

The counterpart of the anterior wedge is the posterior wedge (Fig. 3.2). This lies roughly in the same plane as the anterior wedge, but beyond the ear points. It is formed by the parietal and occipital bones for straight sides, and the mastoid and occipital bones for drop-end sides. Anterior and posterior wedges can be said to have a common 'base' (as in triangles), namely the head width, and point in opposite directions. Whereas the anterior wedge can push the frame forward, the posterior wedge has the opposite effect. The mechanical forces of frame and skull in this area determine whether or not a frame is stable on the wearer's head (see Section 13.5).

Conventional wisdom says that the frame head width shall be 10 mm smaller than the head width. Although Fischbach concurs, he points out that many other factors are involved.

As discussed in Section 13.4, the mass of a glazed frame can easily be estimated provided that one has an accurate scale to weigh the frame, and one can predict the mass of the lenses from the tables provided.

With respect to the surface area of the bridge,

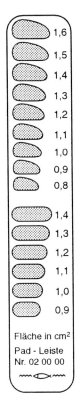

Fläche in cm²
Pad - Leiste
Nr. 02 00 00

Fig. 13.4 Pad area template (courtesy G. Fischbach of H. Meissburger GmbH, Karlsruhe)

Fischbach (1989) differentiates between the pad surface and the pad bearing surface. By means of a pad area template (Fig. 13.4), and the angles associated with the nose, the pressures in the nasal area can be calculated. This facilitates the calculation of the 'reserve' force required for a stable spectacle fit.

Such a fit is not necessarily comfortable. It will depend on the load the skin can comfortably bear. For this purpose Fischbach developed an age-related expression which can be important.

Finally, we must consider the contribution made by friction. Friction may be defined as the force acting in the direction opposite to the movement of one body when the tangential

planes of two bodies slide or roll over another (see Fig. 13.1A and B).

Of particular interest is boundary or greasy friction. Unless specifically cleaned, all surfaces are covered with a very thin film of grease. Because this covers the bearing surface it will prevent contact between the actual surfaces. However, under given conditions such as a heavy load, this film may break down so that contact will take place. This may lead to rubbing and seizure, whereby the surfaces adhere (Hannah & Hillier, 1985), especially with new pads made of silicon material. This can sometimes be observed to occur with the pads of a glazed front and the nasal skin when the front is moved slightly up and down.

The coefficient of friction may be defined as the ratio of the friction force and normal reaction, and depends purely on the nature of the surfaces in contact.

Wolfram (1989) states that the coefficient of friction for skin ranges from 0·1 to 0·6. He quotes a coefficient of about 0·3 for a load of 20 g. Fischbach (1986) carried out his own investigation and found values varying between 0·04 and 0·57 depending on the type of frame material and the state of the skin (greasy, normal or dry). The dryer the skin, the higher the coefficient of friction.

Wolfram (1989) made the following observations:

- the coefficient of friction increases with decreasing loads
- one obtains a larger contact area (and thus greater friction) for softer rather than harder materials
- moisturization of skin causes skin softening and thus an increase in friction
- extensive wetting of the skin results in a decrease of friction
- the phenomenon of skin friction is highly complex and not yet fully understood.

13.8 Simulating the Spectacle Mass

It is very difficult indeed for a first-time spectacle wearer to appreciate what his glazed spectacles are going to feel like, especially after some hours' wear. As shown above, the mass of the front and indeed, of the frame, may be only a fraction of that of the complete pair of spectacles. Hence, the wearer may be unpleasantly surprised when the complete pair is placed on his head.

To overcome this problem, two devices have become available to the dispenser, namely the 'Brillen-Anpass-Gewicht' (spectacle fitting weight) set developed by Hankiewicz & Hankiewicz (1982), and the 'Weight n' See' prescription lens weight simulator (Solomons, 1989) (Fig. 13.5).

The Brillen-Anpass-Gewicht set consists of a pair of machined clamps with a mass of 15 g. By means of a screw, each clamp may be fitted on a side, near to the front. There are additional pairs of weights with masses of 5, 10, 20 and 30 g, and an accessory pair of 5 g which makes it possible to build up intermediate values. Hence, it is possible to simulate the mass of pairs of lenses from 15 g (a pair of +1·00 DS in CR 39 of 54 mm horizontal lens size) to 50 g (a pair of +5·00 DS made in the same size, but of crown glass).

The 'Weight n' See' set (Blitz Enterprises, Fort Lauderdale, FL, USA) consists of six pairs of weights. Each weight is part of a clip which can be easily attached to, and removed from, suitable parts of the frame such as the upper or lower rim, or the side near the front. They are colour coded to represent plastics (red) or glass (blue) lens weights according to groups of back vertex powers. Each half of the pairs of clips has the following mass: light blue 6 g; medium blue 11 g; dark blue 16 g; pink 16 g; medium red 21 g; dark red 26 g. It is more useful to mark the clips with their mass and, by using Tables 13.4 and 13.5 and

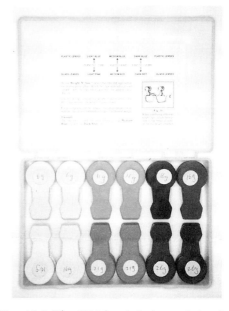

Fig. 13.5 The 'Weight n' See' prescription lens simulator clip-on weights

(combinations of) clips, simulate the expected lens mass, and demonstrate to the prospective wearer the effect of one lens power or type, and another.

13.9 Forces Within a Spectacle Frame

Biessels (1954, 1955) discussed the mechanical forces at work within a spectacle frame (Fig. 13.6). If a side of uniform section were 100 mm long and subjected at its end to a force of 100 cN (or 100 g), the joint would be subjected to a moment of 0·1 m × 100 cN = 10 cN m. At the centre of the bridge, the moments of the right and left sides meet. Hence, the bridge is subjected to 20 cN m (cf. Pople (1987) in Section 13.5). This goes towards explaining why the bridge (Fig. 23.1) and the area of the joints of spectacle

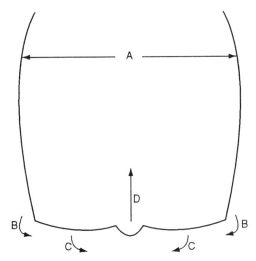

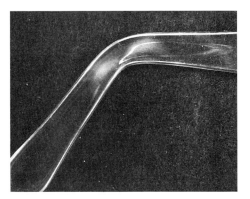

Fig. 13.7 The light areas (made visible by means of polarized light) on either side of the ear point demonstrate the presence of stress caused by deformation of this side. See also Fig. 23.1

Fig. 13.6 The sides of a frame, when worn, are subject to outward-directed forces at the ear points (A). These are transposed into moments (B) around the joint screws. As a result, joints are subject to great force. The rivets of pinned joints pass through holes in the side wires. The holes weaken the side wires and, as a result, the sides tend to break at these points, or just beyond the joint plates. With respect to the front, the forces at (A) have a moment (C) around the centre of the bridge. Because this is furthest away from the points of application (A), the bridge is subjected to the largest force (D). This may cause the bridge to break. Another factor is the deformation of the bridge required to form its curved projection. This causes strain within the plastics material (see Fig. 23.1). To counteract the strain, the bridge is sometimes made thicker than the rims. Metal frames are subject to similar forces in comparable places. These may cause components to bend and/or soldered components to bend or break at the point where they have been soldered (Sperling & Fahrner, 1976)

Sperling & Fahrner (1976) elaborated on this theme (Fig. 13.6). If the bridge of a metal front is not sufficiently sturdy, it may bend forward so that the frame head width increases. This problem is unlikely to arise in a front with a bridge with a brace bar (*bridge brace*). However, the same problem may occur when the junction between joint and rim is not sufficiently sturdy. They also pointed out that some sides are made of very flexible metal. As a result, the side exerts insufficient force through its drop on the mastoid (Figs 13.1B and 13.6). This could also occur with sprung joints, which brings us back to the work of Fischbach (1986), discussed in Section 13.7.

The type of strain described above is also acting at the ear point of the sides (Fig. 13.7). To form the drop of a drop-end side, it needs to be deformed at the ear point. This causes strain in the material itself, because the upper portion of the side is stretched and the lower portion compressed. Furthermore, during wear there is the outward pressure (see Figs 13.1B and 13.6) which causes torque around the ear point and the joint. This strain sometimes causes hairline cracks at the ear point. In old sides and end-covers, this may lead to breakage in the ear point area.

sides are frequently the places where spectacles break (cf. Section 23.3).

Biessels added that when a side is triangularly shaped, a uniform deformation per unit of length will be created along the side. When a force is applied, the straight side will assume the shape of a circle. This would be the best form to prevent breakage.

REFERENCES

Biessels, W.J. (1954–1955). Betere brilaanpassing en brilconstructie. *Oculus, Amsterdam*. Reprinted (1971). Amsterdam: Stichting Ned. Vakopleiding voor Opticiens.

Biessels, W.J. (1955). Neue Gesichtspunkte zur Brillenanpassung. *Süddeutsche Optikerz*. **10** (3), 65–72.

BS 6625 (1992). *Spectacle Frames. Part 2: Specification for Marking.* London: British Standards Institution.

Camau, R. (1985). L'indication du materiau est-elle utile sur les lunettes. *Opticien-Lunetier* No. 379, 46.

Cheswick, S.A. (1992). The weight of bifocal lenses. Final Year Project. London: City University.

Fischbach, G. (1986). *Die Statik in der Brillenanpassung.* Karlsruhe: G. Fischbach (private publication).

Fischbach, G. (1989). *Die Statik in der Brillenanpassung: die Anwendung in der Praxis.* Karlsruhe: G. Fischbach (private publication).

Geldard, F.A. (1972). *The Human Senses.* 2nd edn, Chapters 10 and 11. New York/London: J. Wiley & Sons.

Gottlob, H. (1978). Wie schwer wird die Brille werden? *Deutsche Optikerz*. No. 3, 4–11.

Gunaratnam, C.M.R. (1991). The weight of edged spectacle lenses. Final Year Project. London: City University.

Hannah, J. & Hillier, M.J. (1985). *Applied Mechanics,* p. 50. London: Pitman.

Hankiewicz, G. & Hankiewicz, G. (1982). Das Brillen-Anpass-Gewicht. *Deutsche Optikerz*. **37** (6), 18–24.

Henke, G. & Päsler, U. (1982). Kritische Betrachtungen zu den verschiedenen Methoden der Bestimmung des Glasgewichts gerandeter Brillengläser. *Deutsche Optikerz.*, No. 3, 8–21.

Jalie, M. (1992). An update on low-power aspheric lenses. *Optician* **203** (5334), 28–31.

Käpernick, E. (1982). Die Brille ist eine Federwaage. *Deutsche Optikerz*. No. 11, 53–55.

Maxam, U. (1983). *Brillentechnik.* Berlin: VEB Verlag Technik, p. 52 ff. (reprint 1985).

Norville, F. (1992). Letter to the Editor: Don't miss the real value of aspheric lenses. *Optician* **203** (5337), 10.

Obstfeld, H. (1990). Een kinderbril vereist meer dan een grappig montuurtje. *Oculus, Amsterdam* **52** (4), 11–16.

Obstfeld, H. (1991a). Hoe zwaar weegt een brilleglas? *Oculus, Amsterdam* **53** (1), 5–9.

Obstfeld, H. (1991b). Weight of edged spectacle lenses. *Ophthal. Physiol. Optics* **11** (3), 248–251.

Obstfeld, H. (1992). Letter to the Editor: Lighter uncut not when cuts. *Optician* **202** (5336), 10.

Pople, S. (1987). *Explaining Physics,* 2nd edn, p. 57. Oxford: Oxford University Press.

Solomons, L. (1989). Modern dispensing aids. *Optician* **197** (5186), 21–24.

'Sperling' & Fahrner, D. (1976). Die vier Todsünden beim Herstellen einer Brillenfassung. *Neues Optikerj.* **18** (11), 905–913.

Spooner, J.D. (1942). The effective weight of frames and lenses. *Optician* **104** (2683), 55–58.

Sutter, P. (1937a). Druck- und Kräfteverteilung am Brillensteg. Part 1. *Deutsche Optikerz*. No. 3, 29–30.

Sutter, P. (1937b). Druck- und Kräfteverteilung am Brillensteg. Part 2. *Deutsche Optikerz*. No. 5, 52–53.

Tänzer, P. (1965). Die Statik der Brille. *Augenoptiker* **20** (5), 5–9.

Wolfram, L.J. (1989). Frictional Properties of Skin (Ch 3). In: Leveque, J-L. (ed.), *Cutaneous Investigation in Health and Disease,* p. 49. New York/ Basel: Marcel Dekker.

CHAPTER 14

Cosmetic Dispensing

14.1 Introduction

In this chapter the relationship between body shape, shape of the face, and skin and hair colour will be discussed together with the effects of spectacle frame shapes and colours. It is important to be aware of their inter-relationships and to develop an appreciation thereof. This will enable the dispenser to advise the patient about the most suitable frame for his or her particular face, and to take advantage of optical illusion to improve the patient's appearance. Having referred in the above to spectacle frames in general, it is frequently more accurate to consider the spectacle front instead.

14.2 Shapes

14.2.1 BODY SHAPES

Although the shape of a spectacle frame is not so much related to the form of the wearer's body, it is of basic interest to consider briefly body shapes.

Females generally have a more rounded body shape while that of males is more angular (Figs 14.1 and 14.2). The shape of the face of an individual often has the same characteristics as that of the rest of the body, although there are always exceptions.

Consider Fig. 14.1: what many may consider to be a typical female body shape refers only to the torso, which is hour-glass shaped. When allowing for the effect of the arms, that shape can be described as 'rounded' when the face shape is also round. If the face is more rectangular the shape may be described as a 'soft oblong'. However, when the body is more rectangular and the face rounder, the composite may be described as 'strong oblong'. Both body and face may be more rectangular, or 'oblong'.

The body shapes of males (Fig. 14.2) tend to be less varied and more angular. Together with a round face, the shape could be described as 'oval'. If the face is also angular, the body shape may be described as 'square'; when both torso and face have triangular shapes, the overall shape may be considered as 'angular'.

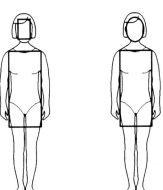
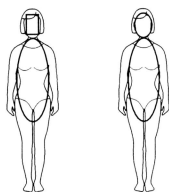

Fig. 14.1 *Female body shapes. From right to left: rounded – soft oblong – stronger oblong – oblong*

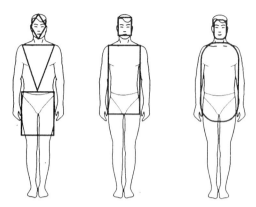

Fig. 14.2 Male body shapes. From right to left: oval – square – angular

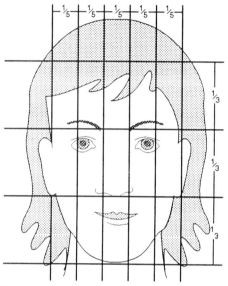

Fig. 14.4 The proportions of the human face (see Section 14.3.2.1)

In principle, the body shape is determined by the structure of the skeletal bones. It may be useful to observe and classify when you first see your patient.

14.2.2 FACE SHAPES

When considering the shape of a face (Figs 14.3 and 14.4) one tends to refer to the portion situated below the level of the eyes. For simplicity, one may talk of oval, round, square and triangular faces (Optyl, undated), but a more appropriate classification of the shape of faces is oval, round, square, diamond, triangular base-up or base-down, and oblong. There are also faces that show a mixture of these features and are, therefore, difficult to classify (Wilson, 1989; Cooney, 1993).

14.3 Cosmetic Aspects

14.3.1 INTRODUCTION

Writers such as Sasieni (1962) have described faces in great detail. With the multitude of lens shapes now available, they are no longer a starting point for the discussion of spectacle frame cosmetics, as in the 1950s (Abel, 1952). In the 1960s 40 or so lens shapes had to be distinguished by students, contrary to BS 3521 (1991) which describes only six generic names for well-known families of lens shapes (see Table 16.1)

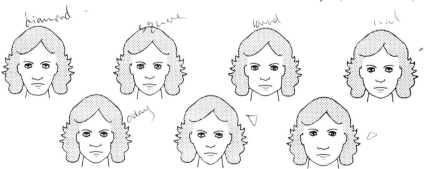

Fig. 14.3 Shapes of faces. From right to left, top row: oval, round, square, diamond. Bottom row: triangular base-down, triangular base-up, oblong

When giving advice on the suitability of a frame, one has to keep three different aspects in mind, namely clinical, mechanical and cosmetic, however, there are also psychological aspects. Clinical aspects lie outside the scope of this book although some are briefly discussed in Chapter 19. Mechanical aspects are considered in Chapters 13 and 16, and psychological aspects are discussed in Chapter 15. The cosmetic aspects will be divided into 'frames and faces' and 'colour'.

14.3.2 FRAMES AND FACES
14.3.2.1 Introduction

When selecting a suitable frame for a particular face one takes into consideration not only the shape of that face but also the relative horizontal and vertical proportions. These consist of the following areas (Fig. 14.4):

- horizontal: temples and eyes (both sides), and nose where each occupies 1/5 of the facial width,
- vertical: forehead, eyes and cheeks/nose, mouth and chin where each occupies 1/3 of the facial height.

Such a face will look perfectly balanced, especially if the shape of the face is oval.

Few people possess these much-desired, classical features. However, the spectacle frame adviser is expected to help to provide ways of creating them! By employing what amounts to optical illusions, this may sometimes be accomplished. For this purpose one has to keep two major rules in mind, namely

(1) **select a frame which has features opposed to the shape of the face it is going to adorn,**
(2) **ensure that the front's brow line follows that of the eyebrows.**

When these rules are observed, the facial features will appear to be better balanced. This may be achieved by observing the following guidelines.

14.3.2.2 Guidelines

The upper rim of a front should follow the brow line, and lie in front of it. The brows should not appear above the rim, or within the lens apertures of the front. This will look 'good' because it is in accordance with the natural arrangement of the facial features. Note there is an exception: sunglass fronts may be larger so that the upper rim may well lie above the brow line, which will be obscured by the dark lenses.

The vertical dimension of the front should be such that the lower rims do not rest on the cheeks when the wearer is not smiling.

An oval face can take many lens shapes provided that Rule 1 is observed, namely avoid oval-shaped lens shapes. Ensure that the front's size is proportional to the face. A low joint (*hinge*) frame and sinuous sides (*temples*) would upset the balance of this face.

A round face needs to be given a more oval appearance, that is, made to look longer and thinner. This may be achieved with a slightly upswept front, or with one having strong vertical features; a square lens shape may also give the desired effect. A clear bridge and high joints with coloured sides will also assist in achieving the desired effect.

A square face will need to be made to look longer. This may be created with roundish lens shapes having delicate feature such as a thin metal rim. It softens any heavy facial features. A horizontal oval lens shape may also be suitable.

A diamond-shaped face needs to be made to look less angular. Hence, a roundish or a squarish front with rounded corners would be suitable. An upswept front may suit some. The front should not be wider than the cheekbones, and the sides should be plain.

A base-down triangular face needs a base-up front such as an upswept shape, an oval shape with a distinctive brow line, or rimless or Supra spectacles. A high joint frame would also give a better balance; the front may be wider than the cheekbones.

A base-up triangular face may be counter-balanced by a pilot or a lightly coloured, squarish lens shape as these tend to distract attention from the upper portion of the face. A low joint frame should also be considered.

An oblong face looks better balanced when its characteristics are modified by a front with strong horizontal features. These may be found in a squarish or in an oval lens shape with strong horizontal lines. A shallow pilot shape may also be suitable. Note that long faces require pro-portionally deeper lens shapes than wide faces and that a fully coloured front appears to shorten a long face more than a two-tone front. A coloured bridge and sides will also help to make the face appear shorter and more oval.

Wide faces look better when fitted with a front with a deep lens shape. Two-tone fronts appear to lengthen wide faces.

A long nose will look shorter, and a thin nose wider when fitted with a front with a low or a clear bridge.

A high bridge (for instance, a keyhole bridge, one with a brow bar, or a dark front with a dark bridge) will make a nose look longer; a dark front with a clear bridge has the opposite effect.

If the nose is pronounced, the front should have an unobtrusive (e.g. colourless) bridge. In this way, the front will distract attention from the nose. A similar effect may be achieved by using a front that is darker or coloured on the temporal side of the rims, and/or in the area of the lugs (*end-pieces*) where a decoration may provide further distraction.

A low bridge will appear to lengthen a short forehead.

Eyes that have a small interpupillary distance (PD) will look further apart when fitted with a front with a clear bridge. A dark bridge helps to 'reduce' the distance between the eyes.

The front's lower rim may be used to conceal 'bags' under the eyes by covering that part of the face.

Avoid extreme lens shapes (round, tapered, sharp angles, octagonal, etc.), in particular when strong cylindrical corrections are required. These shapes do not fit with the natural shape of a face while the cylindrical correction will result in thick lens edges that may accentuate an undesir-able facial feature.

If the level of one eye is higher than that of the other (Section 3.2.2) do not select a dark-rimmed front (Fig. 14.5) and if possible, avoid a small lens. Both features draw attention to the asym-metry. Small differences in monocular PD are not normally perceived as distracting since a symmetrical face is an anathema (Fig. 14.6).

A simple, but effective, tool to use when demonstrating the effect of curved lines on a face is shown in Fig. 14.7.

Note that the crest height, together with the frontal angle, determines the suitability of a lens shape in the nasal area.

A different aspect is the so-called weight of a

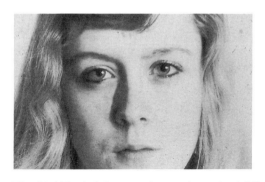 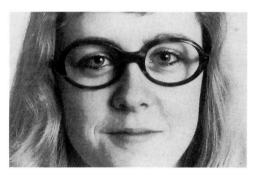

Fig. 14.5 *The dark frame emphasizes the eye-level difference of this face*

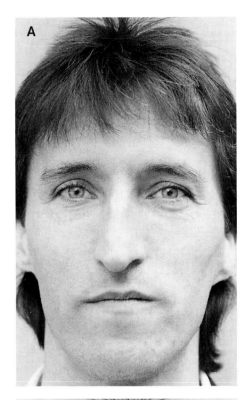

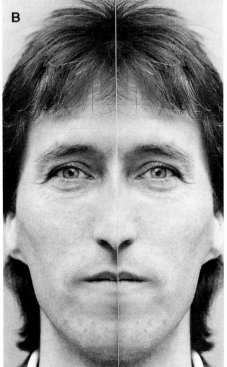

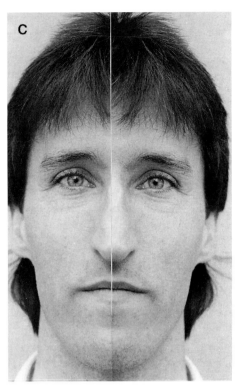

Fig. 14.6 *A perfectly symmetrical face gives many people an uncomfortable feeling because it is so unnatural. A, original photograph; B, right side and mirror; C, left side and mirror.*

frame. This does not refer to the actual mass of the frame, but to the width of the rims, frequently in conjunction with that of the sides. Faces with delicate features, such as those found in women and children, require lighter (thinner) fronts. Faces exhibiting larger or broader features require heavier (thicker) fronts. An exception to the rule is that a man of small stature with large,

Fig. 14.7 *Diagram illustrating the effect of curved lines on a face. The left is a happy face, the middle a sad one and the right gives an impression of indifference*

broad facial features may look better with a lighter weight frame because this will neutralize the rather incongruous head–body relationship.

A dark but thin front tends to give a heavier impression. A two-tone front makes a lighter impression. When in doubt, select a lighter-weight frame.

14.3.3 COLOUR

14.3.3.1 Introduction

With this aspect of the spectacle frame choice we enter another dimension of the realm of psychology. A frame on its own is an incomplete entity. One can only guess at its character in association with the face of its wearer. In other words, the frame must be considered together with its immediate surround – hair, eyes and skin – and their respective colours. In addition, cosmetics are important: eye make-up and lipstick interact strongly with the frame colour. However, one may also have to take account of the next ambit where one may find earrings. The better one tries to integrate these aspects, the more complicated the task appears. Here, experience counts, and experience grows with practice.

A boldly coloured spectacle frame dominates the face, and the overall impression one perceives. Within the context of skin and hair colours, the frame and its colour should neither look lost nor should it dominate because of an unacceptable clash of the colours. In association with clothes, the frames should appear complementary: they should tone in, or create a colourful accent. Most importantly, the spectacle wearer should be content with the combination of colours. This is a matter of taste – a personal and psychological matter. When spectacles were considered no more than a prosthesis they did not need to be an article of beauty. However, that objective can now be achieved simultaneously, and this may enhance the prosthesis to the point that it is also pleasing to the wearer.

It is probably true to say that the number of spectacle wearers who know which spectacle frame colours suit them is small. Only those who are familiar with the use of colour will feel confident to make their own decision. The approving comments of others will, of course, instill confidence. However, many patients arrive with no clear concept of colour (Pritchard, 1976).

This poses the question: why don't they know? There are several reasons. Possibly they have never worn spectacles before and, therefore, have never considered frame shapes and frame colours. Some patients do not feel confident about choosing colours, or think that they have no feelings on the matter. Hence, they are reluctant to name a suitable colour. A further possibility is that they like many colours and can not make up their mind. It may also be difficult for some to imagine how a certain frame and colour would affect their 'looks'. In all these cases the patient is more likely to welcome advice rather than reject it. However, whether the patient will act upon advice is another matter. In addition to psychological influences, there are others, such as cultural. What about the patient who has a colour vision problem?

Based on the research of Johannes Itten and others (see Sections 15.3 and 15.4), a concept was developed during the 1980s that has the objective of identifying the colours, fashion accessories, etc. that make a person look their best. The system makes it possible to select a wardrobe of matching garments and accessories where one has the certain knowledge that the articles acquired will tone in with hair colour and skin colouring and with each other. This system, sometimes referred to as the 'seasonal colour theory', has been described in greater detail by several authors (Jackson, 1981; London & Adams, 1985; Karpinski, 1987; Pertiet, 1987). Others, such as Wilson (1989), follow a slightly different approach, with the same object in mind.

Although the word 'season' is frequently used in descriptions, it must be made clear that this has nothing to do with the seasons of the year as such:

A, B, C and D could have been used instead. However, the names of the seasons give perhaps a more emotive description. Colour tones suitable for Winter and Summer people are basically cool, for Autumn and Spring people they are warm, for Winter and Spring people they are vibrant, and for Autumn and Summer people they are muted or softer.

The issues are hair, eye and skin colour together with the contrasts between these. For our purposes, the following descriptions may be adequate. The suggested colours have been distilled from Kampers (1985), London & Adams (1985), Pertiet (1987), Shafer (1984), and Wilson (1989) together with my own observations. The sequence of colours is not of any particular significance. Note that there are not only clear-cut cases of these seasons, but also all manner of transitional types.

14.3.3.2 Guidelines

People with a dark colouring or strong contrast between the colours of their skin, eyes and hair usually have dark brown, black or blue-black hair. They are characterized as 'Winters', and look best in vibrant colours. They make up the major part of the world population. Their best frame colours are probably stark, cool colours: blueish reds, burgundy, cool blues, emerald green, pinks, black, white, slate grey, grey-beige, very dark brown, silver, and reddish to dull gold.

Fair people have usually less contrast between the colours of these three body components. Their skin is pinkish, and their hair ash brown or ash blond, or grey. They are characterized as 'Summers', and look at their best in softened colours. Their best frame colours are probably subdued, weak (desaturated) colours such as blue-reds, opaque pastel colours, pink, dull silver, reddish light gold, pewter, taupe, rose brown, rose beige, grey navy, blue grey, grey and ash brown.

People with a dark colouring and golden skin undertones usually have red-brown hair, or at least warm red highlights in their hair, while some are auburn or golden brown. They are characterized as 'Autumns', and look at their best in softened colours, like 'Summers'. Their best frame colours are probably cream, orangy reds, olive, amber, golden brown, rust, beige, copper, gold, teal and moss green.

A lighter version of the last group has a fair skin complexion, possibly with freckles, and strawberry red hair, or various golden or blond shades of hair. They are characterized as 'Springs', and look at their best in vibrant colours, like 'Winters'. Their best frame colours are probably orangy reds, beige, cream, ivory, tan, camel, golden brown and gold.

Note that the best way to ascertain whether a particular frame colour is suitable for a given person is to make that person wear a frame of the colour in question. One approach is only to show the person (in the mirror, or whatever other device is used) what the frame looks like on him or her, *after you have decided* that it is a suitable colour. This is a matter of observation; proficiency comes with experience.

14.3.3.3 Further advice
- Avoid frame colour combinations such as blue-yellow, red-green and purple-green;
- avoid striped patterns;
- chose a colour that is a shade lighter than the wearer's hair;
- lighter colours are more suitable for smaller faces;
- a gold colour (metal frame) gives young Caucasians a more mature appearance;
- a reddish gold coloured frame will suit almost any dark-skinned face;
- do not fit a big man who has a dark skin with a light coloured, light-weight frame, and likewise, do not fit a small, fair haired man with a heavy, dark frame;

- use a lighter weight frame to neutralize the incongruous head–body relationship of a small man with large, broad facial features;
- faces with delicate features (as in women and children) require lighter and thinner frames;
- a dark but thin front makes a heavier impression;
- a two-tone front makes a lighter impression than a fully coloured one.

Note that some patients like to go against the rules and recommendations: they either like to make a 'statement' about one aspect or another, or consider such a (second?) pair of frames 'fun' glasses.

14.3.4 TINTED LENSES

Lightly tinted lenses are often referred to as having a cosmetic tint. They are not intended to give any substantial protection against visible radiation and are used only for fashion purposes. They may be marked according to BS 2724 (1987), with protection factors from 1·1 to 2·0. Sunglasses have a protection factor greater than 2·0, and transmit less than 29·1% of the visible radiation incident on them (Obstfeld, 1991). According to the American National Standard ANSI Z80.3 (1986), sunglasses and fashion eyewear intended primarily for cosmetic use have luminous transmittances greater than 40%.

Tinted lenses may be used to disguise deformations and skin blemishes. A graduated tint may solve a particular problem of this nature. If the skin blemish has a colour that differs from the skin colour, the lenses should have a colour not dissimilar to that of the blemish, provided that colour vision and the perception of signal lights are not affected.

Suitable cosmetic lens colours for 'Winters' and 'Summers' are pink and grey, and for 'Autumns' and 'Springs', brown and green.

Yellow lenses should be avoided because they are usually incompatible with hair and skin colours and hence, with a suitable frame colour. Moreover, because they transmit visible light selectively by absorbing blue light, colour vision is usually severely affected, which can be dangerous in connection with colour-coded substances and objects. If worn at all, they should be used only in bright daylight and never for night driving. Chou (personal communication, 1995) goes as far as to say that, because yellow lenses impair identification of coloured traffic lights, they should not be used at all when driving.

14.3.5 SQUINT

A squinting eye, which is corrected by means of a prism, will give the onlooker the impression that the eye deviates even more than without the correction. This can often lead to mistrust of the dispenser by the onlooker, especially when the squinter is a child and the onlooker its parent! This is the result of the unfortunate optical properties of the prism. The squinting eye will look at the image displaced by the prism towards its apex (and thus brought in-line with the deviating eye). Similarly, the onlooker will see that squinting eye displaced towards the apex of the prism, thus showing a greater deviation than without the prism.

To explain the properties of the prism it can be helpful for the dispenser to hold a powerful prism with its base in the same direction as that of the prescribed prism, in front of his own eye. The onlooker will then observe a similar displacement. This demonstrates not only the effect of the prism in general, but also in this particular situation.

Flom (Hirsch, 1968) used a prism in spectacle lenses to achieve a cosmetic improvement of a squinting eye. To the onlooker, an esotropic eye seen through a prism base-in will appear to be displaced towards the apex of the prism, and thus situated nearer to the centre of the palpebral aperture, and the same will be achieved for an exotropic eye seen through a prism base-out, provided the deviation is moderate, the prognosis for a functional cure is poor and the patient normally fixates with one eye.

14.4 Consequences of Fashion

If one follows the above guidelines, it is possible that difficulties will arise as a result of the current or dominant fashion in frames. It may well happen that the style of fashion frames does not suit a particular patient's face; likewise, the fashion colours may be unsuitable for a particular patient. Pertiet (1987) adds that the adviser ought to have developed a feeling, based on knowledge, for the real wishes of the patient. These may have nothing to do with 'fashion', this just being an excuse in that it provided a 'suitable' answer to a question.

When a particular frame shape is just unobtainable, or a frame is not made in a suitable colour, there is little to stop an ophthalmic dispenser from designing a frame with a suitable shape. Consult your frame maker about the availability of plastics frame materials in suitable colours, and have a 'special' frame made for your patient (see Section 12.6.2). It will give great satisfaction to both your patient and yourself!

From time to time articles appear in fashion magazines in which advice is given by one expert or another on spectacle frame selection. This author has looked at a number of such articles, and has not been impressed with some of the advice given, and even less with the photographs and explanations provided. A common fashion magazine trick is to show the 'before look' without make-up, using drab clothing, etc. The 'redesigned you' is than shown with the right make-up, clothing and accessories. Moreover, the choice of frames may be limited because of a link with a particular spectacle frame manufacturing company (Cooney, 1993). Approach such publications with circumspection. Develop your own views and rely on your good judgement in your role of adviser.

REFERENCES

Abel, P. (1952). *Die Grundlagen der Brillenanpassung.* p. 111. Düsseldorf: Verlag W. Schrickel.

ANSI Z80.3 (1986). *American National Standard for Ophthalmics – Nonprescription Sunglasses and Fashion Eyewear – Requirements.* New York: American National Standards Institute, Inc.

BS 2724 (1987). *Sun Glare Eye Protectors for General Use.* London: British Standards Institution.

BS 3521 (1991). *Terms Relating to Ophthalmic Optics and Spectacle Frames. Part 2: Glossary of Terms Relating to Spectacle Frames.* London: British Standards Institution.

Cooney, M.-R. (1993). *Framed: A Step By Step Guide to Looking Fabulous in Frames.* Harrogate (UK): Lambert House Publishing.

Hirsch, M.J. (1968). Prism in spectacle lenses for cosmesis. *Am. J. Optom.* **45** (6), 409–413.

Jackson, C. (1981). *Color Me Beautiful.* Washington (DC): II Acropolis Books Ltd.

Kampers, L. (1985). *Free to be Beautiful.* Florida (South Africa).

Karpinski, K.J. (1987). *The Winner's Style.* Washington (DC): Acropolis Books Ltd.

London, L.E. & Adams, A.H. (1985). *Colour Right, Dress Right.* London: Dorling Kindersley.

Obstfeld, H. (1991). Zonnebrilnormen. *Visus, Holland,* No. 3, 16–20.

Optyl (undated). *Gesichtstypologie/Practical Problems – and How to Solve Them,* p. 32. Haar/München: Optyl Holdings.

Pertiet, S. (1987). Die Farbe in der Brillenberatung, part 4. *Neues Optikerj.* **29** (8), 8–14.

Pritchard, A.E. (1976). Frame selection with respect to colour. Final Year Project. London: City University.

Sasieni, L.S. (1962). *The Principles and Practice of Optical Dispensing and Fitting,* p. 153. London: Hammond & Hammond.

Shafer, B.L. (1984). *Eyeglass Insight.* Enhance-Her Publication (USA).

Wilson, C.N. (1989). *See the World in Style,* p. 8. Silhouette (USA).

CHAPTER 15

Psychology and Spectacles

15.1 What People Feel and Think about Spectacles

People who wear glasses have traditionally been considered by others to appear more intelligent than non-spectacle wearers (Thornton, 1943; Manz & Lück, 1968; Argyle & McHenry, 1971; Boshier, 1975). Jansen (1965) found that men wearing black, library-type spectacles were thought to hold a more prestigious occupation than when not wearing spectacles. However, Knoll (1978) pointed out that such findings applied only when subjects were presented on photographs, and that this effect was generally lost after a 5-minute talk with the subject!

Mitterauer (1985) summarized the feelings of spectacle wearers about their spectacles (Terry & Zimmerman, 1970; Terry & Brady, 1976) as 'restricting, the cause of rejection and socially humiliating. Women in particular, consider spectacles as affecting beauty, generating fear and as a negative influence on their perception of their own body.' Fisher (1970) found that women are more aware of their eyes than men. Elman (1977) reported that the impression of the photograph of a man wearing glasses was that he was a 'follower' and that his personality was softer, gentler and more sensitive than when he was not wearing glasses. Terry (1989) concluded that men wearing glasses may be subject to some negative gender stereotyping, but they may also be judged to be physically more attractive and as possessing 'positive task relevant characteristics'. However, women who wear glasses were more likely to be subject to 'only negative social judg-

ments'. Knoll (1978) stated that it would not take years, but tens of years before people would change their negative opinion about spectacles. However, changes are taking place, as was found in surveys in the Netherlands (Anonymous, 1989): for the statement 'glasses are a handicap', in 1971 50% of older men agreed and 33% of all other groups agreed, whereas in 1989 the figure was 3% for both groups for the statement 'glasses affect one's image' 30% agreed in 1971, but only 15% agreed in 1989.

15.2 Frame Selection

What are the motives for obtaining a new pair of spectacles? When your patient says that they want 'something new', what do they mean?

Dissatisfaction with the present spectacles may be associated with the fact that the frames keep slipping, or are uncomfortable. This feeling is transferred indirectly to the frame style, material and colour: the frame no longer suits. A dispenser should ask why a change is desired.

However, a glazed spectacle frame is not just an optical appliance used for the correction of sight, it has also become a fashion accessory, like clothes. It may be employed to create a particular impression, such as a 'professional' image, or indicate the wearer's social status. Frame features that influence impressions include materials and their combination, colour, texture, size, shape of the front and lens aperture shape, proportions of components such as rims, lug and sides, and

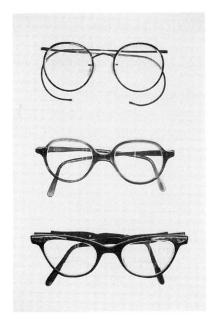 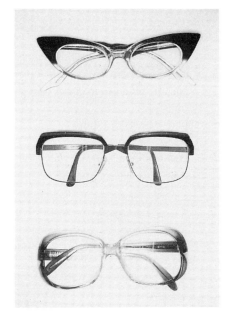

Fig. 15.1 Spectacle frame features that provide different impressions for their wearer

whether the frame has a bulky or neat outline (Fig. 15.1).

How to achieve the impression desired by the wearer will depend on their cultural and educational background, and also upon their personal experiences.

Regional fashion variations were highlighted by Schmacher, an Austrian spectacle frame designer (Blokdijk, 1993). She stated that while frames with large, plastics fronts were worn in North America, Australia, England and South Africa, metal frames with many gold decorations were fashionable in Japan. Similarly, in Italy, France and Spain people preferred plastics frames with small fronts while metal frames with small, round lens apertures were in demand in Scandinavia. Schneider (1958) summarized the aspects of the frame selection process, saying that the dispenser/advisor must

- 'be convinced of the possibility to enhance the beauty of the human face and to accentuate the wearer's personality'

- 'perceive, recognize and know for certain what serves his patient best'
- 'show his endeavour to select the most suitable frame for the collection'
- 'be able to guide the patient in a direction where the patient recognizes him/herself and actively partakes in the selection'
- 'gain the support of the patient's companion (if any)'.

15.3 Colour

15.3.1 INTRODUCTION

A relatively new (1980s) development in fashion is based on the scientific study of the psychological effects of colour. These effects began to be investigated in the 1930s, in Germany. Proponents were Johannes Itten (born 1888, died 1967), a Swiss painter and sculptor, and Frieling (1939). The first application of a colour system to consumer goods was discussed by Birren (1944) in the USA (Bouma, 1971). The effects of colour with respect to spectacle frame selection are discussed in Section 14.3.3.

Pertiet (1987) strongly advised dispensers to acquire some knowledge in this field because they are frequently involved in giving advice on colour. Reading the book by Angeloglou (1982) could provide a start on this subject.

15.3.2 FACTORS INFLUENCING FRAME COLOUR SELECTION

In 1976, Prichard completed a survey that was intended primarily 'to discover whether there is any outstanding factor which influences the choice of a particular colour spectacle frame'. Some of her findings have been condensed into Table 15.1.

TABLE 15.1 *Choice of spectacle frame colour (n, new; p, previous) and hair, eye and skin colour (summarized from Prichard, 1976); only percentages greater than 20 are given in view of the relatively small sample (N = 118)*

	Gold				Brown				Sherry				Black			
	Female		Male		Female		Male		Female		Male		Female		Male	
	n	p	n	p	n	p	n	p	n	p	n	p	n	p	n	p
Hair																
Brown	39	39	37	26	25	32	33	34								
Black	50	20	43	40	33	20	29						20			40
Auburn[1]	25	25						100	25		100		25			
Grey[2]	29			23	43	62	31	38								
Blond[3]	25		29	25	42	58	72	25								
Eyes																
Brown	48	37		27	33	26	45	27							27	
Hazel[4]	29			25	29	50	75	50								
Blue	27	21	35	31	27	36		37								
Grey		25	50	29	50	62	37		25							
Green[5]	37	25	33	33		25	33								33	33
Brown/green[6]									50							
Blue/green	100		33								33					
Brown/blue							100	100								
Skin																
White	35	25	29	25	28		35	34								
Light brown	100	100	50				50	100								
Dark brown[7]	50				50	100										
Yellow[8]			33	50									100			
	Gold				Brown				Gold combi*				Black			
Overall	26	36	24	29	40	30	30	36	5	2	12	9	10	3	16	5

Further details (f, female; m, male):
[1]Blue, f: n: 25; pink, f: n: 25. [2]Grey and greying; gold combination, m: n: 39. [3]Silver, m: p: 25. [4]Silver, m: p: 25. [5]Blue, f: n: 25. [6]Silver, m: n: 100; blue, f: n: 50. [7]Silver, f: n: 100; m: n: 33. [8]Gold combination, m: n: 33, p: 50.
*Gold combination frames: no sherry coloured frames appeared in this section.

TABLE 15.2 *Reasons for frame colour (n, new; p, previous) choice (summary) (percentages, after Prichard, 1976)*

	Total		Female		Male	
	n	p	n	p	n	p
Liked appearance/suited	30	42	22	38	40	46
Suited colouring	13	6	17	12	9	
For a change	11	1	8	2	15	
Don't know	8	8	6	5	11	10
Neutral, matches clothes	7	6	11	7	2	4
Fashionable	2	6	3	7		6

The row marked 'Overall' in Table 15.1 shows how conservative the choice exercised by patients was. As to the reason for choosing the new and the previous frame colour, the relevant percentages were recorded in Table 15.2.

Spectacle wearers appear to start with an open mind. The last two questions in Table 15.3 indicate whether the dispenser should offer help. Clearly, Pertiet's (1987) advice, to learn more about the psychology of colour, is sound.

15.4 Fashion Problems

It has been shown on more than one occasion that, for sunglasses, although a premium was paid for designer-labelled goods, the lenses fitted in such glasses were of inferior quality. Similarly, frame manufacturers may obtain a licence to use a brand name, again allowing increased prices without necessarily having any design input from the fashion house.

Several types of partnership can be formed between frame manufacturers and fashion houses, which can lead to varying quality of products. Dowaliby (1987) described this aspect of fashion for the American market.

TABLE 15.3

Question/ response	Female (%)	Male (%)
Did you have a colour in mind before you came?		
No	57	64
Yes	43	36
Did anyone help you choose your frame?		
No	36	47
Yes	64	53
Did opinions given help?		
Very much	47	38
A lot	50	41
Not much	3	17
Not at all	–	3

REFERENCES

Angeloglou, C. (1982). *Making the Most of Colour*, p. 6–13, 26–29. London: W. Collins Sons.

Anonymous (1989). Collectieve reclame. *Oculus, Amsterdam* **51** (4), 37, 47.

Argyle, M. & McHenry, R. (1971). Do spectacles really affect judgements of intelligence? *Brit. J. Soc. Clin. Psychol.* **10**, 27–29.

Birren, F. (1944). Application of the Ostwald color system to the design of consumer goods. *J. Opt. Soc. Am.* **34**, 396.

Blokdijk, M. (1993). Een ontwerper moet met open ogen door de wereld lopen. *Oculus, Holland* **55** (10), 37–39, 45.

Boshier, R. (1975). A video-tape study on the relationship between wearing spectacles and judgments of intelligence. *Percept. Mot. Skills* **40**, 69–70.

Bouma, P.J. (1971). *Physical Aspects of Colour,* 2nd edn. London/Basingstoke: MacMillan/Philips Technical Library.

Dowaliby, M. (1987). *The Art of Eyewear Dispensing.* Fullerton (CA): Southern California College of Optometry, p. 11.

Elman, D. (1977). Physical characteristics and the perception of masculine traits. *J. Soc. Psychol.* **103**, 157–158.

Fisher, S. (1970). *Body Experience in Fantasy and Behaviour.* New York: Appleton-Century-Crofts.

Frieling, H. (1939). *Die Sprache der Farben.* München/Berlin: R. Oldenburg.

Jansen, J.C.M. (1965). De zwaardere, donkere bril heeft betekenis als status-symbool. *Oculus, Amsterdam* **27** (7), 340–347.

Knoll, H.A. (1978). Eyeglasses and contact lenses: what people think about them. *J. Am. Optom. Assoc.* **49**, 861–866.

Manz, W. & Lück, H.F. (1968). Influence of wearing glasses on personality ratings: crosscultural validation of an old experiment. *Percept. Mot. Skills* **27**, 704.

Mitterauer, B. (1985). *Vom Elend des Brillengestells.* Wien – München: C. Brandstaetter.

Pertlet, S. (1987). Die Farbe in der Brillenberatung. *Neues Optikerj.* **29** (6), 8–12.

Prichard, A.E. (1976). Frame selection with respect to colour. Final Year Project. London: City University.

Schneider, E. (1958). Gedanken zur modischen Brille. *Fachvorträge der WVA-Jahrestagung 1958, Kassel.* 8. Sonderdruck, 66–71.

Terry, R.L. (1989). Eyeglasses and gender stereotypes. *Optom. Vis. Sci.* **66** (10), 694–697.

Terry, R.L. & Brady, C.S. (1976). Effects of framed spectacles and contact lenses on self-ratings of facial attractiveness. *Percept. Mot. Skills* **42**, 789–790.

Terry, R.L. & Zimmerman, D.J. (1970). Anxiety induced by contact lenses and framed spectacles. *J. Am. Optom. Assoc.* **41**, 257–259.

Thornton, G.R. (1943). The effect upon judgments of personality traits of varying a single factor in a photograph. *J. Soc. Psychol.* **18**, 127–148.

CHAPTER 16

Selection, Fitting and Adjusting

16.1 Introduction

While keeping in mind the overriding importance of the facial measurements (Chapter 12) and
what has been discussed in Chapter 13 about the
stability of a spectacle frame on a patient's face,
the selection and later the fitting of a new pair of
spectacles, or the adjustment of an existing pair
may be undertaken. It is imperative to approach
this in a systematic manner, as set out in Section
16.4. Reference is made to the initial selection of
the frame, but this includes neither cosmetic nor
psychological aspects, which were discussed in
Chapters 14 and 15, respectively. Details about
spectacle frames for non-Caucasoids will be
found in Chapter 19 under 'Ethnic Frames'.
Aspects of adjustments and modifications are
also found in Chapter 24. The reader is reminded
of the possible asymmetry of all anatomical
aspects of the head.

16.2 Lens Shapes

From an aesthetic view point, the lens shape,
defined as the outline of the lens periphery with
the nasal side and the horizontal indicated (BS
3521, Part 1, 1991), is dependent on the form of
the wearer's eyebrows, frontal angle of the nose,
vertical distance between eyebrow and cheek
bones, horizontal eye aperture, the semi-temple
width of the head, and the bridge width of the
nose. However, fashion sometimes dictates that
aesthetic aspects be ignored.

The compilers of BS 3521, Part 2 (1991) point
out that the terms listed in Section 3 under the

heading 'Shapes for lenses and apertures in
frames', are either capable of geometrical definition or are accepted generic names for well-
known families of lens shapes (see also Bennett,
1968). As late as the 1960s, some students of
ophthalmic dispensing were taught as many as 40
named lens shapes. However, the proliferation of
lens shapes and the use of lens formers and
electronic lens shape copying equipment, both
employed in conjunction with lens edging equipment, has made a detailed knowledge of lens
shapes superfluous. Hence, in the British Standard mentioned above, only six lens shapes described in Table 16.1 (Fig. 16.1) were defined.
This table includes another two lens shapes
worthy of mention, as specified by Bennett
(1968). Computer-supported spectacle lens
selection made its entry during the late 1980s, and
there are now several packages available. One of
these (Comtrak's Optisoft 3) includes 20 lens
shapes; however, none of these is identified by a
name.

16.3 Frame Measurements

When spectacle frame manufacturers observe BS
6625, Part 2/EN ISO 9456 (1991), spectacle
frame dimensions will be indicated in an identical
manner; as a minimum, a frame shall be marked
with the details set out in Table 16.2, at the
location specified (Fig. 16.2). Moreover, in view
of the problem of identification of the prolifer-
ating frame materials, and their varying characteristics, each component shall be marked as
appropriate. It is also recommended that the

TABLE 16.1 *Lens shapes*

Name	Definition
Contour†	A family of lens shapes resembling the contour of the eye's field of view
Half-eye*	A lens shape for half-eye spectacles
Oval*	Elliptical
Pilot*	A family of lens shapes, essentially triangular, characterized by a nasal cut-away and pronounced fullness in the lower temporal quadrant. This lens shape designated 'Aviator', was designed in the 1930s by the American company Bausch & Lomb, for use in their military aviation sunglasses. Hence, the name 'aviator' as a generic term, is deprecated
P.R.O.†	Pantoscopic round oval; a combination of the round and oval shapes, derived from a semicircle surmounted by a semi-ellipse of the same major diameter
Quadra*	A family of lens shapes, characterized by four recognizable sides of shallow curvature joined by arcs of shorter radius
Round*	Circular
Upswept*	A lens shape in which the upper edge has a marked upward slope towards the temple

*Definitions from BS 3521 (1991) Part 2.
†Definitions by Bennett (1968).

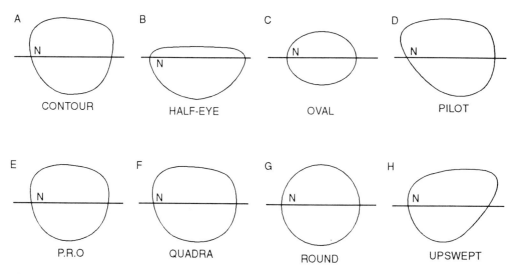

Fig. 16.1 *Lens shapes. Definitions are given in Table 16.1. See Section 16.2*

TABLE 16.2 *Frame measurements according to BS 6625 (1992) and ISO 9456 (1991)*

Position	Measurements
On the front	Horizontal boxed lens size Box symbol (a square in outline) Distance between lenses Bridge width (measurement placed between bridge width symbol / \)
On a side	Overall length of side

The location of the following details is unspecified:
  Manufacturer's or supplier's identification
  Model identification
  Colour identification

mass of a frame of identified size should be made available.

When manufacturers implement this Standard, a huge step forward will have been made with respect to spectacle frame fitting: it will then be possible to take a front with a certain bridge width made by manufacturer A, or a front with the same bridge width but made by manufacturer B, in the certain knowledge that either will fit a patient's nose reasonably well. This was not possible when frames were marked only with the (boxed) distance between lenses because this

measurement has no real bearing on the bridge dimensions.

The sum of bridge width and horizontal lens size does not necessarily equal the frontal width of that front. Hence, the dispenser will have to use their own judgement as to the aesthetic effect of the lens size of a front on its prospective wearer.

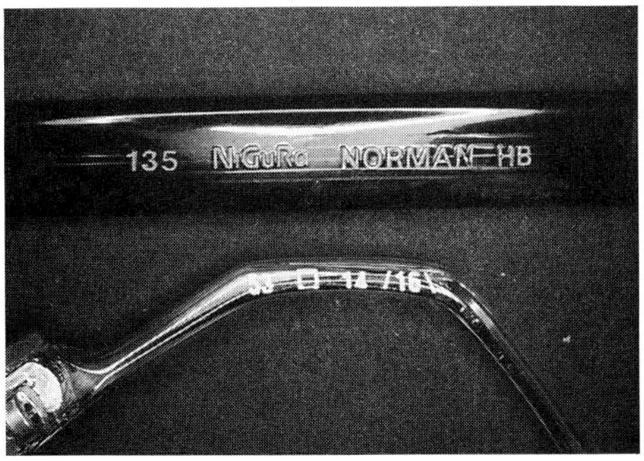

16.4 Frame Selection and Adjustments

Please refer also to Sections 12.3 and 12.4.

16.4.1 THE BRIDGE
This is the crucial part of a frame, not only from a mechanical point of view because it can be considered as a pivot, but also because if a bridge does not fit the spectacles will be neither comfortable nor stable.

The following aspects must be considered (often all at once!): bridge width, distance between rims or distance between pad centres, bridge height, frontal angle (together with splay angle) and angle of crest. However, the last two

Fig. 16.2 *Frame measurements and their specified position according to BS 6625 (1992) and ISO 9456 (1991); see Table 16.2*

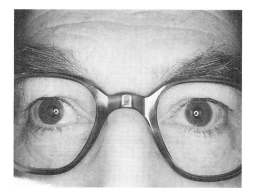

Fig. 16.3 Because the bridge width is too large, the crest rests on the nose

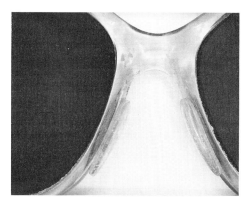

Fig. 16.4 Auxiliary pads, cemented to the nasal bearing surfaces of a plastics front, reduce the bridge width

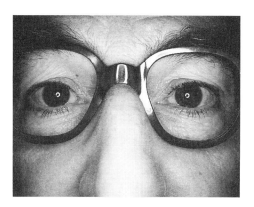

Fig. 16.5 Because the bridge is too narrow (and the frontal angle is too large), the bearing surfaces will lie against the root of the nose rather than against the nasal flanks

dimensions are of secondary importance as they can usually be adjusted or modified. Note that the distance between lenses is of no consequence because it bears no relation to any facial measurement of the prospective spectacle wearer.

If the bridge height is too small and/or the bridge width too large, the front's crest will rest on that of the nose (Fig. 16.3). This does not make for the maximum bearing surface and, hence, the force exerted by the glazed front will bear on a relatively small area. It is therefore likely to cause discomfort. Choosing a front with a smaller bridge width, or a greater bridge height, or filing out the bridge (if possible) to increase the bridge height would serve the purpose. Frames with various bridge/crest heights are shown in Fig. 6.4. Bumping the bridge (Section 10.2) or fitting auxiliary pads (Fig. 16.4) should be considered.

If the front's crest rests on that of the nose, the front's angle of crest must be made to conform fairly closely to that of the nose. This improves comfort remarkably and can be achieved with some careful observation (or use of a facial measurement gauge), and filing.

A bridge which is too narrow (Fig. 16.5) can be stretched by heating and the application of bridge-widening pliers (Fig. 16.6).

It is most important that the bridge width, taken together with the frontal angle, ensures that the bearing surfaces of the bridge lie in close apposition to the nasal flanks in the spectacle plane. If the front is fitted with pads on arms the adjustment may be made with pad adjustment pliers (Fig. 16.7) whereby the splay angle can be adjusted simultaneously. However, in the case of a plastics pad bridge these aspects should be considered more carefully during the frame selection process. The reason is that it is more difficult (and time consuming) to make adjustments afterwards: it would probably involve some filing, smoothing and polishing, to adjust the frontal angle. Note that with a file the latter

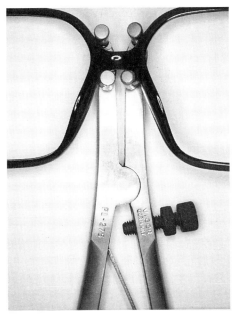

Fig. 16.6 *Bridge widening pliers are used to stretch the heated bridge of a plastics front*

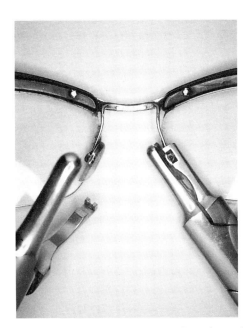

Fig. 16.7 *Pad adjustment pliers grip the pad securely (right) in the recessed portion of the jaw (left)*

can only be increased (provided that there is enough rim material). To reduce the frontal angle, either the lens shape has to be altered, or extra material has to be cemented to the front's bearing surfaces. The latter will have to be followed by filing, smoothing and polishing. In the case of a regular bridge, similar action may have to be taken, but this does not include the splay angle. The splay angle of plastics pads can usually be adjusted by local heating of the pad, followed by pressure applied using the thumb. This does not apply to a saddle bridge: there is usually too much material in the region of the 'pad' and so one cannot deform it (after heating). Hence, filing, smoothing and polishing will be required.

If careful selection of the frame has taken place, and provided that the front is manufactured in a reasonable number of bridge widths, elaborate adjustment exercises are usually not required.

16.4.2 THE FRONT

The frame measurements involved are frontal width, boxed lens size, bridge width, and possibly distance between boxed centres. In general, one may say that the frontal width should be approximately equal to the temple width of the head that it is to adorn. However, fashion dictates may play havoc with this relationship. Fronts for sunglasses may be chosen somewhat wider so that the wearer will benefit from the greater protection this will provide. North (1993) recommended that the frames of spectacles used by vehicle drivers should have thin rims and sides and as large a lens size as possible so that peripheral vision is not restricted (see also DIN 58 216, 1974).

To arrive at the frame measurements suitable for a particular face, consult Section 12.4.2 and in particular Fig. 12.3. It can be shown that the frontal width minus an allowance for the two lugs, equals the distance between centres plus one boxed lens size, and that the distance between centres minus the distance between lenses equals the boxed lens size.

16.4.3 FRONT AND SIDES

The frame measurements associated with the front and sides are angle of let-back, and angle of the side. The angle of let-back is the more important of the two: if it is too small, the front will be propelled forward and the frame will slide down the nose (see Section 13.7). This is a consequence of the mechanics in the relationship between the sides (*temples*) of the frame and the temples of the head. Most heads are wedge-shaped, where the head width is larger than the temple width. Hence, the sides should not touch the temples until the ear point is reached, so that the wedge is inoperative. Even if the temple width were equal to the head width, the sides should be shaped in such a way that they do not touch the temples. See also RAL-RG 915 (1961).

If the angle(s) of let-back need(s) to be increased, the joint(s) need(s) to be filed out (Section 24.2). Note that because asymmetry is a hallmark of the body, the angles of let-back need not be identical. Hence, if a frame is fitted with sprung joints, and if these have an equal spring action when worn, the front may not lie parallel to the frontal plane of the face when unequal angles of let-back are required. The lenses in the front will then have different vertex distances. This may also occur when the patient does not place the frame carefully on his head. Other problems resulting from sprung joints are encountered when such a frame has to be fitted with a pair of heavy lenses. It may then be impossible to stop the frame from slipping because the pressure exerted by the sides is insufficient and cannot be adjusted because the angles of let-back cannot be controlled. It is often not possible to adjust the angle of the side at the joint of frames fitted with sprung joints either. A way around this problem with plastics sides is to

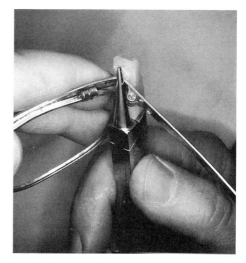

Fig. 16.8 A pair of pliers with a conical and a flat, polyamide jaw, is used to alter the angle of let-back

adjust the side in the vertical plane at a point beyond, but close to the joint. However this is not likely to be possible when dealing with a flat, metal side and, if attempted, the side is more likely to buckle rather than bend.

For fronts with lugs, it may occasionally be better to change the shape or radius of the lug in order to adjust the angle of let-back. For metal fronts this may require the use of special pliers (Fig. 16.8).

The angle of the side and the position of the nose and ears relative to the centre of rotation of the eye, determine the pantoscopic angle (the angle between the optical axis of a lens and visual axis of the eye in the primary position, usually taken to be the horizontal (BS 3521, Part 1, 1991)). This may affect the quality of the retinal image. Older types of joints (*hinges*), with five charniers (*barrels*) or more are very difficult to adjust. One is usually unable to change the inclination of the joint angle. An alternative is then to heat the area of the half-joint to the front (without overheating it so that the pinning or anchorage of the half-joint loosens) and reshape that area with thumb pressure (Fig. 16.9). This may also alter the angle of let-back, which will then have

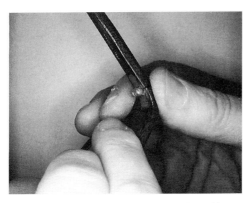

Fig. 16.9 *Applying thumb pressure on a heated lug, to alter the angle of side*

to be adjusted. The joints of some metal fronts are fitted to the rims in such a way that the angle of side cannot be altered at the joints (Fig. 16.10). A possible solution is that discussed for sprung joints (see above).

In exceptional cases, a negative angle of side may be required. With some frames this may be achieved by fitting the right side to the left lug, and vice versa. It will also then be necessary to invert and adjust the drop of each side.

Modern pinless front joints have been designed to be adjustable, by 5° or more, either way. However, the effect of this is usually to reduce the angle of let-back which will then have

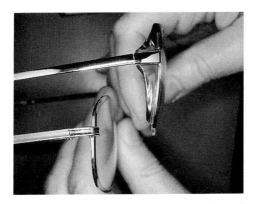

Fig. 16.10 *Examples of metal frames where the angle of side cannot be altered without causing damage, particularly to the rim*

to be increased by means of filing (see Section 24.13.3). Note also that different angles of the side are required when ears are not at the same level.

16.4.4 THE EAR POINT

The position of the ear point, whether measured as front to bend, or length to bend, or overall length and length of drop, should be investigated during selection of the frame. The actual position of the ear point may be affected by the curvature of the front once the lenses have been sprung in, and the front has been given its proper curvature, together with the angle of let-back of the sides and any curvature of the sides in the horizontal plane. However, any variations are usually small.

The ear point of the side should lie neither in front of, nor further away from the face than the top of the root of the ear. When the ear point is situated too far from the front the frame will slide forward; when it is too close to the front the ear point tends to ride up so that the front will start to slide forward while the drop of the side may well cut into the back of the root of the ear (Section 13.5). In either event, its position must be altered.

When the ear point is to be relocated, estimate or measure the length by which the length to bend needs to be increased or decreased. One way of placing the ear point in the correct position is to mark that spot with a marker pen (Fig. 16.11A). A frame heater is then used to warm the ear point before straightening. Next, place your thumb at the marked spot (Fig. 16.11B), and bend the side again. When the side is cool enough, check whether the desired fit has been achieved by placing the spectacles on the wearer's head. Check also whether the downward and inward angles of drop are correct. If a large increase or decrease of the length to bend is required it may be necessary to lengthen or shorten the side (Section 24.14).

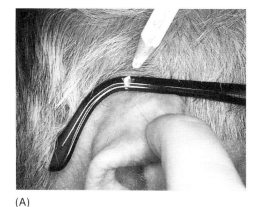

(A)

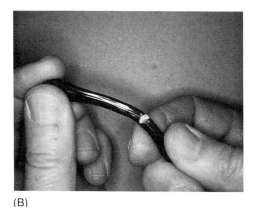

(B)

Fig. 16.11 *A, to alter the position of the ear point, mark its desired position e.g. with a grease pencil; B, the thumb is placed at the marked point and since the area of the bend has been heated, it can be bent*

16.4.5 THE DROP

The aspects to consider are the downward angle of drop, the length of drop, and the inward angle of drop; the shape of the drop can also be of considerable importance.

The downward angle does not usually depart much from 60°, and is, in any case, easily adjustable after the side has been heated around the ear point. The drop should not be too short (RAL-RG 915, 1961) since this is likely to provide too little friction between drop and mastoid to keep a glazed frame in the desired position on the head

(see Section 13.7). If the drop is too short, replacing the whole side with a longer one (provided that it is available), should be considered a priority. When the drop of a plastics side is too long, it can be cut off or filed off, reshaped with a file, smoothed and polished. With a metal side with an end cover (*tip*), it is often possible to reposition the ear point of the end cover (see Section 24.14).

Although one can measure the inward angle of drop, it is more effective to inspect the relationship between the inner aspect of the drop and the mastoid. As explained in Section 13.5, this relationship is very likely to determine the stability of the frame on the head. Having heated the drop, shape it with the fingers so that it follows the convolution of the mastoid; this provides an anchor-hold in it. If the drop's tip protrudes beyond the point where the mastoid curves away, the tip may be shaped to follow this curve also, thus providing an additional hold.

16.4.6 ADJUSTMENTS

When a patient returns for an adjustment to a new or an old pair of spectacles, the above aspects should be checked in the order set out above. Whenever a patient complains about discomfort either on one nasal flank or behind one ear, the mechanics associated with the 'fitting triangle' (Stimson, 1951) should be borne in mind (Fig. 16.12) and the following two features should be checked. First, ascertain whether the discomfort results from misalignment of the pad and nasal flank, or the drop and the mastoid, and correct this if necessary. Second, inspect the contralateral drop or pad, and its alignment with its bearing surface. Note that when the distance between a pad and its contralateral drop is too short, both may cause a reddish impression on the skin, and eventually a sore. However, the wearer may complain only about either the pad or the drop. The discomfort may be relieved by very slightly increasing the distance between pad and ear

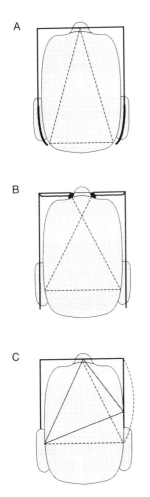

Fig. 16.12 *The 'fitting triangle'. A, the front of a saddle-type bridge fitted with drop-end, curl or straight sides has one 'triangle'; B, a pad bridge front has two triangles placed apex to apex; C, when one side touches a temple, the 'fitting triangle' is asymmetrical, but its symmetry can be restored by adjusting the side so that it is clear of the temple*

point. Slightly decreasing the downward angle of drop may suffice when the drop makes an impression in the groove between ear and mastoid bone.

When the wearer complains about the fit being too loose, but on inspection it is found to be 'just right', one may be reluctant to increase the downward angle of drop. An alternative is

then to effect a minimal decrease in the angle of the side. This will decrease the distance between pad and ear point, thus giving a tighter feel and simultaneously slightly altering the contact areas between pad and nasal flank. This requires careful inspection of the relationship between the frame part and its bearing surface.

16.5 Keeping Stock

Which spectacle frames should one select in order to be able to present a suitable selection of styles to one's patients? This subject has not given rise to many publications.

In larger firms, it is often an experienced person at head office who is responsible for frame purchase. In addition, branch managers may be given the freedom to make selections for their own branch, from collections presented by the representatives of frame manufacturers, importers or wholesale stockists. Individual owners of practices carry their own responsibility.

Hanwell (1993) suggests that regular stock reviews should be carried out to update the range and to ensure that suppliers can meet the demand. The collection should include frames covering the whole spectrum: from inexpensive (which need not be of substandard quality) to more expensive 'fashion' frames. One way of examining one's stock is by selling price for each type (men's, women's and children's frames). Plot selling price against the number of styles in that price group. The ideal curve is that of a gradual slope starting with budget-price frames, gradually increasing in numbers of frames and peaking at a predetermined price. The graph should drop as the premium range of styles is reached. This will highlight any deficiencies that may need to be corrected. In addition, include a few styles that are 'different', at the top end of the range. Try a gimmick-type frame for a period of time, preferably on a 'sale or return' to the manufacturer or wholesaler basis, and await the response.

It is also worthwhile keeping account of the styles that sell well and those that do not. The latter should be replaced with other styles while the former should be kept in the collection. Although the ophthalmic press is a suitable source of information, remember that different countries go through fashion cycles at different times and rates, and that within one country there will also be regional variations (Section 15.2).

16.6 Miscellaneous

To increase the friction of very moist skin a drying powder such as sodium bicarbonate can be applied on the frame bearing surfaces.

A frame, in particular its bridge parts, should not rest on warts, moles or other skin blemishes such as scars caused by the removal of a carcinoma. It may be useful to ask the wearer's general practitioner or surgeon for advice as to which nasal areas to avoid (Archer & Eakin, 1960).

Some groups of people, usually for religious reasons, will not remove their head covering to allow the dispenser to fit the spectacle sides. It is then best to modify the drop of drop end sides into straight sides so that, for instance, a turban may hold the spectacles on the wearer's head; the same may apply to married, orthodox Jewish women who wear a wig. It can be helpful in these cases to curve the ends of the straightened sides inwards so that they will grip around the head, behind the ears. Orthodox Moslem women will remove their head covering or their yashmak (veil) only in private and if attended by a female dispenser. Nuns are usually prepared to remove their head covering.

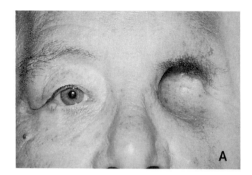

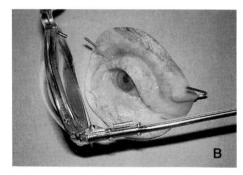

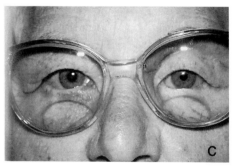

Fig. 16.13 A, photograph of a face with an empty left eye socket; B, the prosthesis shown separated from its frame; C, the face fitted with prosthetic spectacles (photographs courtesy N. Sapp, Moorfields Eye Hospital, London)

Spectacles are sometimes part of a prosthesis (an artificial device used to build up or replace a damaged or missing part of the body). Hence, the dispenser should be prepared to be presented with a pair of spectacles carrying, for instance, an artificial ear, eye or nose (Fig. 16.13). N. Sapp (1993, personal communication) gave the following advice on spectacle frames selected for use with a prosthesis:

(1) Both spectacle lenses should match in weight, be of the same type (that is, both bifocals, etc.) and power so that the magnification of the eye or the prosthesis, as seen by the onlooker, is similar. Note that magnification is sometimes used deliberately, for instance, when the orbit is so shallow that it does not allow an in-depth sculpting of the facial part.
(2) A light-brown spectacle lens tint (not blue or grey) with about 75% transmission, will help to disguise the edge of a prosthesis.

(3) The bridge of the frame should be made of plastics; metal pad bridges make the nasal connection very difficult to hide.
(4) The side wire of plastics sides should not be round in section, but flat so that holes may be drilled and the prosthesis connected to it.
(5) The vertical position of the side with respect to the front should be such that it helps to disguise and aids stability of the prosthesis.

Further information may be gleaned from Watts' (1980, 1992) and Warren's (undated) monographs, and from articles by Staubitz (1982), Priggemeyer (1984), Lloyd & Bode (1985) and Storey (1990).

REFERENCES

Archer, J.E. & Eakin, R.S. (1960). Fitting and adjusting spectacles for the older patient. In: Hirsch, M.J. & Wick, R.A. (eds). *Vision of the Aging Patient*, p. 209. Philadelphia/New York: Chilton.

Bennett, A.G. (1968). *Emsley and Swaine's Ophthalmic Lenses*, Vol. 1, p. 15–19. London: Hatton Press.

BS 3521 (1991). *Terms Relating to Ophthalmic Optics and Spectacle Frames. Part 1: Glossary of Terms Relating to Ophthalmic Lenses.* London: British Standards Institution.

BS 3521 (1991). *Terms Relating to Ophthalmic Optics and Spectacle Frames. Part 2: Glossary of Terms Relating to Spectacle Frames.* London: British Standards Institution.

BS 6625/EN ISO 9456 (1992). *Spectacle Frames. Part 2: Specification for Marking.* London: British Standards Institution.

DIN 58 216 (1974). *Brillen für Fahrzeuglenker; Fassungen und Anpassung.* Berlin: Deutsches Institut für Normung.

Eber, J. (1987). *Anatomische Brillenanpassung*, p. 33. Heidelberg: Verlag Optische Fachveröffentlichungen GmbH.

Hanwell, P. (1993). How to select frames. *Dispensing Optics* **8** (9), 6–8.

Lloyd, W.C. & Bode, D.D. (1985). Prescribing spectacles for anophthalmic patients. *Ann. Ophthalm.* **17**, 426–427.

North, R.V. (1993). *Work and the Eye*, p. 196. Oxford: Oxford University Press.

RAL-RG 915 (1961). *Gütebestimmung im Augenoptikerhandwerk. Individuell angepasste und handwerklich fertiggestellte Korrektionsbrillen.* Berlin: Beuth-Vertrieb GmbH.

Warren, H.S. (undated). *Ocular Prostheses.* London: Ass. Brit. Disp. Opticians.

Watts, E. (1980). *Facial Reconstruction by Prosthetic Means.* London: Ass. Brit. Disp. Opticians.

Watts, E. (1993). Facial prosthesis – a new approach 1992. *Optom. Today*, June 14, p. 25.

Stimson, R.C. (1951). *Ophthalmic Dispensing.* St Louis: Mosby.

Staubitz, F. (1982). Epithesen und deren Montage an Brillenfassungen. *Neues Optikerj.* **24** (5), 37–39.

Storey, J. (1990). The patient with an ocular prosthesis. *Optician* **200** (5279), 22–25.

CHAPTER 17

Paediatric Dispensing

17.1 Introduction

This chapter deals with problems peculiar to children up to the age of about 13. At that age their head has usually reached its adult dimensions. The facial measurements associated with children are discussed in Section 3.3. Note that between the ages of 7 and 14 years the facial characteristics of children with Down's syndrome neither change nor coincide with those of other children. Woodhouse *et al.* (1994) called for a range of frames specially designed for these children to be introduced.

Because the skin of healthy children is in prime condition, it can withstand a remarkable degree of physical insult without permanent damage, with speedy recovery and with adaptation to pain (Eakin, 1964). However, Dishoek & Wal (1984) warned that this relative insensitivity could lead to irritation and malformation of the developing nose and ears.

17.2 Frames for Babies

Currently, ametropic babies are usually fitted with contact lenses. However, if there are contra-indications, spectacles are an alternative.

Babies spend most of the time lying on their back. They tend to 'elevate' their eyes frequently, which requires a lens shape to match. Many babies have high cheek bones as a result of the undeveloped nasal bone. Consequently, the lens shape should be shallow below the horizontal centre line, and protrude high above it. Metal

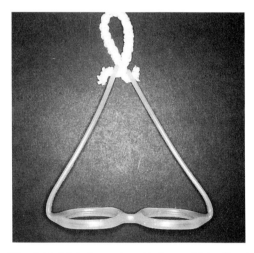

Fig. 17.1 *A jointless, polyamide frame with headband designed for babies (courtesy W.T. Rees Ltd, Wealdstone, UK)*

frames may be manufactured with sides welded to the front (van Doorn, 1994). The sides can be fitted with loop-ends (Fig. 11.24; see Section 17.4). One-piece plastics baby frames are also available (Fig. 17.1)

17.3 Children's Frames

The main features of spectacle frames for children compared with those for adults may be summarized as follows:

(1) the crest height is lower,
(2) the frontal angle is larger,
(3) the splay angle is larger,
(4) the frontal width is smaller,
(5) the angle of side is smaller,

and, as a consequence of the child's smaller cranial features:

(6) the boxed lens size will be smaller and the lens aperture must have a shape that differs from adult designs,
(7) the length to bend and the length of drop will be shorter. In addition, the vertex distance is often very short. As a result of this the, often long, eyelashes may leave an oily substance on the rear surface of the lenses (Lang, 1977).

Because children are continuously growing, one cannot design a spectacle frame for children of a given age. Marks (1961) and Kasparek (1981) considered various aspects of children's frames. Størseth *et al.* (1985) recommended the following characteristics for such frames:

- an oval or round lens aperture
- a saddle or twinned pad bridge
- plastics-covered curl sides (*riding bow temples*)
- large frontal and splay angles
- a negative crest height
- a 0° angle of the side, and fitted with knife-edge surfaced, protective lenses.

It goes without saying that the frame should be cosmetically acceptable (to the parents?), and not too expensive. For the latter reason, 'metal spectacle frames for younger children where it is anticipated that the period of use will not exceed one year' are categorized in BS 6625 as Grade B spectacles frames.

Fixed (as opposed to rocking) pads should be wider at their lower end. This provides a larger bearing surface nearer to the horizontal plane, thus reducing pressure and increasing comfort. Twinned (*twin*) and silicone pads may also be very suitable.

Fahrner (1977) showed a basic lens shape outline for children's frames which takes account of these aspects (Fig. 17.2). It should also be pointed out that children live in a world inhabited

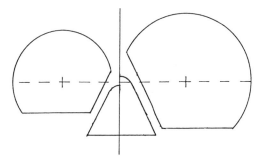

Fig. 17.2 *Basic designs for a child's (left) and an adult's front. The child's distance centration distance (DCD) is 56, and the adult's DCD is 66 mm, requiring 50 and 65 mm uncut lenses, respectively. Modified from Fahrner (1977)*

mainly by, intended for and built by adults. Hence, children have to look upwards (generally about 20° elevation) a great deal of the time, to make eye contact with adults, or simply to look at objects at adult eye level. As a result, children often look through the gap between the upper rims of the frame and their eyebrows (Fig. 17.3). This is of little consequence for myopic children but could have repercussions for esophoric hyperopes in that the esophoria may break down into a squint – an undesirable situation. Moreover, spectacles never slide upwards, they always slip down.

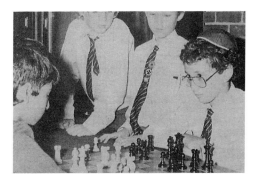

Fig. 17.3 *Children often look over the top of their spectacle front, not only at opponents but even more likely at adults towering above them*

17.4 Dispensing

Some spectacle frames specially designed for very small children are shown in Fig. 17.4. Fronts that are simply scaled-down models of adult fronts are not normally suitable for children's faces, and for their noses in particular (Sasieni, 1954; Veltmann, 1986).

Very small children may be fitted with frames that have loop-end sides. A ribbon is passed through each loop (Fig. 17.5), and tied at the back of the head. For small girls, the ribbon can be tied into a bow on top of their head. Instead of a knot or bow, velcro may be stitched to the ends of the ribbon and used to secure the spectacles. A frame including a 'bridle' is shown in Fig. 17.6. See also

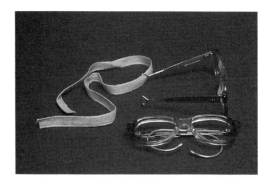

Fig. 17.5 *Pell Optical Co. (Woodford Green, Essex, UK) Model PS 91 consists of a cellulose acetate front which can be provided with curl sides (lower frames) or loop-end sides. In the latter case the spectacles are secured on the baby's head by a ribbon that passes through the loops*

papers by Albrecht (1985) and Earlam & White (1990).

The dispenser may prefer to fit slightly older children with a frame that has curl sides (*riding bow temples*). A simple way to determine the total length required is to take a piece of string, hold it in both hands and let it run from the anticipated position of the back plane of the front over the ear point to the ear lobe of the child's ear. The length of that portion of the string represents the total length of the curl side required. This method

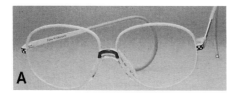

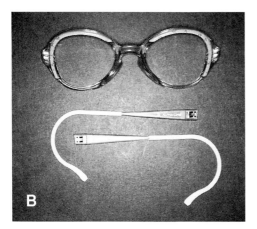

Fig. 17.4 *Sample spectacle fronts for small children. A, Carl Zeiss Model F 6765 is a metal front with plastics bridge. B, Norville Optical Co. (Gloucester, UK) Model Alpha is a two-tone cellulose acetate front with a keyhole bridge and polyamide curl sides; a similar model (Beta) is available with either cellulose acetate drop-end sides or loop-end sides*

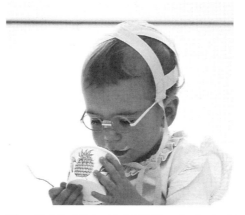

Fig. 17.6 *Carl Zeiss Model 5935 can be fitted with a 'bridle'*

TABLE 17.1 *The weight of positive, edged plastics lenses (Obstfeld, 1996)*

BVP (D)	Description	Uncut diameter (mm)	Mass (g) for boxed lens size	
			48 mm	38 mm
+9·00	Index 1·6	67·5	15 M	11 M
	Hyperaspheric	58·5	12 M	9 M
	CR 39	61·5	15 M	11 M
	CR 39	52·5	8 M	7 M
+5·00	CR 39	60	9 M	7 M
	CR 39	52·5	6	5
+1·00	CR 39	60	5	3
	CR 39	52·5	4	2

M, minibevel

may also be adapted to determine the overall length of a drop-end side.

Schoolchildren are usually provided with frames having drop-end sides (*skull temples*).

Note that the splay angle of children's frames with a plastics pad bridge is not usually made as large as is required to give a comfortable fit to the wearer. The reason is that, if this were done, it would be almost impossible to insert the lenses from behind into the empty front. However, having inserted the lenses, it is a small matter to heat the pads and adjust them with thumb pressure to give the required splay angle (Section 24.7).

Youngsters often engage in games with large and/or fast-moving balls, as in football and racquet sports (see Loran and MacEwen, 1995). If they wear metal spectacle fronts and are hit by the ball, laceration of the skin surrounding the eyes is not uncommon. Although plastics fronts may break, they are unlikely to cause such injury.

The mass of fronts and sides of children's frames is discussed in Sections 13.2 and 13.4, and further details can be found in Tables 13.2 and 13.3.

Because the mass of a glass spectacle lenses is about twice that of a comparable plastics lens, the latter are preferred. The impact resistance of glass lenses, even when toughened, is also less favourable. Lenses made of polycarbonate plastics material, provide the best impact resistance (Obstfeld, 1996). Obstfeld (1996) found for plastics spectacle lenses that

(1) irrespective of power, edged negative lenses of 38 mm boxed lens size have a mass of about 4 g
(2) the mass of edged lenses of 48 mm boxed lens size is 2–4 g greater than that of the equivalent 38 mm lenses, and
(3) lenses of suitable uncut diameter and worked to a knife-edge have the lowest mass.

The mass of positive, edged plastics lenses is given in Table 17.1. Table 13.4 shows the mass of comparable crown glass spectacle lenses.

17.5 Summary

Children's frames should be designed specifically for, and manufactured in sizes that fit their prospective wearers' faces. Dispensers should select frames with an oval or round lens aperture and a saddle bridge with large frontal and splay angles. Frames should be fitted with plastics lenses. Positive lenses should be knife-edge surfaced.

REFERENCES

Albrecht, M. (1985). Specialanfertigung und Anpassung von Kinderbrillen und Kleinstkinderbrillen. *Neues Optiker.* **27** (3), 21–25.

BS 6625 (1985) (Amendment no. 1, 1991). *Specification for Spectacle Frames.* London: British Standards Institution.

Dishoek, E.A. van & Wal, R.J. van der (1984). De bril op de neus. *Oculus, Amsterdam* **46**, 35–37.

Doorn, B. van (1994). De kinderbril van handicap tot mode-item. *Oculus, Amsterdam* **56** (5), 47–49.

Eakin, R.S. (1964). In: Hirsch, M.J. & Wick, R.E. (eds) *Vision of Children*, p. 272. London: Hammond, Hammond & Co.

Earlam, R. & White, K. (1990). Developing a frame for children. *Optician* **200** (5272), 16–18.

Fahrner, D. (1977). Kinderbrillen – Probleme, Lösungsmöglichkeiten. *Neues Optiker.* **19** (7), 579–583.

Kasparek, G. (1981). Anforderungskriterien an Kinderbrillen. *Deutsche Optikerz.*, No. 10, 10–14.

Lang, J. (1977). Die Kinderbrille: Augenärztliche und optische Probleme bei Kindern. *Neues Optiker.* **19**, 575–578.

Loran, D.F.C., & MacEwen, C.J. (1995). *Sports Vision.* Oxford: Butterworth-Heinemann.

Marks, R. (1961). Some factors for consideration in the selection of children's eye wear. *Am. J. Optom. Arch. Am. Acad. Optom.* **38** (4), 185–193.

Obstfeld, H. (1996). Spectacle dispensing Ch. 17. In: Barnard, S. & Edgar, D. (eds) *Pediatric Eye Care*. Oxford: Blackwell Science.

Sasieni, L.S. (1954). Considerations in the design of frames for children. *Optician* **128**, 481–482.

Størseth, G., Lundemo, T. & Lundemo, B. (1985). Barn og briller, 0–7 ar. *Optikeren, Oslo*, No. 4, 15–16.

Veltmann, U. (1986). Stiefkind Kinderbrille. *Augenspiegel*, part 10, 46–55.

Woodhouse, J.M., Hodge, S.J. & Earlam, R.A. (1994). Facial characteristics in children with Down's syndrome and spectacle fitting. *Ophthal. Physiol. Optics* **14** (1), 25–31.

CHAPTER 18

Geriatric Dispensing

18.1 Introduction

Gerontology is the scientific study of the processes of ageing; geriatrics refers to the medical care of old people. Geriatric dispensing deals with the dispensing needs of older spectacle wearers.

18.2 The Skin

The underlying cause of the ageing process is the slowing of the rate of metabolism of the body, which usually takes place over a relatively long period of time. As a result, connective tissue loses its ability to retain water. This causes the characteristic folds and wrinkles of the older person's skin. Selected general systemic changes affect

(1) skeletal tissue resulting in atrophy, distortion of surfaces, and cartilage becoming fibrous and less elastic,
(2) muscular tissue resulting in reduced strength owing to loss of tonus, and impairment of coordination, and
(3) skin, which not only becomes wrinkled, but also flabby, thinner and parchment-like. The effects on the skin result from the degeneration of elastic dermis fibres, the reduction of subcutaneous fat and the atrophy of sebaceous and sweat glands.

Unfortunately, these skin changes can be prominent in the nasal region. Thus, spectacle pads may be separated from the nasal bone only by thin skin. Consequently, abrasion may easily occur and will take longer to heal than in young patients. Skin changes are less of a problem behind the ears because these changes are more commonly limited to dryness and scaliness. Conversely, moles, tumours and other skin irregularities in the areas of touch with the spectacle frame will make fitting much more difficult in that, ideally, the frame should not touch these areas (Archer & Eakin, 1960).

Specific changes of the tissues surrounding the eyes include (Haberich, 1975):

- the early development of so-called 'crow's-feet' (wrinkles in the skin at the outer canthus),
- an increase in the skin folds of the upper eyelid owing to tissue relaxation
- an increase in the skin folds of the lower eyelid allows orbital fatty tissue to penetrate, giving rise to the development of 'bags' under the eyes,
- senile ectropion may cause atrophy of the lid muscles and relaxation of the skin,
- spastic entropion may be caused by dysfunction of the orbicularis muscle,
- small haemorrhages may occur as a result of the fragility of the capillaries of the connective tissue.

Pierce and Morgan (1986) pointed out that simple contact dermatitis may cause increased redness that persists after removal of the spectacles. However, this is not limited to older patients. In extreme cases, spectacle frames may cause pressure sores (painful or diseased spots; see Section 9.3.4. and 9.3.5). They may be classified as (Brocklehurst & Hanley, 1976):

(1) Normal pressure sores which heal within about 6 weeks. In this condition the blood supply is intact and the sore results entirely from a reduced blood flow caused by pressure.

(2) Arteriosclerotic or indolent (painless) ulcers (open sores discharging pus) which take about 16 weeks to heal. These are caused by an impairment of the blood supply which is not only due to vascular disease, but also to pressure.

(3) Terminal ulcers which occur in people who are dying. Such sores do not heal.

Sores may be brought about by three types of pressure, all of which can be caused by spectacle frames (Brocklehurst & Hanley, 1976):

(1) Compression when the compressing force of the bearing surface of the spectacle frame (Section 13.6) is greater then the pressure of the blood within the arterioles and capillaries.

(2) Shearing forces between the nasal skin which is being forced downward by the spectacles (see 'Friction' in Section 13.7), and the stationary nasal bone thus producing stress in the subcutaneous tissues.

(3) Folding of the skin which may obliterate blood vessels.

18.3 Mental State

Archer & Eakin (1960) drew attention to the problems caused by the mental attitude or state of older spectacle wearers, be they first-time or experienced. Not only do both dispenser and patient have to cope with physical limitations and anomalies caused by conditions such as arthritis, palsy or paralysis, but there may also be senility. It is often worthwhile giving your advice not only to the spectacle wearer, but also to a relative or other person who is present. That other per-

son will then be able to remind the spectacle wearer of the advice given and ensure that the wearer takes heed. Written advice is also helpful, especially when memory cannot be relied upon.

18.4 Frame Selection

The above details emphasize the importance of the bridge fitting: the pressure should be distributed over as large an area as possible. Hence, the 'facial' measurements of the nasal area must be taken into account. A saddle bridge frame in a low-density material, together with plastics lenses, will probably provide the best solution. The writer agrees with Dowaliby (1975) who advocated fixed rather than adjustable (rocking) pads, for older patients. Because of their high coefficient of friction, silicon pads should be avoided because they stretch the skin. Stretching is poorly resisted by the skin of older patients.

The spectacle front's lens size should be as small as appears reasonable in view of facial measurements and regardless of fashion. This will help to keep the lens mass small. The frame's mass can be kept small by choosing a front where the frontal width is a little smaller than the temple width. During the final fitting session ensure that the sides do not touch the temples. Selecting a thin frame rather than one with bold features will also help to reduce the weight. Although these recommendations do not amount to major reduction in mass, they may help to alleviate problems. The (semi-)rimless half-eye frame should be considered as a light-weight frame, as should Polymil and Supra styles.

If a pad frame is selected, ensure that the largest possible pads are fitted, or that small plastics pads are modified so as to increase the bearing surface to its maximum. The pads of a metal or combination frame may be replaced by a twinned pad which is likely to be better than 'jumbo'-sized pads. Note that when an older

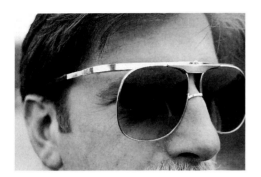

Fig. 18.1 *Suspended spectacle frame which exerts no weight on the nose or ears (patents granted; courtesy Star-Spex Ltd., Douglas, Isle of Man)*

person's metal spectacle front is hit hard, perhaps as a result of an accident, it is more likely to cause laceration of the facial skin than a plastics front.

Although (metal) decorations are usually only small, it can be important to avoid them (remove them) when they are a contributing factor to discomfort and to the prevention or alleviation of pathological developments.

For patients who cannot tolerate any pressure on the nose at all, there are frames that grip around the head (Fig. 18.1 and 19.27B). The temple-rest frame (see Fig. 19.27A) grips at the temples by means of springs.

18.5 Adjustments and Modifications

Pierce & Morgan (1986) made the following recommendations as a general approach to solving problems:

(1) Use temporary or permanent accessories of various kinds that can be applied quickly to the front. These include pads of different sizes, stick-on pad cushions (although some of these tend to deteriorate quickly, particularly when affected by cosmetics and/or perspiration), Usden crutches (see Chapter 19, Cheek rest frames) and twinned pad bridges.
(2) Modify the bridge contour, particularly in fixed pad bridges.
(3) Custom design a 'special' (i.e. handmade) frame that meets the specific requirements of a particular patient.

Option (3) may well be the best. Archer & Eakin (1960) and also Pierce & Morgan (1986) have described various modifications in detail.

For many older people comfort is more important than aesthetics or visual efficiency. Hence, dispensing a comfortable pair of spectacles may well be most important aspect.

REFERENCES

Archer, J.E. & Eakin, R.S. (1960). The fitting and adjusting of spectacles for the older patient. In: Hirsch, M.J., & Wick, R.E. (eds) *Vision of the Ageing Patient,* p. 202. Philadelphia/New York: Chilton.

Brocklehurst, J.C. & Hanley, T. (1976). *Geriatric Medicine for Students,* p. 94. Edinburgh/London: Churchill Livingstone.

Dowaliby, M. (1975). Geriatric ophthalmic dispensing. *Am. J. Optom. Physiol. Optics* **52** (6), 422–427.

Haberich, F.J. (1975). Altern und Gesichtssinn. *Optometrie, Mainz* **23**, 110–120.

Pierce, A.L. & Morgan, M.W. (1986). Fitting and dispensing spectacles for the elderly. In: Rosenbloom, A.A. Jr. & Morgan, M.W. (eds). *Vision and Aging,* p. 253. New York: Professional Press Books – Fairchild.

CHAPTER 19

Special Purpose Frames

There appears to be an unending list of spectacle frames designed for special, and even bizarre, purposes. The largest number of 'specials' may have been catalogued by Müller (1962–65).

The frames described in this chapter include the more common varieties that cannot be described as just serving the purpose of correcting ametropia. A number also alleviate handicaps or medical conditions, while others provide a measure of protection or facilitate observation for specific purposes. Because classification would be subject to debate, they are presented in alphabetical order.

- **Anti-dazzle frames** These are fronts with shields on the side of approaching vehicles (Fig. 19.1A). The shields prevent glare from the vehicle's headlights entering the driver's eyes. However, because the shields must be opaque or made of absorbing material, objects other than light sources are unlikely to be noticed in the dark. Instead of shields, areas of absorbing material have been vacuum-deposited on the lenses' surfaces (Fig. 19.1B). For a review see Phillips & Rutstein (1967).

- **Ankylosing spondylitis frames** (ankylosis: fusion of bones or skeletal parts; spondylitis: inflammation of a vertebra) Wearers of this type of prosthesis suffer from a deformed spine which prevents them from lifting their head to look straight ahead. Kunze (1959) described an arrangement (Fig. 19.2A,B) whereby a pair of mirrors was fitted to a spectacle front and used for looking ahead. The patient could see the floor by looking

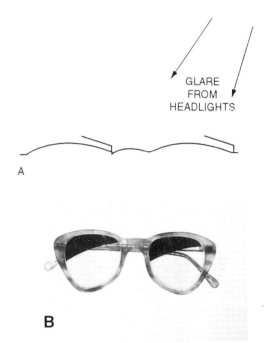

Fig. 19.1 *A, diagram showing a front fitted with shields on the side of approaching cars, thus preventing glare reaching the eyes. B, a front fitted with anti-dazzle lenses. By tilting the head forward, light from an approaching car will be absorbed or reflected by the upper, black area thus preventing dazzle*

between the mirrors. Richer & Hall (1986) described the use of powerful Fresnel prisms, base down, which improved the wearer's mobility by apparently moving his field of view forward. P.J. Turner (personal communication, 1992) inverted recumbent spectacles (Fig. 19.2C) for this purpose.

- **Archery spectacles** See special purpose spectacles, billiards spectacles.

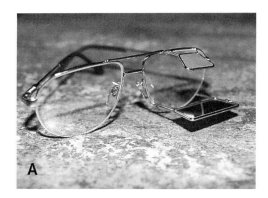

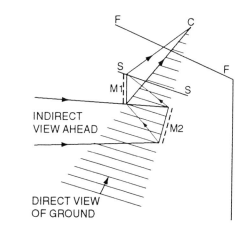

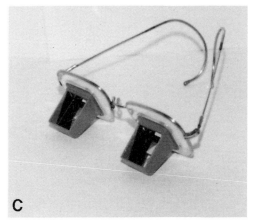

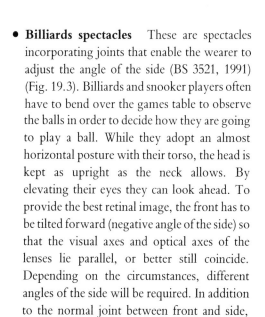

Fig. 19.2 *Ankylosing spondylitis frames. A, a patient who is unable to lift his head can see the ground when looking in between the two mirrors. While looking into the 'upper' mirror, he will see the scene ahead reflected by the 'lower' mirror (courtesy Obrira, Rathenow, Germany). B, ray diagram: C, position of wearer's eye; FF, facial plane; M1, upper mirror; M2, lower mirror; SS, spectacle plane. C, curl sides spectacles fitted with 'inverted' Hamblin prisms as used in recumbent spectacles (courtesy P.J. Turner, Bristol). Compare with Fig. 19.22*

- **Billiards spectacles** These are spectacles incorporating joints that enable the wearer to adjust the angle of the side (BS 3521, 1991) (Fig. 19.3). Billiards and snooker players often have to bend over the games table to observe the balls in order to decide how they are going to play a ball. While they adopt an almost horizontal posture with their torso, the head is kept as upright as the neck allows. By elevating their eyes they can look ahead. To provide the best retinal image, the front has to be tilted forward (negative angle of the side) so that the visual axes and optical axes of the lenses lie parallel, or better still coincide. Depending on the circumstances, different angles of the side will be required. In addition to the normal joint between front and side,

another is provided on the side. This allows the side to be adjusted in the vertical plane, thus facilitating an adjustment to a negative angle of the side. Because of the forward tilt of the front, the vertical lens size may be unusually large. For the same reason the optical centre of each lens must be decentred upwards. The fronts may have unusually low (negative) crest heights. There are billiards spectacles where the front is set at a fixed negative angle of the side.

This type of spectacle is also used for shooting from a prone position (see special purpose spectacles).

- **Cheek rest frames** These frames are for patients who cannot tolerate any pressure on their nose. There are no nasal bearing surfaces

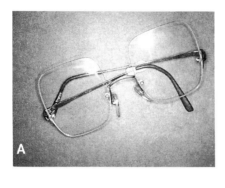
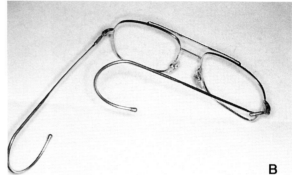
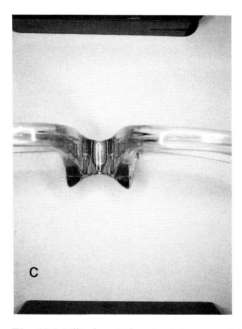
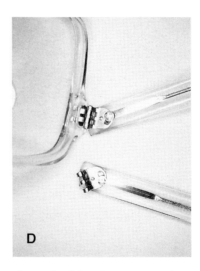

Fig. 19.3 *Billiard spectacles. A, rimless type with a fixed, negative angle of the side. B, a metal frame with a secondary joint on each side; the angle of the side can be made positive or negative. C, inset bridge of the Super-Cue billiard spectacles photographed in the spectacle plane, from below. D, plastic frame showing the adjustable joint providing a negative angle of the side (Super-Cue, courtesy Lesbro, Birmingham, UK).*

on the front. Instead, pad arms (like stilts; *Usden crutches*) are fixed to the lower rims of the front (Fig. 19.4). The arms have pads fitted and these rest on the cheeks. (Springer, 1970). See temple rest frames.

- **Clip-on** An attachment holding an auxiliary lens or lenses in front of spectacles by spring action or by means of hooks (Fig. 19.5) (BS 3521, 1991).

- **Cyclophoria spectacles** Spectacles incorporating a device for rotating one or both fields of view (BS 3521, 1991).

- **Entropion spectacles** (entropion: a condition where the lower eyelid and eyelashes have turned towards the eye) A gallery (see Figs 2.34 and 11.29, and orthopaedic and ptosis frames) is fitted on the lower rim of a front. This exerts a force on the lower lid in

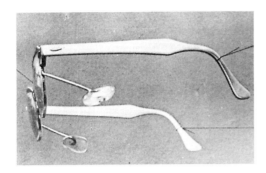

Fig. 19.4 Cheek rest front

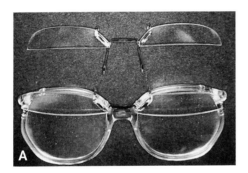

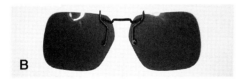

Fig. 19.5 Samples of clip-on attachments. A, upper portion clip-on to provide, for instance, an addition for distance or intermediate vision over a pair of reading glasses. B, preshaped clip-on used to transform spectacles into sunglasses. Clip-ons with extra-large filters that can be cut to shape and size in order to fit onto the front of conventional glasses are also available

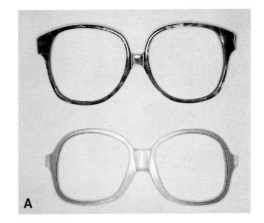

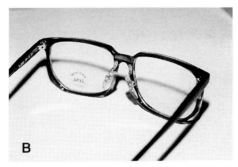

Fig. 19.6 Ethnic frames. A, above: Onyx model 02 (courtesy of M. D. Cooper Promotions, 1A Keats Parade, Church Street, London N9 9DP, UK); below: own design by a Mongoloid student (crest height, −3 mm; frontal angles, right 30°, left 25°). B, plastics front production model fitted with metal pad arms and plastics pads (courtesy Kan Chi-ming, Optometry Section, Hong Kong Polytechnic)

order to keep it in its normal position. If the pressure is too great it may interfere with the drainage of tears, causing the tears to run over the cheek. See orthopaedic spectacles.

- **Ethnic frames**   This term has been used for spectacle frames designed to fit a specific ethnic group (Fig. 19.6). The distinguishing feature of one such range of plastics frames is the keyhole bridge modified to a slot. This helps to reduce the weight of the front. Furthermore, the frontal and splay angles are large and the pads are placed relatively low. A range of plastics frames made in Hong Kong features metal pad arms fitted with rocking pads (Fig. 19.6B). This construction is used in many cases. If no special frames are available, metal frames with rocking or twinned (*twin*) pads are used. See Anonymous (1993) and Cooper (1993).

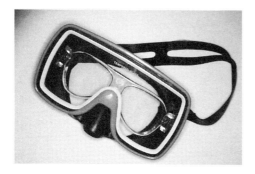

Fig. 19.7 *Face mask fitted with an insert for correction lenses (courtesy Norville Optical Co., Gloucester)*

- **Face masks** (BS 4532, 1969) A face mask enables the wearer to see underwater and prevents water from being inadvertently breathed up the nose (Fig. 19.7). It consists of a piece of transparent material sealed to the face in a watertight manner. BS 4532 specifies not only details about the mask, but also about the eyescreen and headstrap. Flat, corrective lenses may be cemented to the back surface of the eyescreen. Care must be taken to consider the effect of the, often large, vertex distance. See Obstfeld (1982) for technical aspects of vision under water.

- **Fishing spectacles** No special frame is required, but for the sake of completeness, it is mentioned here. Presbyopes may find it convenient to wear a pair of glasses with one very small bifocal segment, set in such a position that it does not interfere with distance vision, e.g. well to one side. This facilitates fixing the fly to the hook. Polarizing lenses enable one to see fish below the water surface.

- **Flip-up frames** There are several variants that have one thing in common: the frames are fitted with a secondary front that can be swivelled upwards (Fig. 19.8). The front surfaces of the lenses in the secondary front will then almost touch the wearer's forehead. The secondary front may be fitted with

protective lenses (e.g. sunlenses), or contain a near or distance vision addition. If the secondary front is connected to the primary front with two joints, it is imperative that the joint screws share the same axis of rotation. If they do not, they will break owing to torsion. Consider fitting glass lenses as they are less likely to mark each other than plastics lenses.

- **Flying frames** Pilots prefer large lens sizes in 'pilot-shaped' (Section 16.2) goggles to obtain as high and wide a view as possible. However, this adds to the weight (of glass lenses; polycarbonate lenses have a number of advantages such as being lightweight and having best demisting (Margrain & Owen, 1996) and impact resistance properties) and to peripheral distortion. Loop-end sides and a browbar help to stabilize frames. This can be important when flying through turbulence and particularly when performing aerobatic manoeuvres. A strap running behind the head will be useful. Spectacle sides should neither interfere with a radio headset nor be uncomfortable to wear. It is wise to see the headset, or oxygen mask, if worn, and assess the whole arrangement. It may be best to let the front rest on such a mask, having removed the pad arms and pads from metal fronts. Helmets, worn as protection in case of an accident or against noise, may cause restriction of the field of view or distortion from visors. They may also cause fogging owing to condensation of water particles and give rise to an uncomfortable fit of frames worn underneath (DeHaan, 1982). A type of goggle for use under a helmet is shown in Fig. 19.9A. Figure 19.9B shows two models in use by the Royal Air Force. See also Rossi (1995).

- **Folding frames** Such frames have additional 'double' joints on the bridge of the front and in each side (Fig. 19.10). The joints in the bridge allow the one half front to be placed against the other, and the joints in each side

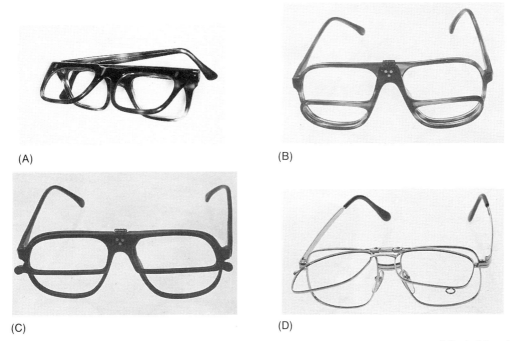

(A)   (B)

(C)   (D)

Fig. 19.8 Flip-up frames. A, full flip-up plastics front. B, lower half flip-up front (courtesy Franel Optical Supply Co., Maitland, FL, USA). C, upper half flip-up front (courtesy Franel Optical Supply Co.). D, full flip-up metal frame (courtesy Franel Optical Supply Co.)

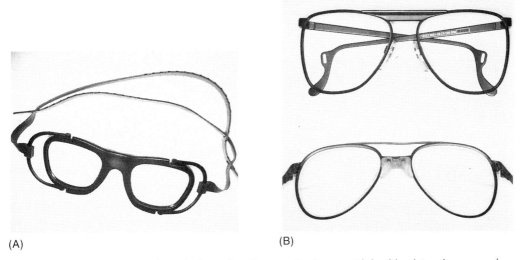

(A)   (B)

Fig. 19.9 Flying frames. A, polyamide flying front for correction lenses, with head band (can be worn under a helmet). B, CFS 9021 (above) and ARS 9013. Both have the same type of sides for use with a head band. The front of the latter is steeply curved, to fit under a face protector, and shows a silicone inset bridge and E-type bifocal lenses (© Crown Copyright/MOD)

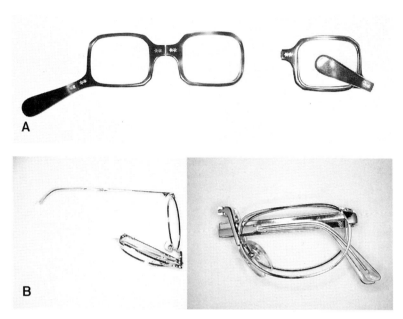

Fig. 19.10 Folding frames. A, plastics with handle (lorgnette type). B, full metal frame (courtesy Lesbro, Birmingham)

allow the parts to be wrapped around the folded front. When folded, a frame may be only a little thicker than 1 cm.

- **Gas mask spectacles**   These were worn under a gas mask or 'gases eye-protector' BS EN

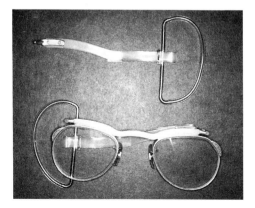

Fig. 19.11 Gas mask spectacles: a metal front fitted with correction lenses and thin polyamide strap-like sides adjustable in length. A loop to fit around the ear is attached to each side

165–168 (1995), to provide a spectacle correction for ametropes. Characteristically, they have thin, flat, pliable sides which cause minimal disturbance to the seal between mask and face (Fig. 19.11). Positive air pressure within the mask is used to keep noxious gases out. However, during exertion the pressure may be reversed. Recently, a number of face masks have been given BS EN 136 (1992) mask leakage certification for use with spectacle inserts (C. Owen & T.H. Margrain, personal communication, 1995). See Stobbe *et al.* (1988) for the effect of facial hair. Also known as respirator spectacles.

- **Golf spectacles**   This is not a special frame, but spectacles for presbyopes so that they can see and write on their score card. A small bifocal segment is usually set well to one side.
- **Hay fever spectacles**   Filtered air is delivered from an air pump to the frame through a fine tube (Fig. 19.12). The air passes through

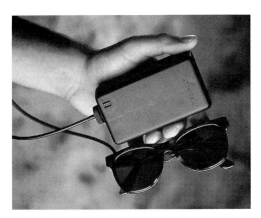

Fig. 19.12 Hay fever spectacles and pump (courtesy of Duncan & Todd, Aberdeen, UK)

the hollow bar of the spectacle front, and is blown downwards through small holes in the bar. Thus, allergens are kept away from the eyes by positive air pressure (Stem & Scott, 1993; Woods & Haycock, 1994).

- **Hearing-aid frames**   These frames have a microphone and sound amplifier incorporated in their side(s) (Fig. 19.13). They are used by people who have hearing difficulties. Band (1991) described four types: 'behind the ear' aids, aids where the sound is conducted by means of air, aids with 'bone-conduction' sides, and cros and bi-cros sides. He discussed their problems and gave practical tips,

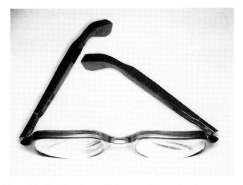

Fig. 19.13 Hearing-aid frames. Note the dimensions of the sides

especially for the bone-conduction types. Forbes (1984) dealt also with the special visual needs of deaf patients.

- **Half-eye spectacles**   Spectacles designed so that either the upper or the lower part of the field of view is outside the periphery of the lens (BS 3521, 1991) (Fig. 19.14).
- **Hemianopia spectacles**   Spectacles incorporating a device that laterally displaces one or both fields of view (BS 3521, 1991) (Fig. 19.15). These are designed to assist patients who suffer from blindness in one-half of the field of view of one eye. In principle, they are designed only to make the patient aware of moving objects in the blind part of the field. He may then direct his gaze in that direction. By means of a mirror device the scene within the blind part of the field is imaged on the seeing side of the eye's field (Kono, 1952; Duszynski, 1955; Mehr & Freid, 1975; Mintz, 1979; Villani, 1977). When a mirror is used, the image produced will be left–right reversed. This may cause another difficulty for the wearer. A double-mirror arrangement will overcome this problem, but is likely to produce a heavier front (Fig. 19.15B). As an alternative a (Fresnel) prism placed over the hemianopic side of the field has been used (Mehr & Freid, 1975; Villani, 1977). Weiss (1990) reported on a patient whose visual fields were reduced to a small central field surrounded by several crescent-shaped peripheral islands of vision. This individual benefited from a pair of single vision bicentric lenses, their dividing lines being placed vertically. Note that during head movements stationary objects imaged by the mirror will appear to move.
- **Industrial eye protection**   BS EN 165–168 (1995) describe the basic requirements. Basic designs as illustrated in BS 7028 (1988) are shown in Fig. 19.16. Since the introduction of industrial eye protection in

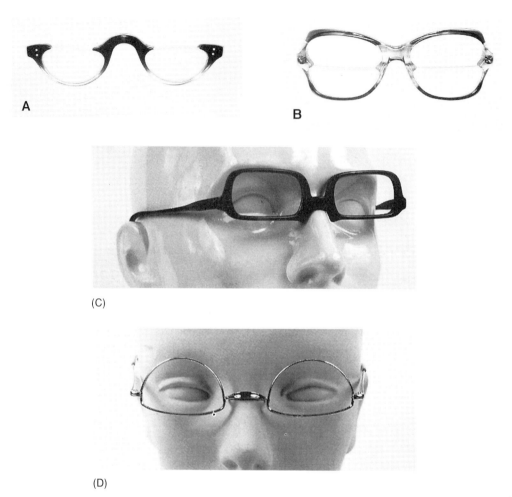

A

B

(C)

(D)

Fig. 19.14 Half-eye spectacles. A, a supra-type with regular bridge. B, a full front where correction lenses can be fitted in either the upper or the lower portion. C, plastics upper half-eye spectacles (courtesy Ursula Hotstegs GmbH, Geldern, Germany). D, metal upper half-eye spectacles (courtesy Ursula Hotstegs GmbH)

1923 (in the UK), admissions to hospital for eye injuries from occupational causes dropped from 71% to 15% by 1980 (MacEwen, 1989). See also ANSI Z87.1 (1989) and CSA 294.3 (1992).

• **Lochbrille** (see pinhole spectacles or similar attachments) These often incorporate sidecups, for use in the after-care of cases of retinal detachment (BS 3521, 1991).

• **Lorgnon** A spectacle lens for occasional use, mounted on a handle, not unlike the appliance shown in Fig. 2.1.

• **Lorgnette** An eyeglass for occasional use, held before the eyes by a handle into which the lenses may fold when not required (BS 3521, 1991) (Fig. 2.19). The dispenser must enquire whether the user is right or left handed and fit lenses accordingly.

• **Make-up frames** These are intended to assist ametropes and presbyopes when

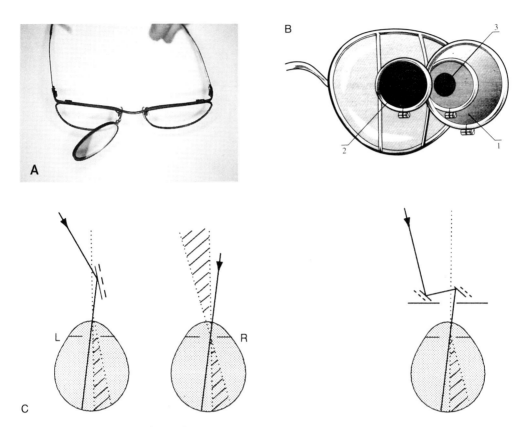

Fig. 19.15 *Hemianopia spectacles. A, front with nasal, semi-silvered mirror (see C, left diagram). B, spectacle front showing: 1, front of temporal mirror; 2, back of nasal mirror; 3, front of nasal mirror, as seen by reflection in temporal mirror (see C, right diagram) (courtesy Obrira, Rathenow, Germany). C, ray paths; shaded areas represent blind portions of the visual fields*

applying eye make-up (Fig. 19.17; see also Fig. 19.27B). Conventionally, they have separate rims that are attached to a frontal bar with hinges so that they can be rotated upwards (or downwards) independently. The eye behind the correcting lens may then be used to observe through a mirror the fellow-eye and its surround. Some contact lens wearers use them when inserting their lenses. Note: use of a mirror may double the observation distance. Also known as vanity frames.

- **Monocle** A single lens, with or without a frame or mount, designed to be held between the brow and the cheek (BS 3521, 1991) (Figs 2.34 and 11.29).

- **Multiple pinhole spectacles** Spectacles fitted with opaque discs that have a number of small apertures, for use in certain cases of low visual acuity (BS 3521, 1991). See lochbrille, pinhole spectacles.

- **Orthoscopic spectacles** A binocular magnifying device consisting of convex lenses with prismatic effect, base-in. Thus, near objects can be observed binocularly without having to converge (Fig. 19.18A). A similar device consists of a front that may be fitted with correcting lenses, and a pair of prisms at a

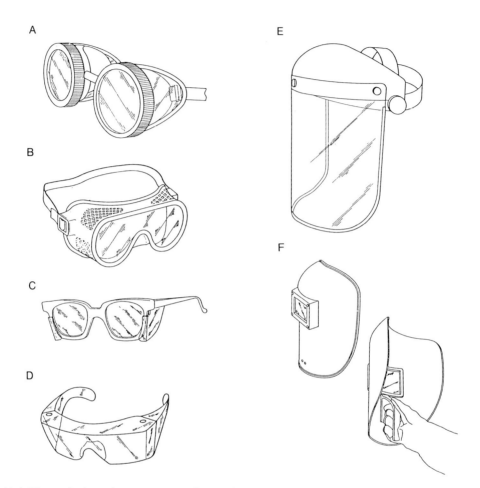

Fig. 19.16 *Types of industrial eye protectors as illustrated in BS 7028. A, cup-type goggles; B, box-type goggles; C, spectacles (including prescription spectacles); D, eye shields; E, face screens or shields; F, welding face screens*

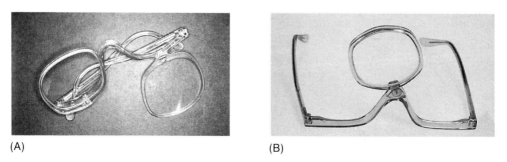

(A)   (B)

Fig. 19.17 *Make-up frames. A, a low joint, plastics frame with the left lens rotated forward allowing access to the left eye (if the frame had been worn). B, low joint, plastics frame with a single rim which may be rotated in front of either eye (Uni-site, courtesy of Franel Optical Supply Co., Maitland, FL, USA)*

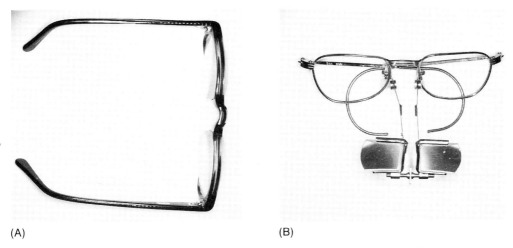

Fig. 19.18 *Orthoscopic spectacles. A, a pair of powerful positive lenses, prism base-in, fitted in a plastics frame. B, the front of the metal frame may be fitted with a correction; the distance between the prisms can be adjusted, and the prisms may be flipped up*

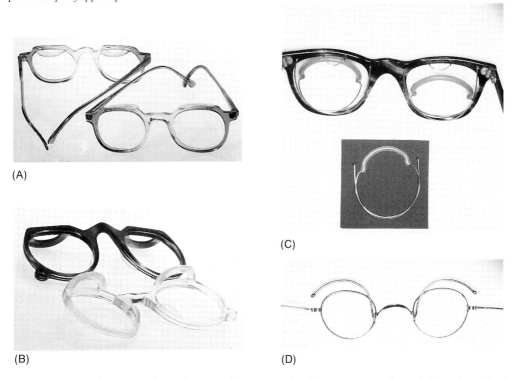

Fig. 19.19 *Ptosis frames. A, plastics frames with ptosis crutches (TS-1, courtesy of Franel Optical Supply Co. Maitland, FL, USA). B, plastics lorgnettes with ptosis crutches ('Earless', courtesy of Franel Optical Supply Co). C, the plastics frame shows a 'parked' (left) and a free 'floating' ptosis crutch fitted to the back of the front; below: an unattached floating crutch showing the silicone sleeve which will be in touch with the drooping eyelid (courtesy Maxian Optical Services, Glanrhyd, Ystradgynlais, Swansea, UK). D, a pair of conventional 'spring' crutches fitted to a metal frame*

short distance in front of the spectacle front. The centration distance of the prisms may be adjustable, and the prisms may also be flipped up (Fig. 19.18B).

- **Orthopaedic spectacles**   Spectacles fitted with attachments designed to relieve certain non-optical conditions, e.g. entropion and ptosis (BS 3521, 1991). See entropion and ptosis frames.

- **Pinhole spectacles**   Spectacles fitted with an opaque disc with a small aperture of the order of 1 or 2 mm before one or both eyes (BS 3521, 1991). See lochbrille, multiple pinhole spectacles.

- **Ptosis frames**   (ptosis: drooping of the upper eyelid) The front carries a gallery on the upper part of its back plane. The gallery runs parallel and at a distance from the back plane. It must exert enough force on the skin of the upper lid to raise it so that it clears the patient's pupil. When a gallery is fixed to the nasal and the temporal sides of the front, it is called a fixed gallery (Fig. 19.19). A 'spring gallery', often made of piano wire, is fixed only on the nasal side, its end usually being protected with a small ball (Fig. 19.19D). In view of the mechanics involved, it is wise first to get a frame with an optimum fit and adjust it fully. It is then easier to determine the position and length of the gallery. Instead of ptosis frames, ptosis contact lenses can be used. See entropion and orthopaedic spectacles. See also Moss (1982).

- **Quizzer**   A front to which a handle is attached (Fig. 19.20). Used briefly. See lorgnette.

- **Respirator spectacles**   See gas mask spectacles.

- **Reversible spectacles**   Spectacles which are designed to be worn with either lens before either eye (BS 3521, 1991) (Fig. 19.21). When a presbyopic patient is essentially monocular, the distance correction may be fitted in one rim of a front and the near correction in the other. Such fronts are fitted with a bridge that can be fitted on the nose in more than one way (swivelling W-bridge, X-bridge, fixed metal pad bridge). The sides may have joints than can rotate through 180° so that the front (glazed with flat lenses) may fit on the face back-to-front. Alternatively, the sides' butts may revolve so that the frame will fit upside down.

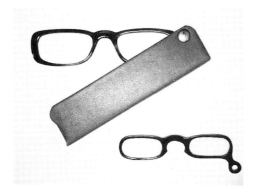

Fig. 19.20 Quizzers. The handle of the upper is its case. A ribbon which runs through the hole in the handle of the lower sample is attached to the wearer's clothing, thus preventing it from damage if dropped. See lorgnette

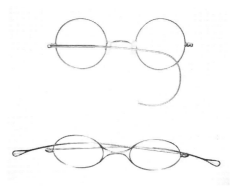

Fig. 19.21 Reversible spectacles: a frame with a X-bridge and loop-end sides (below) and a round eye frame with a bridge where the pads are placed vertically. The side has a hollow butt within which the remainder of the curl side can rotate

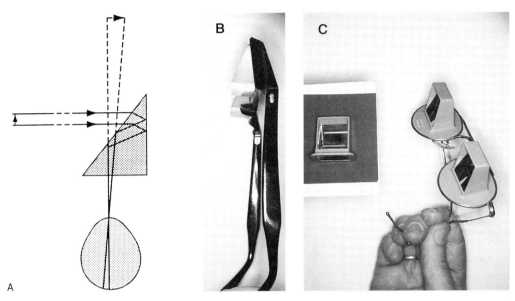

Fig. 19.22 *Recumbent spectacles. A, the patient lies on their back and looks at the ceiling. Diagram showing the manner in which the light rays from an object placed along a line parallel to the body of the wearer are rotated through 90° so that the object appears against the ceiling. B, an appliance with a pair of prisms. C, a metal frame with a pair of Hamblin prism holders; inset: view into a holder showing the prism (compare with Fig. 19.2C)*

- **Recumbent spectacles** These spectacles are primarily intended to enable a recumbent person to read in comfort by displacing the field of view (BS 3521, 1991) (Fig. 19.22). They may be used by bedridden patients to allow them to read without having to hold the reading matter above their head. They are fitted with either small reflecting prisms or with mirrors. An optical correction may be fitted between prism or mirror and the eye. The images produced by prisms may show coloured fringes owing to chromatic aberration (see Smith *et al.*, 1990). The front of the frame must be rigid and the optical components very carefully aligned to avoid diplopia. To cater for a variety of postures the front is usually fitted with joints or a device facilitating adjustment of the angle of the side.
- **Shooting spectacles** See special purpose spectacles, billiards spectacles, archery spectacles.

- **Snooker spectacles** See billiards and special purpose spectacles.
- **Special purpose spectacles** These spectacles are often of special shape and have lenses that are decentred or tilted to give suitable

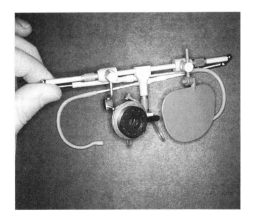

Fig. 19.23 *Special purpose spectacles. Note the diaphragm in front of the right lens, and the occluder on the left side*

centration for use in archery, billiards, shooting, etc., and for special occupations (BS 3521, 1991) (Fig. 19.23).

- **Spectacle magnifier**   This is a magnifier, in the form of spectacles, that is mounted or held close to the eye and designed to improve near vision (Fig. 19.24; BS 7522, 1993 and ANSI Z80.9, 1986).

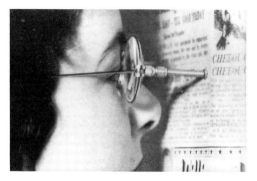

Fig. 19.24 *Spectacle magnifier. A spacer attached to the front keeps the reading matter at the required distance*

- **Sports frames**★   There are two basic models (Fig. 19.25). One has protective and corrective lenses fitted in the spectacle front (as in goggles). The other consists of a face plate covering both eyes, behind which corrective lenses have been fitted. The lenses may be

---

★While going to press, a draft document ISO/TC 172/ SC 7 N 228 had been published, entitled 'Ophthalmic optics – Spectacles with prescription lenses for use in sports – Safety requirements and testing' and based on DIN 5334 : 1993 – 11.

Fig. 19.25 *Sports frames. A, front with absorbing eye shield, the length of the side and the shape of the curl are adjustable; (below) insert with correction lenses. B, jointless polycarbonate frame with head strap and silicone saddle bridge insert. C, ski goggles with U.V. and visible radiation absorbing eye shield, air vents and head strap; inset: insert for correction lenses*

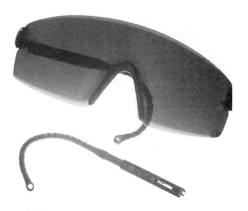

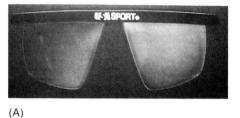

(A)

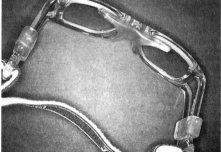
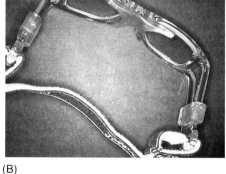

(B)

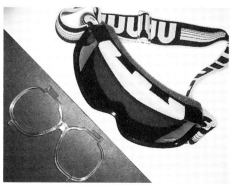

(C)

placed in a separate holder (resembling a front) which is connected to the frame, or they may be cemented to the back surface of the face plate. The latter construction is often used in diving or swimming goggles. Instead of conventional sides some sports frames have a strap that passes behind the head. Since the early 1980s eye injuries caused by sports have increased dramatically, often because many sportsmen do not realize the risks involved (Jones, 1987). For particular applications consult AS/NZS 4066 (1992), ASTM F803–3 (1983), BS EN 174 (1996), BS 4110 (1979), CSA P400-M (1982), CSA Z262.2 -M (1990), DIN 58 216 (1980) and Obstfeld & Pope (1995).

- **Stenopaeic spectacles** These spectacles are masked so as to permit vision only through a slit (BS 3521, 1991).

- **Swimming goggles** (surface) BS 5883 (1980) refers to goggles having individual cup-type lenses incorporating an eye seal, designed for surface swimming only (Fig. 19.26). BS

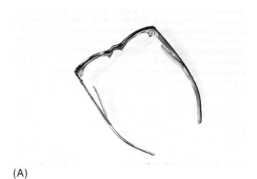

(A)

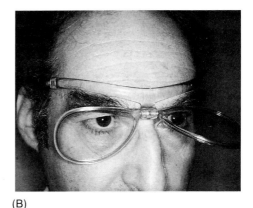

(B)

Fig. 19.27 Temple rest frames. A, this supra front has sides fitted with springs that press against the wearer's temples. B, each rim of this model can be rotated upwards, thus providing access to the eye; the sides surround the head

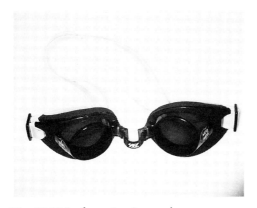

Fig. 19.26 Surface swimming goggles

5883 provides details about the lenses, eye seal, headstrap and bridge strap together with methods of test. See Obstfeld (1982) for technical aspects of vision under water.

- **Telemicroscope** See spectacle magnifier.

- **Temple rest frames** These are for patients who cannot tolerate pressure on the nose. There are no nasal bearing surfaces at all. Instead, spring-loaded flat pads are fitted on the inner surface of each side. During wear the pads press against the temples of the wearer (Fig. 19.27). The pressure should be adjusted to the minimum required to keep the front in the desired position. Therefore, the frames must be sturdy. See cheek rest frames (see also Fig. 18.1).

- **Trial frame** A spectacle frame with variable adjustments for the distance between the optical centres of the lenses, side length, crest height, etc. Each rim consists of one or more cells into which 'trial' lenses may be placed during a refraction (the process of measuring and correcting the refractive error of the eyes) (Fig. 21.1).

- **Trigeminal frames**   When a branch of the trigeminal nerve has been severed, the sensations of touch and heat will be lost to the eye. As a consequence, the blink reflex will be lost. To protect the eye from foreign bodies, etc., a shield is fitted which protrudes from the back plane of the front and fits snugly against the face (Fig. 19.28).
- **Vanity frames**   See make-up frames.

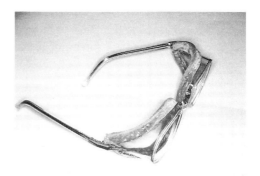

Fig. 19.28 *Trigeminal frames: the space in front of each eye is enclosed by a cup into which a lens can be fitted. In this appliance the rim touching the skin is lined with fabric*

REFERENCES

Anonymous (1993). Do minorities need special frames? *Optician* **205**(5387), 11.

ANSI Z87.1 (1989). *American National Standard Practice for Occupational and Educational Eye and Face Protection.* New York: American National Standards Institute, Inc.

ANSI Z80.9 (1986). *American National Standards for Ophthalmics – low vision aids.* New York: American National Standards Institute, Inc.

AS/NZS 4066 (1992). *Eye Protection in Racquet Sports.* Homebush (NSW), Wellington: Standards Association of Australia.

ASTM Standard F803-3 (1983). *Standard Specification for Eye Protectors for Use by Players of Racquet Sports.* Philadelphia: American Society for the Testing of Materials.

Band, C. (1991). See hear! A review of hearing-aid spectacles. *Optician* **201**(5296), 27–30.

BS 3521 (1991). *Terms Relating to Ophthalmic Optics and Spectacle Frames. Part 1: Glossary of Terms Relating to Ophthalmic Lenses.* London: British Standards Institution.

BS 3521 (1991). *Terms Relating to Ophthalmic Optics and Spectacle Frames. Part 2: Glossary of Terms Relating to Spectacle Frames.* London: British Standards Institution.

BS 4110 (1979). *Specification for Eye-protectors for Vehicle Users.* London: British Standards Institution.

BS 4532 (1969). *Specification for Snorkels and Face Masks.* London: British Standards Institution.

BS 5883 (1980). *Specification for Surface Swimming Goggles.* London: British Standards Institution.

BS 7028 (1988). *Guide for Selection, Use and Maintenance of Eye-protection for Industrial and Other Uses.* London: British Standards Institution.

BS 7522 (1993). *Low Vision Aids. Part 2: Specification for Spectacle Magnifiers and Similar Devices.* London: British Standards Institution.

BS EN 136 (1992). *Part 10: Specification for Full Face Mask for Respiratory Protective Devices.* London: British Standards Institution.

BS EN 165 (1995). *Personal Eye Protection – Vocabulary.* London: British Standards Institution.

BS EN 166 (1995). *Personal Eye Protection – Specification.* London: British Standards Institution.

BS EN 167 (1995). *Personal Eye Protection – Optical Test Methods.* London: British Standards Institution.

BS EN 168 (1995)/ISO 4855 (1981). *Personal Eye Protection – Non-optical Test Methods.* London: British Standards Institution.

BS EN 174 (1996). *Personal Eye Protection – Ski Goggles for Downhill Skiing.* London: British Standards Institution.

Cooper, M.D. (1993). Letter to the Editor: Different fit, different view. *Optician* **205**(5388), 14.

CSA P400-M (1982). *Racquet Sports Eye Protection.* Ottawa (Ont.): Canadian Standards Association.

CSA 294.3 (1992). *Industrial Eye and Face Protections.* (National Standards). Ottawa (Ont.): Canadian Standards Association.

CSA Z262.2-M (1990). *Face Protector and Visors for Ice Hockey Players.* Ottawa (Ont.): Canadian Standards Association.

DeHaan, W.V. (1982). *Optometrist's and Ophthalmologist's Guide to Pilot's Vision*, p. 157. Boulder, CO: American Trend Publ. Co.

DIN 58 216 (1980). *Brillen für Fahrzeugführer, Teil 1.* Berlin: Deutsches Institut für Normung.

Duszynski, L.R. (1955). Hemianopsia dichroic mirror device. *Am. J. Ophthal.* **39**(6), 876–878.

Forbes, P.L. (1984). Dispensing to the hard of hearing. *Ophthal. Optician* **24**, 398–399.

Jones, N.P. (1987). Eye injuries in sport: an increasing problem. *Br. J. Sports Med.* **21**, 168–170.

Kono (1952). *Rare Visual Aids.* Woodside, NY: Kono Manufacturing Co.

Kunze, O. (1959). Die Zeiss-Kyphosenbrille als Korrektionsmittel bei Wirbelsäulenversteifung. *Mschr. Feinmech. Opt., Köln*, **76**(6), 187–188.

MacEwen, C.J. (1989). Eye injuries: a prospective survey of 5671 cases. *Br. J. Ophthal.* **73**, 888–894.

Margrain, T.H. & Owen, L. (1996). The misting characteristics of spectacle lenses. *Ophthal. Physiol. Optics* **16**(2), 108–114.

Mehr, E.B. & Freid, A.N. (1975). *Low Vision Care.* Chicago: Professional Press.

Mintz, M.J. (1979). A mirror for hemianopia. *Am. J. Ophthal.* **88**(4), 768.

Moss, H.L. (1982). Prosthesis for blepharoptosis and blepharospasm. *J. Am. Optom. Ass.* **53**(8), 661–667.

Müller, K. (1962a). Brillen. Versuch einer umfassenden Darstellung aller Arten und Formen. *Augenoptiker* (6), 30–31.

Müller, K. (1962b). Brillen. Versuch einer umfassenden Darstellung aller Arten und Formen. *Augenoptiker* (10), 28–29.

Müller, K. (1963a). Brillen. Versuch einer umfassenden Darstellung aller Arten und Formen. *Augenoptiker* (2), 18–20.

Müller, K. (1963b). Brillen. Versuch einer umfassenden Darstellung aller Arten und Formen. *Augenoptiker* (4), 24–26.

Müller, K. (1963c). Brillen. Versuch einer umfassenden Darstellung aller Arten und Formen. *Augenoptike* (7), 22–23.

Müller, K. (1963d). Brillen. Versuch einer umfassenden Darstellung aller Arten und Formen. *Augenoptiker* (12), 30–32.

Müller, K. (1964a). Brillen. Versuch einer umfassenden Darstellung aller Arten und Formen. *Augenoptiker* (4), 18–19.

Müller, K. (1964b). Brillen. Versuch einer umfassenden Darstellung aller Arten und Formen. *Augenoptiker* (9), 54–55.

Müller, K. (1964c). Brillen. Versuch einer umfassenden Darstellung aller Arten und Formen. *Augenoptiker* (12), 50.

Müller, K. (1965a). Brillen. Versuch einer umfassenden Darstellung aller Arten und Formen. *Augenoptiker* (4) 44.

Müller, K. (1965b). Brillen. Versuch einer umfassenden Darstellung aller Arten und Formen. *Augenoptiker* (9), 56–58.

Obstfeld, H. (1982). Vision under water, Ch. 21. In: *Optics in Vision*, 2nd edn. London: Butterworths.

Obstfeld, H. & Pope, R. (1995). Spectacle correction of sports vision, pp. 117–127. In: Loran, D.F.C. & MacEwen, C.J. (eds) *Sports Vision*. Oxford: Butterworth–Heinemann.

Phillips, A.J. & Rutstein, A. (1967). Amber night driving spectacles. *Br. J. Physiol. Optics* **24**(3), 161–205.

Richer, S.P. & Hall, T. (1986). Mobility spectacles for a patient with ankylosing spondylitis. *Am. J. Optom. Physiol. Optics* **63**(11), 927–930.

Rossi, A. (1995). Flying high. *Optician* **210**(5515), 20–22.

Smith, G., Johnston, A.W. & Maddocks, J.D. (1990). The NAP prism. *Optom. & Vis Sci.* **67**(2), 133–137.

Springer, D.A. (1970). Custom modification of a frame to allow a patient with cancer of the nose to comfortably wear spectacles – a case report. *Am. J. Optom. Arch. Am. Acad. Optom.* **47**(10), 798–800.

Stem, M.A. & Scott, G.J.T. (1993). *A Pilot Study of Protective Spectacles for Hay Fever Sufferers.* Report of Asthma and Allergy Research Unit, Leicester General Hospital, UK.

Stobbe, T.J., Da Roza, R.A. & Watkins, M.A. (1988). Facial hair and respirator fit: a review of the literature. *Am. Ind. Hyg. Ass. J.* **49**, 199–204.

Villani, S. (1977). Domande del lettore. *Luce e immagini, Firenze* **31**(1), 2–3.

Weiss, N. J. (1990). An unusual application of prisms for field enhancement. *J. Am. Optom. Assoc.* **61**(4), 291–293.

Woods, D.R. & Haycock, A. (1994). Evaluation of a mechanical, non-drug, device (airshield [TM] spectacles) for the prevention of hay fever symptoms. In: *The Health Report*, Issue 1, Jan. Auckland (NZ): Health Consultancy Group Ltd.

CHAPTER 20

Vertex Distance

20.1 Introduction

The distance between the visual point of a lens (the point where the visual axis of the patient's eye intersects the back surface of the correcting spectacle lens) and the corneal apex is called the vertex distance (BS 3521, Part 1, 1991). It is frequently incorrectly referred to as the back vertex distance: because there is no such thing as a front vertex distance, the word 'back' is redundant.

The vertex distance should be measured along the visual axis. The radius of curvature of the back surface of the spectacle lens is normally much longer than the distance from distance visual point to the centre of rotation of the eye (Fig. 20.1). Hence, the vertex distance for distance vision is usually smaller than that for near vision. As a result of a change in effectivity at the corneal vertex of the incident vergence, some apparent accommodation may be experienced, but only for more extreme spectacle lens powers.

A vertex distance should be stated on a prescription if a meridional power exceeds 5.00 D

(BS 3521, Part 3, 1991). The reason for this requirement appears to be the following. If such a prescription were to be used for contact lenses where the vertex distance reduces, for all practical purposes, to nil, the back vertex power of the contact lens will have to differ from that of the spectacle lens to provide an optimum correction. If a 5.00 D spectacle lens corrects an eye at a vertex distance of 10 mm, the power of a contact lens will have to differ from that power by 0.25 D. When the vertex distance is reduced, positive spectacle lenses will have to be increased in power, and negative lenses decreased. This is in order to satisfy the requirement for clear distance vision: the second principal focus of the spectacle lens should coincide with the far point of the eye (Fig. 20.2). For astigmatic eyes, each of the two far points requires a second focal point of the spectacle lens to coincides with it; hence, the reference to a meridional power. In near vision, the image point produced by the spectacle lens of a near object point must conjugate with the retina by means of some intermediate point such as the

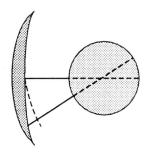

Fig. 20.1 The vertex distance varies with the direction of gaze

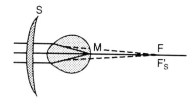

Fig. 20.2 An ametropic eye will be corrected for distance vision when the second principal focus F'_s of the spectacle lens S coincides with the far point F of the eye, because far point and macula M of the eye are conjugate points

near point. Note that the greater the spectacle lens power, the greater the importance of the vertex distance because of the greater change in effectivity of that lens at the corneal vertex, for the same change in vertex distance. (For a detailed treatment of these aspects, see for instance Obstfeld, 1982, Chapters 9, 14 and 16).

20.2 Measuring the Vertex Distance

A parameter that increases in importance the more powerful a lens is, is its sagitta, or 'sag'. If this were ignored, the vertex distance may be several millimetres longer than anticipated. Any calculation will then be based on an inaccurate starting point and will lead to an inaccurate result. This problem may be solved in a variety of ways that vary in accuracy.

One can calculate the sag of a lens provided that the back surface radius can be established and the cord of the sag, which could be assumed to be equal to the lens size of the front, is known. If the previous correcting lens for that eye had the same power or was of similar power, one can try to estimate the sag of the old lens with a rule or measure it with a depth gauge. Table 20.1 provides the sags for a series of back surface powers, as measured with a lens measure (*lens clock*), for different refractive indices. This Table makes it possible to estimate the sag from the lens measure reading and the horizontal lens size (or diameter). By adding this value to the distance measured between cornea and back plane of the front, the approximate vertex distance can be determined.

TABLE 20.1 Sagitta (sag) depth (mm) for various refractive indices and diameters

Lens measure/ surface power (D)	Diameter (mm; $n = 1.490$)			Diameter (mm; $n = 1.523$)			Diameter (mm; $n = 1.56$)			Diameter (mm; $n = 1.6$)			Diameter (mm; $n = 1.7$)			Diameter (mm; $n = 1.8$)			Diameter (mm; $n = 1.9$)		
	40	50	60	40	50	60	40	50	60	40	50	60	40	50	60	40	50	60	40	50	60
1	0	1	1	0	1	1	0	1	1	0	1	1	0	0	1	0	0	1	0	0	1
2	1	1	2	1	1	2	1	1	2	1	1	2	1	1	1	1	1	1	0	1	1
3	1	2	3	1	2	3	1	2	2	1	2	2	1	1	2	1	1	2	1	1	2
4	2	3	4	2	2	3	1	2	3	1	2	3	1	2	3	1	2	2	1	1	2
5	2	3	5	2	3	4	2	3	4	2	3	4	1	2	3	1	2	3	1	2	3
6	2	4	6	2	4	5	2	3	5	2	3	5	2	3	4	2	2	3	1	2	3
7	3	5	7	3	4	6	3	4	6	2	4	5	2	3	5	2	3	4	2	2	4
8	3	5	8	3	5	7	3	5	7	3	4	6	2	4	5	2	3	5	2	3	4
9	4	6	9	4	6	8	3	5	8	3	5	7	3	4	6	2	4	5	2	3	5
10	4	7	10	4	6	9	4	6	9	3	5	8	3	5	7	3	4	6	2	4	5
11	5	8	12	4	7	11	4	7	10	4	6	9	3	5	8	3	4	6	2	4	6
12	5	9	13	5	8	12	5	7	11	4	7	10	4	6	8	3	5	7	3	4	6
13	6	9	15	5	9	13	5	8	12	5	7	11	4	6	9	3	5	8	3	5	7
14	6	11	17	6	10	15	5	9	14	5	8	12	4	7	10	4	6	9	3	5	7
15	7	12	20	6	11	17	6	10	15	5	9	14	5	7	11	4	6	9	3	5	8
16	7	13	24	7	12	20	6	11	17	6	10	15	5	8	12	4	7	10	4	6	9
17	8	14	–	7	13	24	7	11	19	6	10	17	5	8	13	4	7	11	4	6	9
18	9	16	–	8	14	–	7	13	23	7	11	19	6	9	14	5	8	12	4	7	10
19	10	19	–	9	16	–	8	14	–	7	12	22	6	10	15	5	8	13	4	7	11
20	10	–	–	9	18	–	8	15	–	8	13	30	6	11	17	5	9	14	5	8	11

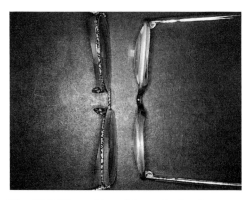

Fig. 20.3 *The position of the peak of a glazed lens bevel affects the vertex distance. Left front: BE −9.50 D. The peak of the upper lens bevel is placed too close to the front surface. This makes for a shorter vertex distance than that of the lower lens where the peak is placed too close to the centre of the bevel. Right front: BE +8.25 D. Upper lens protrudes as a result of incorrect glazing*

Although one can specify the base curve of the new lens, a difference may occur as a result of edging: will the bevel be placed closer or further from the back vertex than in the old lens? (See Fig. 20.3.)

To measure the vertex distance of a glazed front, determine the distance from the *front* vertex of the spectacle lens to the corneal apex and reduce it by the centre thickness of the lens (Fig. 20.4).

Henker (1924) pointed out that it is not possible to measure the vertex distance accurately with a simple millimetre rule and the dispenser's eye (Fig. 20.5). To avoid a parallax error, the dispenser's eye must move to the second sighting position, over a distance equal to the unknown vertex distance. The vertex distance scale mounted on some trial frames (Fig. 20.6) would require such a movement. However, one can try

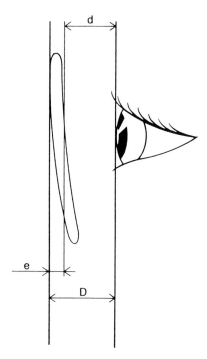

Fig. 20.4 *A practical way of measuring the vertex distance d of a glazed lens: measure the distance D between the lens' front surface and cornea, and subtract the centre thickness e. (Diagram courtesy of Essilor Ltd)*

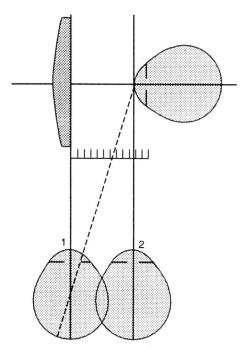

Fig. 20.5 *To measure the vertex distance accurately with a millimetre rule, the dispenser's eye must be moved between positions 1 and 2, in order to avoid parallax*

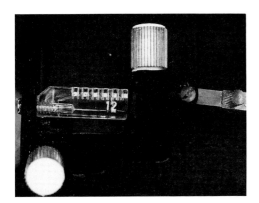

Fig. 20.6 *The vertex distance measuring scale of a trial frame*

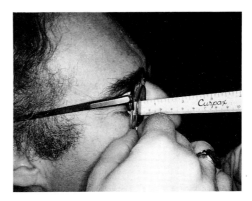

Fig. 20.7 *A millimetre rule is passed through a vertical slit in a piece of cardboard (stenopaiec slit). The slit is held against the empty front of the frame and the rule touches the patient's closed eyelid. The rule shows a measurement of 12 mm, so the vertex distance will be 14 mm; no account is taken of the position and thickness of the actual spectacle lens*

to reduce this error by moving one's eye a centimetre or so.

A more accurate method is to use a stenopaeic slit and a millimetre rule. The disc containing the slit may be held against the front of the spectacle frame selected for the patient. Having instructed the patient to close his eye and to expect his eyelid to be touched, pass the rule through the slit and read off how far the rule has moved beyond the disc at the point where it touches the eyelid (Fig. 20.7). Add a 2 mm allowance for the lid thickness and make a further allowance if the beginning of

the rule does not coincide with the zero of its scale. Allow also for the sag of the lens and for the increased vertex distance, if the spectacles will be used mainly for near vision, as discussed above.

The Wessely keratometer (Fig. 20.8) was designed by Professor Karl Wessely (1874–1953; professor of ophthalmology at Munich) to measure the diameter of the cornea and pupil. It can also be used to measure the vertex distance

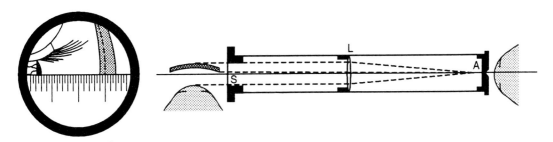

Fig. 20.8 *The Wessely keratometer. The ray diagram shows how rays from the spectacle lens and corneal apex pass through a semi-circular aperture S situated above a millimetre scale (see inset). Having been refracted by the lens L the rays pass through the pinhole at A (magnification ×2.5). Inset: the distance between the cornea (left) and the front surface of the lens measures 14 mm. Allow for the centre thickness of the lens to obtain the vertex distance. (Diagrams by permission of* Optician)

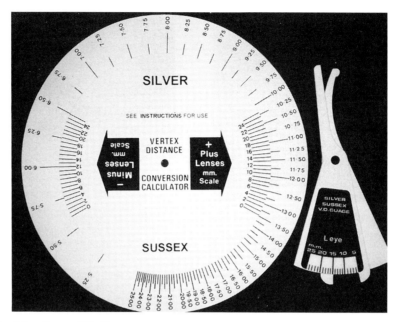

Fig. 20.9 *The Silver/Sussex VD Gauge*

(Anonymous, 1957). Its optical principle is that of a telecentric system. It consists of a millimetre scale situated approximately in the focal plane of the lens. The rays from the scale, the corneal vertex and the edge of the spectacle lens or the rim of the spectacle front will all be seen clearly through the use of a pinhole.

The Rayner Vertex Distance Measuring Set (*distometer*) is an instrument which is placed between spectacle lens or front and eyelid, the eye having been closed beforehand. When the button is pressed, a small arm moves towards the eyelid. On reaching the eyelid, the button is released and retracted while the cursor remains stationary on the scale. Allow for the eyelid thickness (2 mm). A vertex power converter is provided as part of the set; this is a disc-shaped nomogram which gives the power change resulting from a change in vertex distance. A similar device, the Silver/Sussex VD Gauge, is marketed by Sussex Vision (1994) (Fig. 20.9).

Obal (1949) designed a combined vertex and sag meter. In the 1970s the German company

Oculus marketed a set of parallax-free corneal vertex distance gauges, suitable for use in trial frame or glazed spectacles.

There are a number of pupillary distance (PD) rules and larger PD measuring devices that can also be used to measure the vertex distance. These include the Essilor Reflection Pupillometer (Fig. 20.10) and the Rodenstock Reiner Interpupillary Gauge (see Section 21.3.3; Fig. 21.6). Steel & Walsh (1994) described how, by adding a millimetre grid and a pointer, a slitlamp can be used to measure the vertex distance including the sagitta. By focusing at the back surface of the spectacle lens and the front surface of the cornea, they achieved an accuracy of ± 0.5 mm.

20.3 Calculations

The sag may be calculated from the equation

$$s = r - (r^2 - y^2)^{1/2}$$

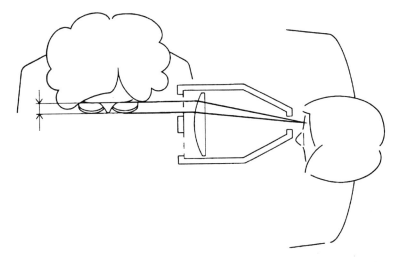

Fig. 20.10 *The Essilor Reflection Pupillometer can also be used to measure the vertex distance (diagram courtesy of Essilor Ltd)*

where s = sag, r = radius of curvature of the lens' back surface and y = half the length of the cord, all expressed in millimetres (Fig. 20.11). See Table 20.1.

A simple way to calculate the power of a correcting lens when the vertex distance has (to be) changed is as follows:

(1) Start with sign and (meridional) power of lens (D),

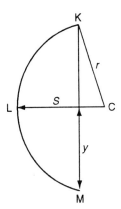

Fig. 20.11 *The relationship between the sag s of the curved surface KLM, the radius of curvature r and the half-cord y. C is the centre of curvature of the surface*

(2) calculate its focal length (mm),
(3) subtract vertex distance change if *vertex* distance is reduced; add *change* if it is increased (allow for sign of focal length); value obtained is new focal length,
(4) calculate (meridional) power of lens (D).

If the lens is astigmatic, repeat the above for the second meridional power.

- **Example 1** A $-15{\cdot}00$ DS trial case lens corrects an eye at 15 mm. It can be fitted at a vertex distance of 10 mm, in a carefully chosen spectacle frame. The required back vertex power may be calculated thus:

(1) trial case lens power	$-15{\cdot}00$ D
(2) focal length	$-66{\cdot}67$ mm
(3) reduction in vertex distance: subtract	5 mm
new focal length	$-71{\cdot}67$ mm
(4) theoretical back vertex power	$-13{\cdot}95$ D
practical lens power	-14.00 D

- **Example 2** A patient corrected by a -15.00 DS at 10 mm in his present frame,

Spectacle frames and their dispensing

TABLE 20.2 Changes in power for variations in vertex distance

Substitute the power below if a plus lens is moved **FURTHER** or a minus lens is moved **NEARER** by (mm)						Power at original position	Substitute the power below if a plus lens is moved **NEARER** or a minus lens is moved **FURTHER** by (mm)					
6	5	4	3	2	1	position	1	2	3	4	5	6
4·85	4·88	4·90	4·93	4·95	4·98	5·00	5·03	5·05	5·08	5·10	5·13	5·15
5·32	5·35	5·38	5·41	5·44	5·47	5·50	5·53	5·56	5·59	5·62	5·66	5·69
5·79	5·83	5·86	5·89	5·93	5·96	6·00	6·04	6·07	6·11	6·15	6·19	6·22
6·26	6·30	6·34	6·38	6·42	6·46	6·50	6·54	6·59	6·63	6·67	6·72	6·76
6·72	6·76	6·81	6·86	6·90	6·95	7·00	7·05	7·10	7·15	7·20	7·25	7·31
7·18	7·23	7·28	7·33	7·39	7·44	7·50	7·56	7·61	7·67	7·73	7·79	7·85
7·63	7·69	7·75	7·81	7·87	7·94	8·00	8·06	8·13	8·20	8·26	8·33	8·40
8·09	8·15	8·22	8·29	8·36	8·43	8·50	8·57	8·65	8·72	8·80	8·88	8·96
8·54	8·61	8·69	8·76	8·84	8·92	9·00	9·08	9·17	9·25	9·34	9·42	9·51
8·99	9·07	9·15	9·24	9·32	9·41	9·50	9·59	9·68	9·78	9·88	9·97	10·07
9·43	9·52	9·62	9·71	9·80	9·90	10·00	10·10	10·20	10·31	10·41	10·53	10·64
9·88	9·98	10·08	10·18	10·28	10·39	10·50	10·61	10·73	10·84	10·96	11·08	11·21
10·32	10·43	10·54	10·65	10·76	10·88	11·00	11·12	11·25	11·38	11·51	11·64	11·78
10·76	10·87	10·99	11·12	11·24	11·37	11·50	11·63	11·77	11·91	12·05	12·20	12·35
11·19	11·32	11·45	11·58	11·72	11·86	12·00	12·15	12·30	12·45	12·61	12·77	12·93
11·63	11·76	11·90	12·05	12·20	12·35	12·50	12·66	12·82	12·99	13·16	13·33	13·51
12·06	12·21	12·36	12·51	12·67	12·83	13·00	13·17	13·35	13·53	13·71	13·90	14·10
12·49	12·65	12·81	12·97	13·15	13·32	13·50	13·68	13·87	14·07	14·27	14·48	14·69
12·92	13·08	13·26	13·44	13·62	13·81	14·00	14·20	14·40	14·61	14·83	15·05	15·28
13·34	13·52	13·71	13·90	14·09	14·29	14·50	14·71	14·93	15·16	15·39	15·63	15·88
13·76	13·95	14·15	14·35	14·56	14·78	15·00	15·23	15·46	15·71	15·96	16·22	16·48
14·18	14·39	14·60	14·81	15·03	15·26	15·50	15·74	16·00	16·26	16·52	16·80	17·09
14·60	14·81	15·04	15·27	15·50	15·75	16·00	16·26	16·53	16·81	17·09	17·39	17·70
15·01	15·24	15·48	15·72	15·97	16·23	16·50	16·78	17·06	17·36	17·67	17·98	18·31
15·43	15·67	15·92	16·18	16·44	16·72	17·00	17·29	17·60	17·91	18·24	18·58	18·93
15·84	16·09	16·36	16·63	16·91	17·20	17·50	17·81	18·13	18·47	18·82	19·18	19·55
16·25	16·51	16·79	17·08	17·37	17·68	18·00	18·33	18·67	19·03	19·40	19·78	20·18
16·65	16·93	17·23	17·53	17·84	18·16	18·50	18·85	19·21	19·59	19·98	20·39	20·81
17·06	17·35	17·66	17·98	18·30	18·65	19·00	19·37	19·75	20·15	20·56	20·99	21·44
17·46	17·77	18·09	18·43	18·77	19·13	19·50	19·89	20·29	20·71	21·15	21·61	22·08
17·86	18·18	18·52	18·87	19·23	19·61	20·00	20·41	20·83	21·28	21·74	22·22	22·73
18·25	18·59	18·95	19·31	19·69	20·09	20·50	20·93	21·38	21·84	22·33	22·84	23·38
18·65	19·00	19·37	19·76	20·15	20·57	21·00	21·45	21·92	22·41	22·93	23·46	24·03
19·04	19·41	19·80	20·20	20·61	21·05	21·50	21·97	22·47	22·98	23·52	24·09	24·68
19·43	19·82	20·22	20·64	21·07	21·53	22·00	22·49	23·01	23·55	24·12	24·72	25·35
20·21	20·63	21·06	21·52	21·99	22·48	23·00	23·54	24·11	24·70	25·33	25·99	26·68
20·98	21·43	21·90	22·39	22·90	23·44	24·00	24·59	25·21	25·86	26·55	27·27	28·04

desires a larger frame. As a result the vertex distance will increase to 15 mm. The dispenser wants to make the patient aware of the increased lens power required. His calculation runs as follows:

(1) present lens power	−15.00 D	
(2) focal length	−66.67 mm	
(3) increase in vertex distance: add	5 mm	
new focal length	−61·67 mm	

(4) theoretical back vertex power −16·21 D
practical lens power −16·25 D

Table 20.2 gives the changed (meridional) power of the lens based on a change in vertex distance. Similar tables, or tables giving the change per dioptre, have been provided by Zeiss (1963), Fleck *et al.* (1970) and Griffiths (1994).

REFERENCES

Anonymous (1957). A new optical measuring instrument. *Optician* **134** (3471), 325–326.

BS 3521 (1991). *Terms Relating to Ophthalmic Optics and Spectacle Frames. Part 1: Glossary of Terms Relating to Ophthalmic Lenses and Spectacle Frames.* London: British Standards Institution.

BS 3521 (1991). *Terms Relating to Ophthalmic Optics and Spectacle Frames. Part 3: Specification for the Presentation of Prescriptions and Prescription Orders for Ophthalmic Lenses.* London: British Standards Institution.

Fleck, H., Heynig, J., Mütze, K. & Schwarz, G. (1970). *Sehhilfenanpassung.* Berlin: VEB Verlag Technik, p. 106.

Griffiths, A.I. (1994). *Practical dispensing,* p. 170. London: Assoc. British Dispensing Opticians.

Henker, O. (1924). *Introduction to the Theory of Spectacles* p. 79. Jena: School of Optics.

Obal, A. (1949). Gerät zur Messung der Hornhautscheitel – Glas – Distanz. *Bericht deutsch. Ophthalm. Ges.* **55**, 384–388.

Obstfeld, H. (1982). *Optics in Vision,* 2nd edn. London: Butterworths.

Steel, S.E. & Walsh, G. (1994). Use of a slit lamp to measure back vertex distance. *Ophthalm. physiol. Optics* **14**(2), 213–215.

Sussex Vision (1994). Vertex distance gauge & conversion disc. Lancing, W. Sussex, UK: Sussex Vision (brochure).

Zeiss, C. (1963). *Handbuch für Augenoptik,* pp. 50–54. Oberkochen: Zeiss.

CHAPTER 21

PD – Measurement and Centration Distances

21.1 Distance PD/Distance CD

21.1.1 INTRODUCTION

The pupillary distance, more properly described as the interpupillary distance, may be defined as the distance between the centres of the pupils of a pair of eyes. For practical reasons, it is usually measured in the plane of the spectacle frame while the eyes fixate a distant object at eye level. This measurement is denoted 'distance PD', or more frequently, just PD. The monocular PD (MPD) is the distance between the midline of the nose and the right or the left pupil centre. If the MPDs are unequal each recorded measurement must be preceded by 'right' or 'left'.

The centration distance (CD) is defined as the specified horizontal distance between the right and left centration point (BS 3521, Part 1, 1991). The latter is the point where the optical centre is to be located (BS 3521, Part 1, 1991). The monocular centration distance (MCD) must be specified for each lens if the MCDs are unequal. This is of particular importance for high-powered and progressive power lenses (Section 21.1.2).

Before discussing further details, some reference lines associated with the eye must be defined (Fig. 21.1):

(1) Optical axis: the imaginary line joining the centres of curvature of the refracting surfaces of the eye.

(2) Visual axis: the imaginary line joining the object of regard and the foveola of the eye's retina, and passing through the nodal points of its optical system. Because the nodal points lie very closely together (Obstfeld, 1982), they may be considered as coincident for the present purposes.

(3) Pupillary axis: the imaginary line passing through the centre of the (entrance) pupil of the eye, perpendicular to the surface of the cornea.

The angle between the optical and visual axes is denoted 'angle α' (Fig. 21.1). It commonly

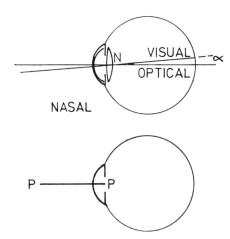

Fig. 21.1 *Above: a horizontal section through a diagrammatic human eye showing the visual and optical axes and also the angle a situated between these axes; N, nodal point. Below: P–P, pupillary axis which passes through the pupil centre*

subtends 5° (Millodot, 1990). The visual axis lies usually to the nasal side of the optical axis; its value is then preceded by a positive sign. It is given a negative sign if the visual axis lies on the temporal side of the optical axis. The two axes need not lie in a horizontal plane.

Because the visual axes of a pair of eyes fixating a distant object at eye level may be assumed to lie parallel, their distance, whether measured in the spectacle plane, pupillary plane or at the centres of rotation of the eyes, will be a constant for a given person. This is of relevance for the centration distance of glazed lenses (Sections 21.13 and 21.14).

21.1.2 REASONS FOR CENTRING LENSES
The reasons for measuring and recording the PD are as follows. Under normal conditions, a corrected ametropic eye while directed at a distant object at eye level, may be considered to form a centred optical system with insignificant image and chromatic aberrations. Such a system has a common axis, that is, the visual axis and the optical axis of the spectacle lens or of the correcting lens system coincide. Therefore, the position of the visual axis, and that of the optical centre of the lens (system) must be determined carefully in order to be able to approximate to such a centred system.

If an eye does not look through the optical centre of its spectacle lens, rays of light reach it after prismatic deviation. This has the effect of apparently displacing the object of regard.

Because the eyes are seldom stationary the status of the 'centre of rotation' of the eye must be considered. Following research by Fry & Hill (1962), whose findings agree with Emsley's (1955), the centre of rotation is commonly accepted to be situated about 15 mm behind the corneal vertex and 1.5 mm nasally to the line of sight. The latter is the imaginary line joining the observed object and the centre of the pupil.

The centre of rotation should lie on the axis of the centred system when the eye occupies the primary position, that is, when both eyes are directed at a distant object situated on the midline of the eyes at eye level, and the head is held erect. If one now measures the PD, it is assumed to represent the distance between the centres of rotation of the eyes. A critical review and comment was written by Riedl (1991).

Conventional 'best form' spectacle lenses whose curvatures are computed to eliminate or minimize a stated image defect or defects under defined conditions (BS 3521, Part 1, 1991), have been designed on the basis of a notional distance of 25 mm or so between the centre of rotation of the eye and the back vertex of the lens.

Under conditions of binocular vision, when the eyes are rotated together to observe an object, the relationship between the two centres of rotation of a pair of corrected, ametropic eyes becomes important. From a practical point of view, one should be concerned about the absence or presence of prismatic power (defined as the measure of the deviation of a ray of light as a result of passing through a specified point on a lens or prism; BS 3521, Part 1, 1991). This is absent only when an eye's visual axis passes through the optical centre of a lens. Hence, this is the most desirable arrangement (Villani, 1971; Joseph, 1982). In the majority of cases prescriptions for spectacles stipulate such an arrangement, although it is sometimes a matter of inference, as is demonstrated by the quote that follows the definition of centration distance (BS 3521, Part 1, 1991): 'NOTE. If an inter-pupillary distance only is stated this is taken to be the centration distance'. However, if a certain amount of prismatic power is required, it is usually specified with respect to the PD which must be known anyway.

Prentice (1890) taught that the prismatic power of a lens is directly proportional to its power and the (horizontal) distance between its optical centre and the pupil centre. Unprescribed horizontal prismatic power, prism base-out (requiring convergence of the visual axes) gives much less frequent cause for complaints than prism base-in (which requires divergence). An unprescribed vertical prismatic difference of as little as one prism dioptre may lead to difficulties with binocular vision. The vertical centration of anisometropic prescriptions and of pairs of powerful spectacle lenses is therefore important.

21.2 Measuring the Distance PD

Methods of measuring the PD may be divided into objective and subjective methods. The former are more frequently used. Subjective measurements require cooperation of the patient who needs to make accurate observations. This requires explanation by the practitioner which may be misunderstood. Furthermore, the patient may not be successful in completing the task, resulting in an erroneous result. Because subjective PD measurements can also be time consuming, practitioners tend not to employ them.

The practitioner has a number of options when measuring the PD objectively (Fig. 21.2). He can attempt to locate the pupil centres visually and measure the distance between them. If the pupils are not irregularly shaped, and the borders between pupils and irides are clearly visible, this method can be successfully employed. Because the centre of the apparently black pupil is not a 'landmark', its position can only be estimated. It is frequently more satisfactory to measure from the edge of one pupil to the corresponding edge of the other (for instance, from 'nine o'clock' in

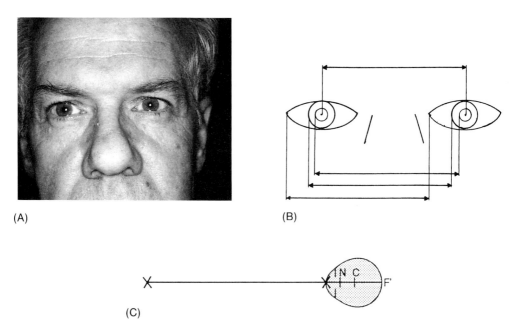

(A)

(B)

(C)

Fig. 21.2 *A, the photograph illustrates the options available to the practitioner to determine the patient's PD: B, (distances from below to above) between corresponding points on the canthi, iris (limbal) borders, pupil borders and between the catoptric images; C, the light source X is, to the dispenser/onlooker, imaged as x in the cornea when the foveola F' is directed at the light source – the centre of rotation C and nodal point N lie also on the imaginary line connecting the aforementioned points*

one eye to 'nine o'clock' in the other). However, when the irides are heavily pigmented, it can be practically impossible to determine the positions of the pupil edges. Because irides are seldom irregularly shaped, many practitioners measure from one outer iris edge (limbus) to the corresponding edge of the other. Another approach is based on the fact that the average horizontal diameter of the limbus measures 11 mm; the distance between the inner edges of the right and left limbus can be measured, and 11 mm added. This, too, will give the distance between the pupil centres. Better still, add only 9 mm, and this will give approximately the visual axes distance (see Section 21.3.3). This method may also be used when pupils are irregularly shaped or unequal in size. With respect to the latter, Sasieni (1962) suggested taking the mean of two measurements, namely of the distance between the right hand pupil edges and the left hand pupil edges.

If the patient is uncooperative (for instance, a child), or the eyes have a squint, one may have to resort to measuring the distance between the outer canthus of one (closed) eye and the inner canthus of the other (Fig. 21.3). Alternatively, one can measure the distance between the catoptric images.

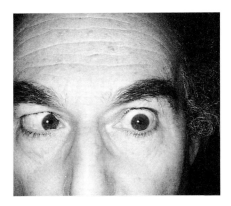

Fig. 21.3 *In the case of a squint the PD may be taken as the distance between the corresponding points of the canthi or the distance between the catoptric images*

Von Haugwitz (1981) and Hutchinson (1984) review the development of early instrumentation back to about 1880.

21.3 Objective Methods of Measuring the Distance PD

21.3.1 INTRODUCTION
Because it is not practical to measure the PD in the plane of the pupils themselves, the measurement is usually taken in a plane at a small distance in front of the eyes. This plane will more or less coincide with that eventually occupied by the front of the spectacle frame. Hence, it will be referred to as the spectacle plane. It usually lies parallel to the plane of the patient's face. The distance between a pupil and the spectacle plane is approximately equal to the vertex distance.

21.3.2 GENERAL REQUIREMENTS
Before any PD measurement is taken, the following preconditions should be satisfied:

(1) Patient and dispenser should be seated facing each other squarely.
(2) The patient's eyes should be well-illuminated, but glare must be avoided.
(3) The patient's and dispenser's eyes should be at the same level. This is best achieved by seating the patient on a chair while the dispenser is seated on an adjustable stool.

21.3.3 EYE-TO-EYE METHOD
This appears to be the simplest method since the only equipment required is a millimetre rule. The latter is usually called a PD rule (Fig. 21.4). The method has been ascribed to Viktorin, a German master optician who practised around the beginning of the twentieth century (Müller, 1965; see also Hardy, 1930).

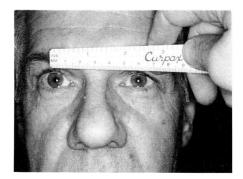

Fig. 21.4 *A PD rule held in the spectacle plane is steadied against the patient's forehead*

The procedure is as follows:

(1) The dispenser closes their right eye and/or points at their left eye while instructing the patient to look with both eyes at his open, left eye.
(2) The PD rule is placed in the patient's spectacle plane while steadying the hand by holding the rule lightly against the patient's forehead (Fig. 21.4). For further support, place the elbow on the table.
(3) Adjust the position of the rule until the zero of its scale is seen in line with either the patient's right pupil centre/pupil edge/iris edge or limbus.
(4) The dispenser closes the patient's left eye, opens their right eye and/or points at their right eye while instructing the patient to look with both eyes at the dispenser's right eye.
(5) The dispenser reads the position of either the patient's left pupil centre/pupil edge/iris edge on the rule's scale. This reading represents the distance PD.
(6) Go back to (3) to check that the zero-position is still in line with the right eye's chosen feature. If it is, record the PD measured; if not, start from the beginning.

The basis for this method relies on the fact that the PD (of adults) does not vary by many milli-

metres (see Table 21.1), one may assume that in (3) and (5), above, the pupillary or visual axes of patient and dispenser coincide, and because their PDs are almost the same in these two positions, the axes will lie parallel provided that there is a reasonable distance between the two.

The following circumstances can give rise to errors during the use of a PD rule (Mattison-Shupnick, 1980):

(1) Parallax due to a difference in patient's and practitioner's PD.
(2) Anisocoria (unequal pupil diameters in a pair of eyes).
(3) Difference in visual axes distance and pupil centres distance.
(4) Asymmetry of the face.
(5) Invisible pupil margins in patients with dark irides.
(6) Vertical differences in the position of a pair of eyes.
(7) Poor reproducibility of the measurement.
(8) Lateral head or rule movement during the measurement.
(9) Uncertainty about the position of the near point while measuring the near PD (see Chapter 22).

If the general requirements (Section 21.3.2) are adhered to, it can be shown that, even in an extreme case (distance between centres of rotation of patient's eyes 50 mm; distance between patient's centres of rotation and spectacle plane 25 mm; distance between centres of rotation of patient and dispenser 400 mm; distance between centres of rotation of dispenser's eyes 70 mm), the parallax error amounts to little more than 1 mm. A serious error can occur if either person moves during the process, and a smaller one if the patient does not look at the dispenser's pupil centre, but slightly to one side.

However, not every dispenser can close one eye only, as is required for this method. Hence, Brooks & Borish (1979) suggest that the most

TABLE 21.1 (Inter)pupillary distance of various groups of adults (distance PD, measurements in millimetres)

	Range	Average	Mean (M + F)	SD	Reference
European					
	59–71·5		64·5		Babalola & Szajnzicht (1960)
	58–72	F 60–61			Sasieni (1962)
		M 63–64			
	59–71		64·11		Pirbhai (1965)
		UF 61·89		2·90	Virdee (1989)
		UM 65·08		3·29	
German					
F	56–70	62·5			Rünz (1978)
M	58–72	65·0			
	64–68				Kasparek (1981)
F	56–66				Fleck et al. (1960)
M	62–72				
F	56–68	64			Fleck et al. (1970)
M	60–76	66			
French					
	54–77				Darras (1982)
F	54–72	60			
M	56–76	64			
African					
MF?	63–80		70		Banks (1968)
	62–72		69·5		Pirbhai (1965)
West African					
MF?	63–72		69·6		Babalola & Szanjzicht (1960)
West Indian					
MF?	61–69		67		Banks (1968)
Chinese					
	60–70		64·72		Pirbhai (1965)
American					
			63·5	10·5	Shepard (1942)
MP	60–71	A	65·7	3·17	Hofstetter (1972)
FU	57–67		61·5	3·08	
MU	60–70	A	64·4	3·07	

F, female; M, male; SD, standard deviation; P, private optometry practice; U, university optometry clinic; A, 5th to 95th percentile.

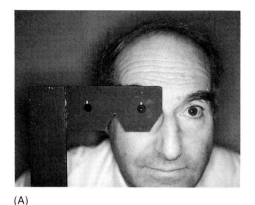 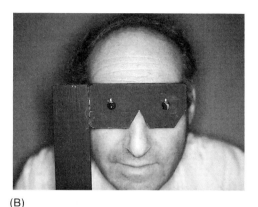

(A)   (B)

Fig. 21.5 This device, which sits on a stand (not shown), is suitable for use by a uniocular dispenser, to measure a patient's distance PD. The distance between the white fixation marks (above the apertures) is 64 mm. Modified after Waters (1952). See Section 21.3.3. A, first, the patient is instructed to fixate the white mark above the aperture in front of the dispenser's sighting (right) eye. The dispenser can now line up the zero of a millimetre scale with a landmark on the patient's right eye. B, having transferred his sighting eye to the other aperture, and having instructed the patient to fixate on the mark above that aperture, the dispenser can determine the position of the equivalent landmark of the patient's left eye on the scale

professional solution for the dispenser is then to close one eye by covering it with the palm of one hand, as this appears to be a natural part of the technique.

Waters (1952) suggested a solution for dispensers with one blind or amblyopic eye (Fig. 21.5). Two holes, 1 cm diameter, are drilled in a piece of wood fixed on a stand. The centres must be 64 mm apart. A fixation mark is placed above each hole on the side facing the patient. The PD rule is held in the patient's spectacle plane. With the device placed between patient and dispenser, the former is instructed to look at the right fixation mark while the dispenser uses his or her 'good' eye to look through the hole below the fixation mark in order to line up the PD rule. The dispenser then moves the 'good' eye to the other hole while the patient fixates the mark above it; a reading is then taken. This method ensures a reasonable result.

The PD of a patient with a squint may be measured by first covering the patient's (say) left eye and lining up the PD rule with a chosen point on the right eye, observed by the dispenser's left eye. Next, uncover the left eye, cover the other eye and take a reading of that eye's matching point on the rule with the right eye.

The Grolman (1977) and Baaken (Anonymous, undated) devices are used with the eye-to-eye method. Both methods involve a measuring device which is fixed to the spectacle front of the frame selected for the patient so that measurements are made in the spectacle plane. The Baaken device can be used, together with an adjustable double-mirror centring device, to determine the near-vision centration distance (Anonymous, 1986).

The Rodenstock (1975) Reiner Interpupillary Gauge (Fig. 21.6) is held in the spectacle plane and the adjustable scales are projected in the pupillary plane, by means of a semi-silvered mirror. The cursors are circular, and may be set either concentric with the pupil edge (if visible) or with the limbus.

Fleck *et al.* (1970) showed a transparent platelet made of thin plastics that can be fixed in the

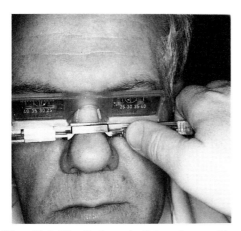

Fig. 21.6 *The Rodenstock Reiner Interpupillary Gauge in use. The millimetre scales reflected in the semi-silvered mirrors in front of the patient's eyes facilitate measurement of the monocular PDs. In addition, the conventional PD is provided on another scale. The gauge can also be used to measure the vertex distance*

lens aperture of the spectacle front. Horizontal and vertical millimetre scales make it possible to determine the position of the pupil with respect to, for instance, the boxed centre of the lens shape of the front.

21.3.4 CENTRING DISCS

Trial cases often contain one or more centring discs: these are discs placed in the trial frame to facilitate adjustment for correct centration (BS 3521, Part 1, 1991) which carry a cross at their geometrical centre, similar to centring rules (Fig. 21.7). The latter are devices consisting of one

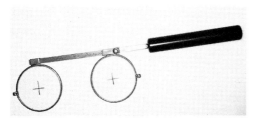

Fig. 21.7 *A rule fitted with 'centring discs'*

fixed centring disc and another which slides along a bar to which a handle is attached. They can be used in conjunction with the eye–to–eye method (Section 21.3.3).

21.3.5 TELESCOPIC DEVICES

Telescopic devices employ a collimating system. This is arranged (1) to let parallel rays of light emerge from the eye-piece, by placing the object in the first focal plane of a positive lens, and (2) with devices for the measurement of the PD, the patient's eye may be placed close to the positive lens and selected parallel rays originating from the eye will, after refraction by the lens, be converged to focus in the plane of a pinhole (eyepiece). The dispenser observes the patient's eye through the pinhole.

There are two distinctly different optical arrangements. One has a collimator system for each eye (Fig. 21.8). The other (Fig. 21.9) has one large collimator lens with a diameter approaching the width of a spectacle front. Whereas the first type requires the dispenser to take a scale reading with each eye, the second allows readings to be taken with one eye only. Hence, it is suitable for monocular dispensers. The latter system is used in the Essilor and the Bausch & Lomb PD Gauges (Figs 21.9 and 21.10) and the spectacle fitting instrument of Schenk (Fleck *et al.*, 1970). Each type has an optical system that is telecentric on the patient's side, thus avoiding parallax errors when reading the scale(s). The scale(s) and the patient's eye(s) are imaged by the lens(es) at distance. Using a single collimator, Hahn (Darras, 1982) designed a coincidence PD meter. Unfortunately, it is not possible to measure MPDs with this instrument.

Although telescopic devices present an improvement over PD rules where parallax errors are difficult to avoid, all have in common the problem of having to judge the position of the pupil centre. Kochniss (1991) reported that this

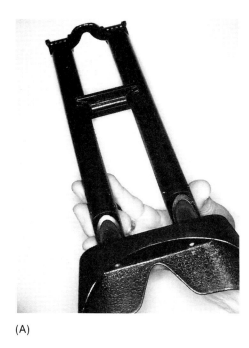

(A)

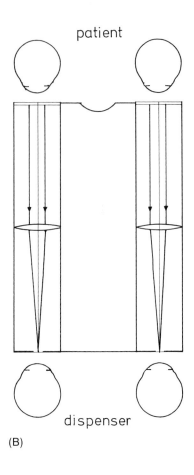

(B)

Fig. 21.8 A, *Carl Zeiss Jena telescopic monocular PD-measuring instrument. The 'bridge' on the far side fits over the patient's nose. An occluder fitted in the bar on the patient's side obscures one eye or the other. B, ray diagram showing the collimator system fitted in each tube*

can be accurately determined with the Rodenstock PD Meter. Another advantage of telescopic devices is that because the patient sees the pinhole(s) images straight ahead with each eye, convergence is suppressed.

In general, instruments are placed on the patient's nose where they may slide sideways if the instrument's bearing surface does not fit the patient's bridge properly. This can affect the accuracy of the MPD measurement by several millimetres.

Some instruments are provided with a shutter which acts as an occluder. This makes it possible to measure separately the distance between the midline of the nose and the pupil centre of each eye. In addition to providing the MPD for high

and progressive power lenses, the occluder is also useful when the patient has a squint.

Instruments provided with two sliding vertical hair lines facilitate the estimation of the position of each pupil centre. By mechanical or electronic means, the MPDs and also the distance PD (or the near CD; Section 21.7), are provided. These instruments can also be used to determine the diameters of pupil, iris or cornea. Some may also be used as vertex distance gauges (Section 20.2).

21.3.6 CORNEAL REFLECTION DEVICES
This method of measurement of the PD makes use of the first Purkinje or catoptic image (Obstfeld, 1982) of the cornea. For this purpose, a

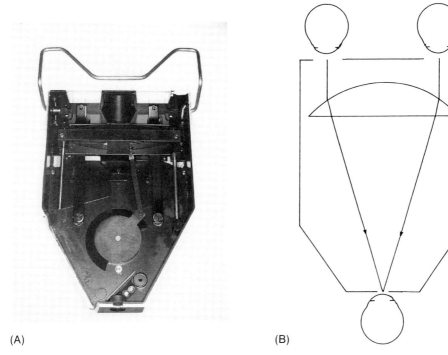

(A) (B)

Fig. 21.9 A, photograph of the inside of an Essilor corneal reflection pupillometer. The large disc seen near the front is connected with the collimator. When the disc is rotated, the collimator slides along the two horizontal bars away from or towards the patient's eyes. On the far side are the 'windows' in front of the patient's eyes, and the forehead guard. B, ray diagram showing how the one eye of the practitioner can (successively) observe the eyes of the patient, through the large collimator lens

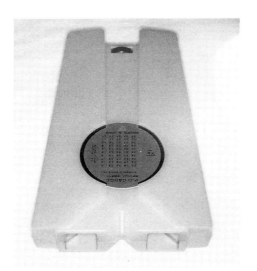

Fig. 21.10 The Bausch & Lomb PD gauge seen from the patient's side. The table printed on the disc provides bifocal insets based on the monocular PD

small light source is placed in front of the eye and the patient is instructed to observe it. As a result, the foveola, centre of rotation of the eye, nodal point and light source are lined up on the visual axis of the eye. For all practical purposes, the visual axis will now intersect the cornea at the point where the corneal reflection of the light source appears to be situated (Figs 21.2 and 21.3). This point does not usually coincide with the pupil centre.

To measure the distance PD, the single light source may be presented optically (Fig. 21.11) to each eye separately and for distance vision, apparently at infinity. The reading is taken by the dispenser with one eye. Examples are the Essel/ Essilor (Anonymous, 1971; Alexandre, 1974)

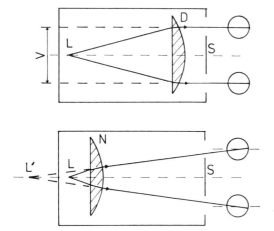

Fig. 21.11 *Ray diagram of a corneal reflection PD meter. Above: for distance vision, the light source L appears at infinity through the collimator lens placed at D (compare with Fig. 21.9A). S, Spectacle plane which contains a cursor in each window. The cursor is moved to coincide with the corneal reflection. V, visual axes distance. Below: for near vision, the light source L is imaged at L' by the collimator lens which has been moved to N. The eyes converge at L'*

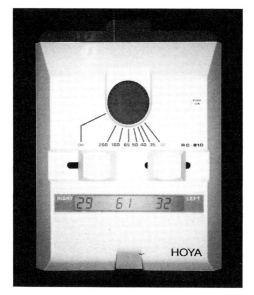

Fig. 21.12 *The Hoya corneal reflection PD meter provides a digital display of the monocular (29, 32) and binocular PDs*

and the Hoya corneal reflection PD meters (Fig. 21.12).

The following technique, which employs a retinoscope or direct ophthalmoscope (modified from Anderson, 1954), is based on the same principle:

(1) Fit the spectacle frame selected on the patient's head, and remove it once adjusted.
(2) Fit the lens apertures of the front with either dummy lenses, clear (preferably not tinted) formers (as used with automatic lens edging machines), or fit a strip of clear, self-adhesive tape vertically across the apertures.
(3) Place the frame on the patient's head.
(4) The dispenser should now ensure that the midlines of the patient's head and their own coincide, and that the spectacle plane is perpendicular to these midlines.
(5) Switch on instrument and observe with the left eye the patient's right eye through the sighthole.
(6) Instruct the patient to look at the (apparent) light source of the instrument.
(7) Use a finely pointed marking pen to place a mark coinciding with the corneal reflection on the dummy lens or tape.
(8) Without altering the position of his body, the dispenser should transfer the instrument to their right eye and repeat points (5) and (6).
(9) Remove the frame from the patient's head, and measure the distance between the marks. This represents the distance between the visual axes for the patient for distance vision. The MPDs may be determined relative to the vertical symmetry line of the front.

Note that it may be advisable to reduce the ambient illumination. Instead of a retinoscope or ophthalmoscope, a small light source, such as used in a pen torch (*penlight*), may be employed. However, this light source cannot be held on the line coinciding with visual axes of patient and dispenser. It is usually held below or to the side of the dispenser's head. This may reduce the accuracy of the resulting measurement because of parallax.

While taking PD measurements with several corneal reflection pupillometers, B.R. Chou and the author found that the corneal reflections of a pair of eyes could not be seen by looking from one to the other, because the eye relief of the instruments was too short. Therefore, the dispenser must move their eye sideways while looking through the pinhole. This may introduce errors.

Readers interested in the development of corneal reflection devices are referred to Sasieni (1962) who described a number of, now historic, instruments.

21.4 Subjective Methods of Measuring the Distance PD

Subjective methods invariably employ pinhole discs (Fig. 21.13). These are opaque discs with a small circular central aperture (BS 3521, Part 1, 1991). Having determined the patient's prescription, a pinhole disc is slipped into the right-hand cell of the trial frame worn by the patient. An identical device is placed in front of the other eye. If the pinholes are not centred on the visual axes, the patient will see a blurred image of each pinhole superimposed on a distant fixation object. While adjusting the horizontal position of each pinhole their images will start to overlap and then coincide. When the patient reports the latter stage, the distance between the pinhole centres will be equal to the distance between the visual axes (Anonymous, 1957; Unger, (1957).

This method can be employed with the Baaken system (Anonymous, undated) and Knobloch's (1982) device (Fig. 21.14), as follows:

(1) Instruct the patient to look at a distant fixation object while wearing his distance correction.
(2) Roughly precentre the pinhole discs with respect to the horizontal and vertical meridians of the pupils of each eye.
(3) Cover one eye and ask the patient whether the fixation object appears centrally within the blurred outline of the pinhole. Adjust the position of the pinhole until the object appears centrally in the pinhole's outline.
(4) Repeat this procedure for the other eye.

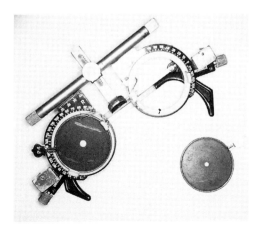

Fig. 21.13 *A pinhole disc (below right) and another fitted in the cell of a trial frame*

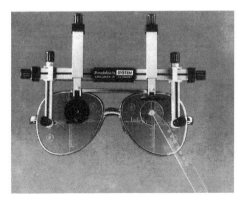

Fig. 21.14 *Knobloch's KMS device fitted onto a spectacle front*

(5) Uncover the eye and, by alternately covering the pinholes in front of each eye, the patient will easily notice small differences in the positions of object and pinholes. (Without alternately covering the pinholes, patients will still be able to tell whether the images of the pinholes coincide perfectly, or whether their positions need adjustment to achieve this.)

Emsley (1953) suggested a technique where chromostereopsis is used to measure the visual axes distance. Patients can usually observe a small apparent difference in distance (stereopsis) between the red and green parts of a distant object, set against a black background. However, when a red–green target is observed through a pinhole, the stereoscopic effect disappears when the pinhole lies on the visual axis. This method was tested by McCormack & McGill (1982) following the steps set out in the previous paragraph.

In 1977 Obstfeld designed a student laboratory experiment based on Ivanoff's (1953) experimental arrangement for the measurement of the chromatic aberration of the human eye. The distant target consisted of a small square, the upper half of which was green and the lower half red. When looking through a pinhole which is not centred on the visual axis of the eye concerned, the vertical edges of the red section appear out of alignment with the vertical edges of the green section. By adjusting the position of the pinhole along the horizontal meridian, the vertical edges may be aligned. At this point the pinhole will lie on the visual axis of the eye. The procedure may be repeated for the other eye. Inserting the pinholes in a trial frame provides a readily available device when employed with a suitable red–green test, as used for subjective refraction. In this manner the monocular visual axes distances may be determined. Because it employs vernier acuity, it is a very sensitive test,

provided that the patient's head is carefully steadied during the procedure.

21.5 Distance PD: Comments

Several reports (Backman, 1972; Hoeft, 1980; Darras, 1982) concluded that the Essilor Corneal Reflection PD meter provided the most reliable measurements. It was thought that the smaller measurements obtained with a rule were due to involuntary convergence when the dispenser is seated relatively close to the patient.

The PD is usually larger than the visual axes distance. This is caused by the angle α (Section 21.1.1). Backman (1972) and Hoeft et al. (1980) recorded a difference of 2 mm, which is in agreement with Villani's (1971) observation and similar to the results obtained with Obstfeld's experimental setup reported in the previous section. McCormack & McGill (1982) calculated that the difference should be 0.95 mm and found that the results obtained with their method gave significantly less variability than results obtained with a rule. The method is advocated for use with patients that have high refractive errors or low tolerance to unintended prismatic powers and when dispensing progressive power lenses.

Both Fleck et al. (1960) and Darras (1982) report asymmetry in MPD, in 80–90% of patients, with a maximum of 5 mm. The left MPD is usually smaller than the right. Harvey (1982) pointed out that there are differences in the PD as a result of gender, preselection requirements of the sample and trends in body size.

It is important to observe the patient's posture from the moment the dispenser sets eyes on him, particularly at times when the patient is at ease. This makes it possible to take into account head tilts (whether sideways, forwards or backwards).

Because people with squints tend to use one eye at a time, it is usually advisable to centre the lenses as if the eyes were operating together under normal conditions of binocular vision. If this is not done, unnecessary prismatic and unaesthetic glazing problems are created. An exception is the case where the patient is accustomed to a particular centration of the lenses.

Table 21.1 shows that the range of distance PD measurements for adult Caucasians does not vary greatly, that the mean value for males and females lies around 65 mm, that the average PD of females is 3–4 mm smaller than that of males, and that the measurements for Mongoloids and Caucasians are very similar. However, the measurements for Negroids are larger than for both other groups. The measurements obtained for the 'American' sample agree with the Caucasian measurements, and the standard deviations of both groups based on university optometry clinics are in good agreement (see also Section 3.2.3 and Tables 3.2 and 3.4–3.6).

21.6 The Near PD

The near PD, or interpupillary distance for near vision, may be defined as the horizontal distance between the pupil centres or visual axes of a pair of eyes measured in the pupillary plane when these eyes observe a near fixation point. Note the fundamental difference when compared with the distance PD: the latter does not vary according to the plane of measurement (centres of rotation of the eyes, pupillary plane, spectacle plane) whereas the near PD will vary with the distance of the object. Because the near PD can be of some practical use only for contact lens wearers, I do not devote much text to it.

Hardy (1930), referring to Watt (1929), wrote: 'A reading PD ought never to be taken with a rule. It can be calculated if the distance PD, working distance, and distance between lens plane and centres of rotation are known'. Note that this quotation refers to the lens plane and not

the pupillary plane. This discrepancy has long been a source of confusion and inaccuracy.

21.7 The Near CD

The near centration distance, near CD, may be defined on the basis of the (distance) CD as the distance between the right and left centration point during near vision. As this refers to the centration points of the spectacle lenses, the near CD applies in the spectacle plane.

The distance between patient and fixation point should be specified. Although it is seldom measured and recorded in practice, it is essential when dealing with high-powered corrections and high additions, since this factor determines the amount of convergence required and hence, the near centration distance of the lenses.

As a rule one can say that lenses used for near vision are centred correctly when the optical axes of the lenses pass through the centres of rotation of the eyes of the spectacle wearer during near vision. This will not occur when the wearer uses distance correction, nor is it likely to occur when the wearer uses multifocal lenses.

Note that most corrected non-presbyopic ametropes use their distance glasses for near vision too. Corrected hyperopes cope with unprescribed prism base-out, requiring more convergence than when the lenses are centred for near vision. Similarly, corrected myopes adapt to more prism base-in, requiring less convergence. Hence, when single vision reading glasses are used for near vision, the lenses should be centred with this in mind if this is the *first* reading prescription and the addition is more than, for example, 1 D. If the addition is less, the wearer is unlikely to experience difficulty in adapting to the new accommodation–convergence relationship, nor will this occur with subsequently prescribed reading glasses.

For the actual image formation and further

details about accommodation and convergence in corrected ametropes see Obstfeld (1982), and for a more detailed examination of the centration of spectacle lenses and near vision see Obstfeld (1990). Note that the purpose of insetting the segments of multifocal lenses is to ensure that, during reading, the fields of vision through the segments coincide (BS 3521, Part 1, 1991).

21.8 Measuring the Near CD

21.8.1 THE SINGLE EYE METHOD

Using a millimetre rule, PD rule, or the Rodenstock Reiner Interpupillary Gauge (see Section 21.3.3), the procedure is as follows:

(1) The dispenser places himself or herself at the required near vision distance from the patient. A rule of, for instance, 50 cm, placed or fixed flat on the dispensing table, should be used to be able to measure this distance with some accuracy. The dispenser's preferred or dominant eye should be placed on the midline of the patient's face, that is, opposite the patient's nose. The other eye may be closed. Furthermore, the general requirements stated in Section 21.3.2 should be observed.

(2) The dispenser instructs the patient to look with both eyes at the former's one sighting eye.

(3) The dispenser places the PD rule in the patient's spectacle plane while steadying the hand holding the rule against the patient's forehead. For further support, rest the elbow on the table top.

(4) Adjust the position of the rule until the zero of its scale is situated in line with the patient's right pupil centre/pupil edge/iris edge or limbus.

(5) The dispenser looks at the patient's left eye and notes the position of the equivalent part

of the left eye on the rule's scale. This reading represents the near CD, which should be recorded.

21.8.2 IMPROVED SINGLE EYE METHOD

Michaels (1985; based on Anderson, 1954) described an improvement on the above method which he considered to be the simplest. A small light source, such as that of a pentorch, is held by the patient at the required working/reading distance. The dispenser places their preferred eye just above the light source and observes the corneal reflections of this source (Figs 21.2, 21.3 and 21.15). By measuring the distance between the corneal reflections in the spectacle plane with a PD or similar rule, the visual axes distance in the spectacle plane for near vision is measured. As Michaels points out, this method may also be used to measure the near MCDs starting from the nasal midpoint. See also Section 22.5.

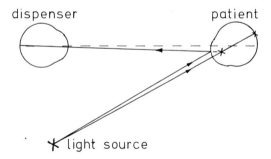

dispenser   patient

light source

Fig. 21.15. *Ray diagram showing the position of the catoptric image x of the light source X, as seen by the dispenser*

21.8.3 TO CALCULATE THE DISTANCE PD OR MPD

It is now possible to arrive at the distance PD or MPD. Table 21.2, based on the similar triangles in Fig. 21.16, shows the number of millimetres to be added to the near (monocular) visual axes (or axis) distance to find the distance (monocular)

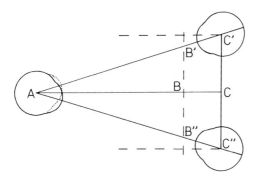

Fig. 21.16 *Diagram for the calculation of the distance PD or MPD (see Section 21.8.3 and Table 21.2). A, centre of rotation of the dispenser's eye; B, middle of spectacle plane where B' and B'' represent the near centration points; C' C C'' represents the plane passing through the patient's eyes' centres of rotation; ABC, midline between the patient's eyes*

visual axes (or axis) distance. Study of Table 21.2 shows that the figures may be simplified to facilitate memorization.

The single eye method can also be used for this purpose (Darras, 1982) provided that the dispenser's eye is placed accurately on the midline of the patient's face and the position of the

midline along the scale is noted along with the near CD. By adding the appropriate value found in Table 21.2, the MPDs and distance PD can be obtained.

21.8.4 TO MEASURE NEAR CD AND DISTANCE PD OR MPD

A more efficient way based on the eye-to-eye method (see Section 21.3.3) follows the steps described for distance vision, up to and including step 3. The dispenser then reads with their left eye the position of the patient's left eye's reference feature on the scale. This reading represents the near CD, and is memorized. Now, steps (4) and (5) (Section 21.3.3) are followed to obtain the distance PD. Both measurements are then recorded in the order distance PD/near CD (for example 64/60).

Note that the last method does not allow for the measurement of unequal MPDs. However, the following permits this. Figure 21.17 is a diagram showing the theoretical calculation of the near CD based on the distance PD and the near fixation distance, or of the distance PD based

TABLE 21.2 *Number of millimetres to be added to the near (monocular) visual axes (or axis) distance (VAD) to obtain the distance visual axes (or axis) distance*

Viewing distance	VAD		Monocular VAD	
	Near	**Distance**	**Near**	**Distance**
300 mm	55	+5	27·5	+2·5
	60	+5	30	+2·5
	65	+6	32·5	+3
	70	+6	35	+3
400	55	+3	27·5	+1·5
	60	+4	30	+2
	65	+4	32·5	+2
	70	+5	35	+2·5
Simplified				
300		+5·5	}	+2·5
400		+4		

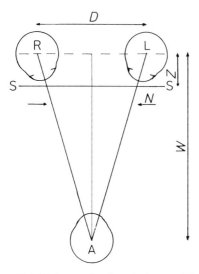

Fig. 21.17 *Diagram for the calculation of the near CD based on the distance PD (see Section 21.8.4). A, centre of rotation of dispenser's eye; D, distance between centres of rotation of patient's eye; L, left eye's centre of rotation; N, near centration distance (CD); SS, spectacle plane; W, near vision distance measured to the eyes' centres of rotation; Z, distance between spectacle plane and centres of rotation of patient's eyes, and assumed to measure 27 mm*

on the near CD, in the spectacle plane. In this diagram there are two parallel planes, namely one through the centres of rotation R and L, the other representing the spectacle plane. The planes form the bases of two similar triangles having their apex A at the centre of rotation A of the dispenser's eye. The distance Z between the two parallel planes is an unknown quantity. However, by adding 13 mm to the vertex distance of the spectacles (minimally 8 mm which represents eyelash length plus eyelid thickness – practically 14 mm or more), one assumes $Z = 27$ mm (Gerstman, 1973, assumed 28.6 mm):

$$D/N = W/(W - Z)$$

or

$$N = D (W - Z) / W$$

where D = distance PD, N = near CD, and W = near vision distance measured to the eyes' centres of rotation; all distances are expressed in millimetres. If the MPDs are unequal, the above equation can be used by substituting the appropriate MPD for either D or N (see also Section 22.5).

21.9 Tables for PD and Near CD

Not all PD meters allow the near CD to be measured. Instead, a table may be provided giving the near CD for stated near vision distances, based on the distance PD. Brooks & Borish (1979) provided corresponding distance and near MPDs for the 40 cm (16 inches) distance. Henker (1924), Bennett (1968) and Darras (1982) provided tables showing the relationship between distance PD and the near CD at given near vision distances. Table 21.3 (after Clayton, 1977) does not materially differ from the one published by Zeiss (1983). All tables show the same figures with small variations in the more extreme values of the PD range.

21.10 Insetting of Multifocal Segments

Although reasons associated with the convergence of the visual axes during near vision are frequently proffered, it must be stressed that the only purpose of insetting multifocal segments is to ensure that the right and left reading fields coincide (BS 3521, Part 1, 1991).

The geometrical inset of a multifocal lens is defined (BS 3521, Part 1, 1991) as the distance between vertical lines through the distance centration point and the midpoint of the segment diameter. This measurement is commonly obtained from the following equation:

inset per segment = (distance CD − near CD)/2

In the case of unequal MPDs, this equation is modified to a calculation for each inset:

$$inset = distance\ MCD - near\ MCD$$

The optical inset is defined (BS 3521, Part 1, 1991) as the horizontal displacement relative to the distance centration point of the near or intermediate optical centre, any prescribed prism being neutralized. As Jalie (1984) pointed out, the optical inset is seldom considered. It is assumed that patients can cope with unintentional horizontal prismatic powers during near vision. The major exceptions are cases where different amounts of prismatic correction are required for distance and near vision.

Ellerbrock (1948) and Biessels (1954) have considered the effect of the distance prescription and addition, as has Scott Sterling (see Waters,

TABLE 21.3 *Centration distances (after Clayton, 1977)*

Distance (6 m or more)	Intermediate		Near	
	900 mm (violin)	500 mm (piano)	400 mm (desk)	300 mm (book)
52	50	49	48	47
53	51	50	49	48
54	52	51	50	49
55	53	52	51	50
56	54	53	52	51
57	55	54	53	52
58	56	55	53·5	52·5
59	57	56	54	53
60	58	57	55	54
61	59	58	56	55
62	60	59	57	56
63	61	59·5	58	57
64	62	60·5	59	58
65	63	61	60	59
66	64	62	61	60
67	65	63	62	61
68	66	64	63	62
69	67	65	64	63
70	68	66	65	64
71	69	67	66	65
72	70	68	67	66
73	71	69	68	67
74	72	70	69	68
75	73	71	69·5	68·5
76	74	72	70	69

Note: the average distance at which visual display units and text (hard copy) tend to be placed is 60 cm (Burns, personal communication, 1989).

TABLE 21.4 Bifocal geometrical insets for reading distance 40 cm (add 0.4 mm for 30 cm distance); after Scott Sterling of Bausch & Lomb Optical Co.

MCD − BVP		MCD − BVP		Inset (mm)
mm	D	mm	D	
35	+10			2·7
35	+7	32	+10	2·5
35	−2	28	+8	2·0
32	−10	28	−3	1·5
		28	−10	1·3

MCD, monocular centration distance for distance vision.
BVP, back vertex power of the spectacle lens for distance vision, along the horizontal meridian.

1952; Table 21.4). The basis for the calculation was discussed by Obstfeld, 1990; Stek & Smitt (1963) considered the required convergence, while Diepes (1981) included the workshop centering equipment. Gerstman (1973) examined a number of guidelines and decided that the simplest means of determining the inset for distance CDs between 62 and 68 mm is to inset the optical centre of each reading lens or the geometrical centre of each bifocal segment by 0·75 mm for each dioptre of object vergence at the spectacle plane. For instance, if the object distance were 20 cm, the object vergence would be 5 D and the inset 5 × 0·75 = 3·75 mm per lens. For distance CDs outside the range mentioned, Gerstman's (1973) table should be consulted.

Earlam & North (1988) held the opinion that it is neither necessary nor desirable 'to measure a near centration distance as it is fraught with inaccuracies and can easily be calculated'; Stollenwerk (1994) concurred. Earlam & North (1988) calculated approximate values of insets (Table 21.5) which do not deviate materially from the

TABLE 21.5 Calculated inset for an object distance of 0.33 m (after Earlam & North, 1988)

Distance PD (mm)	Inset for each lens (mm)
60	2
64–66	2·5
70	3

values given by Kozol (1958), Zeiss (1963) and Gerstman (1973). The final arbiter is the patient – does he appreciate an imperfection in the overlap of the fields of vision, or not? I have not heard of a complaint about the horizontal overlap of the fields of view and have suggested four reasons (Obstfeld, 1990):

- The retinal image of the segment border would be around −65 D and, therefore, out of focus.
- The visual acuity of the retina, upon which the segment border is imaged, may be so low that the lens wearer will not be able to observe the object.
- The patient's attention is not normally centred on observing the segment border.
- The segment border will be projected as a shadow on the otherwise well-illuminated retina and, thus, not be noticed.

The situation differs in progressive power lenses. Segmented lenses provide a good retinal image in almost all parts of the segment (but see Reiner, 1972). The size of the near vision portions of progressive lenses varies according to the design philosophy (and the manufacturer's ability to execute it) while the progression between distance and near portions is usually no more than a narrow channel. It may then become imperative to use the near MCDs accurately so that the visual axes will travel through those portions of each lens not having any, or exhibiting only minimal amounts of aberrations.

This applies to a much lesser extent to the distance portions: these tend to have a much larger area that is free from aberrations than the remainder of the lens, although there are progressive lens designs where aberrations do encroach onto the distance portion. Hence, in the case of progressive power lenses it can be argued that the distance MCDs should be based on the near MCDs, and not the other way around. However, note that the inset of progressive lenses is fixed by the manufacturer (usually at 2 or 2.5 mm per lens) so that the distance MCD is obtained by adding the inset to the near MCD.

Stollenwerk (1994) described a method to determine whether to inset the segment of a multifocal lens for use by a uniocular patient. The method was to cut out a narrow column of newspaper print, seat the patient at a table and ask them to read the column after it has been placed on the table top in front of them. When the patient places the column of print in line with their body's midline, their functioning eye will have converged and a conventional inset will be suitable. However, if the column of print is placed directly in line with their functioning eye, it has not converged. A multifocal lens with a segment which has not been inset should then be ordered and fitted in the patient's spectacles.

21.11 Determining the Near CD

Gillet (personal communication, cited by Darras, 1982) described a method of marking the near CD using a plane mirror placed on the fitting table. When the spectacle frame to be glazed with progressive lenses (presently fitted with dummy lenses, self-adhesive strips or platelets) is placed on the patient's face, he or she is instructed to fixate a mark on the surface of the mirror. The dispenser observes the patient's reflection in the mirror, and marks the position of the pupil centre on each dummy lens, strip or platelet. However, there are two problems: it is difficult to ensure that the patient does not look at the dispenser in the mirror, but fixates the mark on the mirror, and it is also difficult for the dispenser to place the mark accurately on the lens (or substitute) because they have to move their hand in a mirror-reversed fashion.

In 1981 Rodenstock introduced an internally illuminated near centering unit based on the same principle, and produced self-adhesive platelets that could be fitted on the spectacle frame's front. The dispenser could then mark the platelets while looking through the mirror, at the position of the corneal reflection.

In the early 1980s Essilor (1981) introduced the Near Vision Mirror MVP based on this principle. It consists of an adjustable mirror with a fixation cross and a clip-on lorgnette which is fixed on the spectacle frame selected for the patient. The clip-on lorgnette has a cursor in front of each lens aperture. These are adjusted by the dispenser while looking at the patient's face through the mirror, and set to coincide with the corneal reflection of a small, bright light source fitted close to the mirror. The cursor overcomes the problem associated with having to place a mark by hand, by means of a mirror. The lorgnette can also be used to determine the distance PD by applying the eye-to-eye method.

Lewis (1983) sought to create a more natural situation, having noticed that patients use different head tilts while reading. He developed his Reflex Book, Graticule Spex and Accuracy Stickers. The 'book' is a box which contains a light source that gives rise to a corneal reflection, and has a small mirror fitted on either side. The special frame may be substituted by the patient's chosen spectacles fitted with the graticule (a horizontal millimetre scale). The sticker is placed against the graticule to indicate the position of the corneal reflection seen by the dispenser through one of the mirrors. This facilitates the measurement of the near MCD, taking account of the patient's normal head tilt.

21.12 Major Equipment

Over the years, a number of table instruments for the measurement of the PD have been commercially available. Fleck *et al.* (1970) describe the fitting instrument of Schenk and the Centrograph or 'Centering Unit according to Reiner', produced by Oculus (Reiner, 1973, 1974). Carl

Zeiss (Oberkochen) also marketed a Lens Fitting Instrument (Zeiss, 1963).

Essel (Anonymous, 1968) introduced the Centromatic – Posimatic system. The Centromatic instrument (Fig. 21.18) contains a distance and a near fixation device. The operator can observe the patient's eyes by means of a telescopic system. Photographs of the corneal reflections of the eyes are taken during distance and near fixation, thus providing distance and near PDs, and recorded by means of a built-in instant

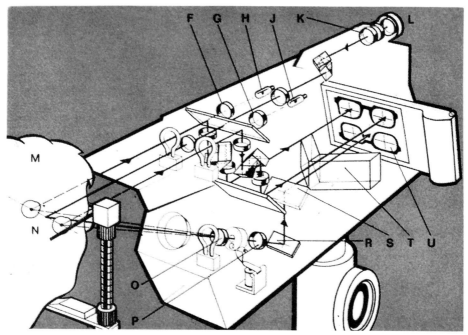

Fig. 21.18 *Ray diagram of the Essel Centromatic instrument. The patient is seated at M and looks at two fixation lights, H and J, placed at the foci of lenses F and G. Hence, the lights appear at infinity. The dispenser, situated at L, observes the position of the subject's eyes through a telescope. The eye piece of this telescope is the lens system at K. The optical axis of the telescope is lined up with the middle of the patient's face. The instrument can be adjusted so that the patient's face, with spectacle frame, can be centred easily. By means of two identical optical systems, each eye and its surrounding spectacle rim is imaged on the upper portion of the film at U. For near vision, the light rays emitted by the fixation lights H and J, are reflected by the corneas at N. The rays pass through the objective lenses O and P, and are deflected by the mirrors R and S. Having passed through the deviation system T, they form an inverted image on the lower portion of the film at U. This instrument provides a permanent photographic record of the positions of the corneal reflections relative to the spectacle rims, for distance and near vision. In combination with the Posimatic system (not shown), uncut spectacle lenses can be accurately centred on the corneal reflections, before edging (courtesey Essilor)*

camera. The photographic record may then be used in the Posimatic instrument, a lens centring unit for the centration of uncut spectacle lenses. A problem with the Centromatic instrument is that the patient's head has to be placed in a head rest. Hence, no account can be taken of the effect of head tilt.

Essilor subsequently (1981) developed the Photocentron. This instrument instantly produces a photographic record of the corneal reflections of the eyes, observing an object apparently placed at infinity. The photograph may be used as a record of the frame (or presented to the patient with the practice address printed on it). The photograph may be used in the Posicentron lens centring unit.

Hemmer (1979) designed an instrument that facilitates the determination of the near visual points whereby the head remains unrestrained. A projection system which images a cross on the patient's forehead is employed to ensure that the patient's eyes are situated at a distance of 40 cm. The distance of the corneal reflections of two small fluorescent tubes is measured and provides the near CD.

Maxam (1985) described two fitting instruments, adding that they had only been used in the preparation of special optical aids.

Kochniss (1987) described a method whereby the distance PD and MPDs are first measured with a reflection PD meter, and marked on centring platelets in the frame selected for the patient. The markings are then checked with the eye-to-eye method. In turn, this is verified by means of a television camera placed 6 m from the patient, taking advantage of the inherent magnification of the monitor.

Göhringer (1989) employed a video-camera linked to a computer. This facilitated not only the determination of the (monocular) PD, but also the segment height and uncut lens size.

21.13 Specifying Centration Distances

When ordering a pair of single vision spectacles from a prescription house it is irrelevant to specify whether the measurement given is the distance CD or near CD since this information is of no consequence to the glaser. With respect to segmented multifocal lenses it is advisable to state either the distance and the near CD, or the distance CD and the inset where the near CD becomes redundant.

When the distance between centres of a front differs from the centration distance, it is sufficient to state the latter on the order form. Any required decentration to obtain the desired centration distance should be determined by the glaser. It should, therefore, not be entered on the order form thus preventing any misunderstanding.

In certain cases, such as anisometropia and aphakia, the vertical centration of the optical centres for near vision may be specified with respect to the horizontal centre line. This is done in order to reduce or to neutralize a vertical prismatic difference between the two eyes. It may also be done to reduce the prismatic power at level with the near visual point thus reducing the degradation of the image (of mainly horizontal lines) experienced when looking off-centre through lenses with a low V-value (Fonseka & Obstfeld, 1995). See also Grolman (1969).

When aspheric lenses are ordered, the vertical centration may be specified to ensure that the wearer looks through the non-aspheric portion of the lenses.

21.14 Tolerances

Using the highest absolute powers, the following optical centration tolerances are given in BS

2738 (1989) per lens: horizontally: 0·12 prism dioptre + 1·0 mm; vertically: 0·12 prism dioptre + 0·5 mm (for lenses other than progressive power lenses) and 0·12 prism dioptre + 0·75 mm (for progressive power lenses); for any pair of lenses in a spectacle frame the tolerances are: horizontally: 1·0 prism dioptre; vertically: 0·25 prism dioptre.

J. Campbell (personal communication, 1992) suggested that it may be more practical to calcu-late the actual tolerance in millimetres, for indi-vidual lenses from the following equations: horizontally: $1·2/F + 1$; vertically: $1·2/F + 0·5$ (for non-progressive lenses), $1.2/F + 0.75$ (for progressive lenses), where F = highest absolute lens power in dioptres.

Note that the tolerance of the geometrical inset of a multifocal lens is ±0.5 mm per glazed lens.

REFERENCES

Alexandre, M. (1974). Measuring monocular PDs. *Optician* **167**(4323), 4, 13.

Anderson, A.L. (1954). Accurate clinical means of measuring intervisual axis distance. *A.M.A. Arch. Ophthal.* **52**(3), 349–352.

Anonymous (undated). *The Baaken Frame Fitting and Centering System.* Dutenhofen (D): Oculus (brochure).

Anonymous (1957). A P.D. measuring device. *Optician* **134**(3471), 319.

Anonymous (1968). Le Centromatic–Posimatic. *Opticien–Lunetier* No. 184, 19–20.

Anonymous (1971). Corneal reflection pupillometer. *Optician* **161**(4174), 28.

Anonymous (1986). *Der Zentrierspiegel.* p. 12. Wetzlar-Dutenhofen (D): Oculus-Optikgeräte GmbH.

Babalola, J. & Szajnzicht, E. (1960). Ocular characteristics in West Africans and Europeans: a comparison of two groups. *Brit. J. Physiol. Optics* **17**(1), 27–35.

Backman, H. (1972). Inter-pupillary distance measurement. *Am. J. Optom.* **49**, 264–266.

Banks, R. (1968). Facial measurements of the Negro. Final Year Project. London: City University.

Bennett, A.G. (1968). *Emsley and Swaine's Ophthalmic Lenses*, p. 167. London: Hatton Press.

Biessels, W.J. (1954). De moderne brilmonturen en de 'P.D.', part II: de centrering van de nabij-bril. *Oculus, Amsterdam* No. 2 (Reprinted 1971 by Stichting Nederlandse Vakopleiding voor Opticiens, Amsterdam).

Brooks, C.W. & Borish, I.M. (1979). *System for Ophthalmic Dispensing.* Chicago: Professional Press.

BS 2738 (1989). *Spectacle lenses. Part 1: Specification for Tolerances on Optical Properties of Mounted Spectacle Lenses.* London: British Standards Institution.

BS 3521 (1991). *Terms Relating to Ophthalmic Optics and Spectacle Lenses. Part 1: Glossary of Terms Relating to Ophthalmic Lenses.* London: British Standards Institution.

BS 3521 (1991). *Terms Relating to Ophthalmic Optics and Spectacle Lenses. Part 2: Glossary of Terms Relating to Ophthalmic Lenses.* London: British Standards Institution.

Clayton, G.H. (1977). *Spectacle Frame Dispensing*, 2nd edn, p. 52. London: Association of Dispensing Opticians.

Darras, C. (1982). *La Tête et ses Mesures*, 3rd edn, pp. 76, 78. Paris: Centre de protection oculaire.

Diepes, H. (1981). Centrage des lunettes. *Opticien–Lunetier* No. 335, 76–91.

Earlam, R. & North, R. (1988). Non-aesthetic criteria for frame selection. In: Edwards, K. & Llewellyn, R. (eds), *Optometry*, p. 519. London: Butterworths.

Ellerbrock, V.J. (1948). A clinical evaluation of compensation for vertical imbalances. *Am. J. Optom.* **25**(7), 309–325.

Emsley, H.H. (1953). *Visual Optics*, Vol. 2, pp. 54–55. London: Hatton Press.

Emsley, H.H. (1955). *Visual Optics*, Vol. 1, 5th edn, p. 355. London: Hatton Press.

Essilor (1981). *Photocentron Technical Brochure.* Paris: Essilor International.

Fleck, H., Heynig, J. & Mütze, K. (1960). *Die Praxis der Brillenanpassung.* Leipzig: VEB Fachbuchverlag.

Fleck, H., Heynig, J., Mütze, K. & Schwarz, G. (1970). *Sehhilfenanpassung.* Berlin: VEB Verlag Technik.

Fonseka, C.M.R. & Obstfeld, M. (1995). Effect of the constringence of afocal prismatic lenses on monocular acuity and contrast sensitivity. *Ophthal. Physiol. Optics* **15**, 73–78.

Fry, G.A. & Hill, W.W. (1962). The center of rotation of the eye. *Am. J. Optom.* **39**(11), 581–595.

Gerstman, D.R. (1973). Ophthalmic lens decentration as a function of reading distance. *Brit. J. Physiol. Optics* **28**(1), 34–37.

Göhringer, W. (1989). *Eine neue Messmethode für die optische Anpassung mit Hilfe eines PC. Deutsche Optikerz.* No. 1, 17–19.

Grolman, B. (1969). An analog device for lens fitting. *Am. J. Optom.* **46**(11), 810–818.

Grolman (1977). *Fitting System Instruction Manual.* Southbridge (MA): American Optical Corporation.

Hardy, W.E. (1930). Obtaining the intraocular distance. *Optician & Sci. Instrum. Maker* **79**, 231–232, 239.

Harvey, R.S. (1982). Some statistics of interpupillary distance. *Optician* **184**, 29, Nov. 12.

Haugwitz, T. von. (1981). *Ophthalmologisch-optische Untersuchungsgeräte. Bücherei des Augenarztes,* pp. 111–114. Stuttgart: F. Enke.

Hemmer, F.G.M. (1979). De Fysio P.D. *Oculus, Amsterdam* No. 12, 45–47.

Henker, O. (1924). *Introduction to the Theory of Spectacles,* p. 311. Jena: Jena School of Optics.

Hoeft, W.M., Martin, J. & Lee, T. (1980). Three ways to measure PD: how they measure up. *Rev. Optom.* **117**(1), 53–56.

Hofstetter, H.W. (1972). Interpupillary distances – adult populations. *J. Am. Optom. Ass.* **43**(11), 1151–1155.

Hutchinson, J.R. (1984). Survey of inter-ocular distance measuring methods and devices. Final Year Project. London: City University.

Ivanoff, A. (1953). *Les Aberrations de l'Oeil.* Paris: Revue d'Optique.

Jalie, M. (1984). *Principles of Ophthalmic Lenses,* 4th edn, p. 159. London: Association of Dispensing Opticians.

Joseph, T.K. (1982). The Kerala decentration meter. A new method and device for fitting the optical centre of spectacle lenses in the visual axis. *Acta Ophthalm., Copenhagen* **60** (Suppl. 151).

Kasparek, G. (1981). Anforderungskriterien an Kinderbrillen. *Deutsche Optikerz.* No. 10, 10–14.

Knobloch, B. (1982). Das Messsystem KMS – eine neue Zentrier- und Anpasshilfe. *Optometrie, Mainz,* No. 1, 34–38.

Kochniss, T. (1987). Die Zentrierung von Brillengläsern in der Praxis des Augenoptikers. *Neues Optikerj.* **29**(4), 8–13.

Kochniss, Th. (1991). *(Monokulare)* PD-Messung in der Praxis des Augenoptikers: Erfahrungen mit dem neuen Rodenstock PD-Meter. *Neues Optikerj.* **33**(12), 22–23.

Kozol, F. (1958). *Ophthalmic Fitting and Adjusting,* p. 104. Philadelphia: Chilton.

Lewis, R. (1983). *The Conquest of Presbyopia.* Maroubra, Australia: R. & M. Lewis.

Mattison-Shupnick, M. (1980). Comparing methods and techniques for interocular distance measurements. *Optom. Monthly* **71**, Dec. 12.

Maxam, U. (1985). *Brillentechnik,* pp. 217, 223. Berlin: VEB Verlag Technik.

McCormack, G. & McGill, E. (1982). Measurement of interpupillary distance with chromostereopsis. *Am. J. Optom.* **59**, 60–66.

Michaels, D.D. (1985). *Visual Optics and Refraction,* 3rd edn, p. 573. St Louis: Mosby.

Millodot, M. (1990). *Dictionary of Optometry,* 2nd edn. London: Butterworths.

Müller, K. (1965). Versuch einer umfassenden Darstellung aller Arten und Formen. *Augenoptiker,* No. 9, 56.

Obstfeld, H. (1982). *Optics in Vision,* 2nd edn. London: Butterworths.

Obstfeld, H. (1990). The importance of lens centration. *Optician* **199**(5238), 37–44.

Pirbhai, M. (1965). The facial measurements of three racial groups. *Manufact. Optician* **18**(15), 684–690.

Prentice, C.F. (1890). A metric system of numbering and measuring prisms. The relation of the prism–dioptry to the lens–dioptry of refractions. *Arch. Ophthalm. (N.Y.)* **19**, 128–135.

Reiner, J. (1972). *Auge und Brille,* p. 76. Stuttgart: F. Enke Verlag.

Reiner, J. (1973). Vereinfachung der Arbeitsgänge bei Anpassung, Zentrierung und Anfertigung der Brillen. 23. Sonderdruck der Wissenschaftlichen Vereinigung der Augenoptiker.

Reiner, J. (1974). Neue Geräte zur Anpassung und Zentrierung von Brillengläsern. *Augenoptiker* **29**(3), 9–13.

Riedl, H.W. (1991). Der Hauptfixierstrahl – ein augenoptisches Märchen. *Neues Optikerj.* **33**(7/8), 30–32.

Rodenstock (1975). Rodenstock (Reiner) Interpupillary Gauge. München/Hamburg: Rodenstock Instrumente (brochure).

Rünz, E. (1978). Die Modellentwicklung in der Augenoptik unter Berücksichtigung der Belastbarkeit der Haut. *Augenoptiker* **33**(4), 9–17.

Sasieni, L.S. (1962). *Principles and Practice of Optical Dispensing and Fitting.* London: Hammond, Hammond & Co.

Shepard, C. (1942). *Optometric Science and Practice.* Chicago: W.R. Wolfe. Cited by Michaels (1985).

Stek, A.W. & Smitt, J.H. (1963). Decentratie van de nabijheidsdelen van dubbelfocusglazen. *Oculus, Amsterdam* No. 2, 70–78.

Stollenwerk, G. (1994). Horizontale centrering van multifocale glazen. *Oculus, Holland* **56**(10), 17–27 (translated from *Neues Optikerj.* **36**, 1).

Unger, M. (1957). A new method of measuring interpupillary distance. *A.M.A. Arch. Ophthal.* **58**(2), 257–258.

Villani, S. (1971). Not interpupillary distance but visual axis distance. *Atti Fond. G. Ronchi* **26**, 281–298.

Virdee, S. (1989). An analysis of dispensing clinic records. Final Year Project. London: City University.

Waters, E.H. (1952). *Ophthalmic Mechanics,* Vol. 1, p. 234–238. Corpus Christi, TX: Waters.

Watt, N. (1929). Spectacle fitting – an analysis of common faults. *Optician & Sci. Instrum. Maker* **78**(2013), 165–166.

Zeiss (1963). *Handbuch für Augenoptik,* p. 42. Oberkochen: C. Zeiss.

Zeiss (1983). *Handbook of Ophthalmic Optics,* p. 151. Oberkochen: C. Zeiss.

CHAPTER 22

Segment Top Position and Progression Height

22.1 Introduction

22.1.1 DEFINITIONS

In BS 3521, Part 1, (1991) the following definitions are given of terms encountered in this chapter:

- **Distance portion (DP)**   That portion of a lens having the correction for distance vision.
- **Dividing line**   The boundary line between two adjacent portions of a bifocal or multifocal lens.
- **Field of view**   A general term denoting the maximum angular extent of vision through an optical appliance under given conditions.
- **Fitting cross**   A reference point (indicated by two intersecting lines) on a progressive addition power lens which is specified by the manufacturer and is usually coincident with the start of the progression.
- **Intermediate portion**   That portion of a trifocal or multifocal lens having the correction for vision at ranges intermediate between distance and near.
- **Near portion (NP)/reading portion**   That portion of a lens having the correction for near vision.
- **Pantoscopic angle**   The angle between the optical axis of a lens and the visual axis of the eye in the primary position, usually taken to be the horizontal.
- **Jump**   This is the displacement of the image of an object which occurs when viewing across the borderline between two portions of different power in a bifocal or trifocal lens.
- **Prism thinning**   A process, sometimes applied to progressive power lenses and E-style bifocals, where vertical prism is worked across the whole lens in order to reduce the thickness in the distance portion.
- **Progression**   The zone covering the transition between the near and distance portions of a progressive addition power lens.
- **Progression height**   The vertical distance of the fitting cross above or below the horizontal centre line.
- **Segment**   A supplementary lens added to the main lens by cementing or fusing, or a supplementary surface on the main lens, for the purpose of providing the desired difference in power.
- **Segment height**   The vertical distance of the segment top above the horizontal tangent to the lens periphery at its lowest point (including the bevel's peak).
- **Segment top**   The point of contact of the curve of the segment with its horizontal tangent or, in the case of a straight-topped segment, the midpoint of the straight top.
- **Segment top position**   The vertical distance of the segment top above or below the horizontal centre line and assumed to apply to the highest segment of a multifocal lens.
- **Visual point**   Point of intersection of the eye's visual axis with the back surface of the lens.

22.1.2 REQUIREMENTS AND OBSERVATIONS

Whatever the type of segmented multifocal lenses fitted in the spectacle wearer's frame (and provided the wearer has normal binocular vision):

(1) each near visual point should lie well within its segment;
(2) the segments should not interfere or encroach on the fields of view during distance vision;
(3) they should be positioned such that (intermediate and) near vision through the segments is comfortable;
(4) the fields of view seen through the segments should coincide.

Abel (1952) stressed that any measurement of the segment top position (STP) cannot be carried out accurately unless the frame has been fitted properly, including adjustment of the angle of the side.

Epting & Morgret (1964) refer to the 'pantoscopic tilt' (but see definition of pantoscopic angle in Section 22.1.1) when the top of the glasses tilt outward, and the 'retroscopic tilt' when the bottom of the glasses tilt outward.

Brooks & Borish (1979) wrote that the inclination of the front may be anything from 4 to 18° from the vertical, allowing the visual axes to pass through the optical centres 'when the gaze is directed ahead towards the ground at approximately walking observation distance. This presents a reasonably angled plane for both distance viewing and reading. In addition, the angle has a more appropriate cosmetic effect when viewed from the side'. Hill & Kroemer (1986) found that, under this condition, the visual axes were usually 10–15° depressed.

The vertical lens size of the front must be sufficiently deep to accommodate distance (intermediate) and near portions that are of useful size to the needs of the patient (Table 22.1).

TABLE 22.1 *Minimum segment heights of multi-focal lenses and minimum vertical lens sizes of fronts to be glazed with multifocal lenses (after Darras, 1982)*

Type	Minimum segment height (mm)	Minimum vertical lens size (mm)
Bifocal	14	30
Trifocal	17	33
Progressive lenses	22	37

The dividing line(s) between distance (intermediate, if applicable) and near portions of segmented lenses, are usually noticeable to the wearer. Although it can be argued that an area roughly equal to the prevailing pupil height (Fig. 22.1) cannot be used for vision, this is not the experience of this presbyopic writer. With at least low-powered additions one can see objects at any distance through any portion of the lens fairly well. However, there is a ghosting effect when the pupil straddles the dividing line: close to the clear image of the object, there appears to be a second which is (slightly) blurred. When the wearer then moves their head from side to side, they will notice that one image appears to be stationary while the other image moves. The direction of movement depends on the image

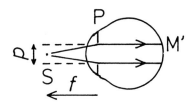

Fig. 22.1 *The segment top at S lies in the first focal plane of the eye and is imaged as a blur circle in the retinal plane M'. f, First focal length of the eye; p, pupil diameter; P, entrance pupil*

which is perceived to be stationary. By means of a small head movement up or down, apparently stationary and moving images may be exchanged. The dividing line itself is not seen (Section 21.10) but the position of the blurred/sharp images suggests its position.

With increasing addition power, the blurred image will become more and more defocused. Because this is a step-by-step process which increases every time the power of the addition is increased, most patients tend to be little bothered by it.

22.2 The Segment Top Position

22.2.1 INTRODUCTION

Previously, a rule of thumb was frequently used for the segment top position (Abel, 1952; Holmes *et al.*, 1958), such as '2 mm below' (the horizontal centre line). Darras (1982) stressed that there is no such thing as a universal STP, that each case is a particular one, that each presbyope must be provided for in a way that is suitable to his or her needs and that an STP is not final. Hence, there are no hard and fast rules for the STP of segmented multifocal lenses or the progression height of progressive lenses, only general recommendations. These must be adapted to the needs of the individual wearer by the dispenser. By discussing with the prospective wearer the circumstances under which they will use the glasses, an insight will be obtained of specific requirements. This will provide not only information on which to base the choice of multifocal lens for a first-time wearer, but also for the position of the segment top.

22.2.2 FACTORS
22.2.2.1 Type of multifocal lens
Segmented and progressive power lenses require

fundamentally different approaches. The STP of bifocal lenses will depend on:

(1) the shape of the segment;
(2) the position of the optical centre of the near portion, although this is commonly only considered when a problem has arisen, or different prismatic effects are required for distance and near vision;
(3) jump.

Dowaliby (1988) wrote that 'practitioners feel that the reduction of image jump ... is more critical'. This writer agrees with Uhlmann (1969) that this aspect is overemphasized since spectacle wearers do not seem to be bothered by it. He added that vision of the floor, staircase, etc., is always hampered by the near portion and that this is the cause of complaints.

22.2.2.3 Head posture
Different postures may be adopted during distance and during near vision, and patients are seldom conscious of them. It is useful to observe the patient from the moment they arrive so that one can study these postures without the patient being aware of it. Make the patient walk to a window and look outside, or ask them to look from a distant to a near object.

For postures during near vision, ask the patient to read, draw or write something and observe them. Note, for instance, whether the patient bends their head over the page, or depresses eyes and chin, or only their eyes; the last is required when using many types of near portions.

Some people tend to hold their head such that their nose points upwards. The segment top of multifocal lenses will then have to be placed a little lower in order to avoid interfering with their distance vision (Fig. 22.2). Although some tall people tilt their head forward, because of their length, the segment top may still have to be

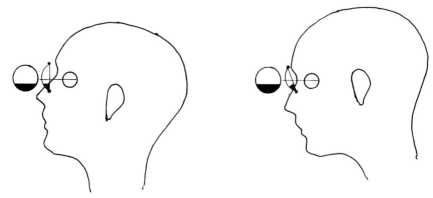

Fig. 22.2 *Left: bifocal wearers of average stature who tend to have a 'nose in the air' posture, require relatively low-placed segment tops. Right: because tall people tend to tilt their head forward which requires an inclination of the spectacle plane, their bifocals also need to be placed low. Circles show similar fields of view through near portion (black) and distance portion*

placed relatively low. Conversely, a very short person (including children) will need a higher segment top, but while driving a car this person may have to tilt his head downward for clear distance vision (Homes, 1958). Because that posture may well be inconvenient and uncomfortable on longer car journeys, a separate pair of (single vision?) driving glasses might be required.

22.2.2.3 The nature of work and its distance

Many patients need to use multifocal lenses to be able to carry out their job and hobbies. The ideal would be to observe the wearer during these activities. Unfortunately, this is not usually practical. Hence, one has to rely on the wearer imitating such postures. Do not overlook that the new glasses may have a higher addition than before and thus, possibly, a shorter working distance and reduced depth of field.

22.2.2.4 The degree of ametropia

The greater the ametropia, the higher the segment top should be placed, is one of Darras' (1982) general rules. This will provide more

comfortable near vision because the visual axis will run very close to the optical centre of the distance portion. Hence, the retinal image will hardly be affected by aberrations (see Reiner, 1972). This is of particular importance when correcting aphakics and anisometropes, and when lens materials with a low V-value (subject to more chromatic aberration) are used. Fonseka & Obstfeld (1995) found that the retinal image of objects containing high spatial frequencies (fine detail) is significantly degraded when the image formation takes place off axis. By looking through such lenses or lens portions close to their optical centre(s), the aberrations are minimized.

22.2.2.5 The power of the addition

The (apparent) far point of a low addition will appear to lie higher in the field of view than that of a higher addition (Fig. 22.3). Hence, the higher the addition, the lower the segment top may be placed; however, the higher the ametropia, the higher the position of the segment top (see Section 22.2.2.4). Note that the position of the (apparent) near point depends on the amplitude of accommodation.

The size of the field of view depends on the

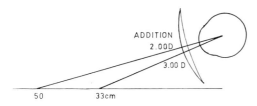

Fig. 22.3 The (apparent) far point of a lower addition (say, at 50 cm from the spectacle lens) will appear to lie higher in the field of view than that of a higher addition. Accommodation will have the same effect as increasing the addition

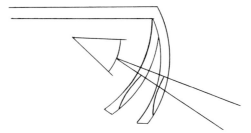

Fig. 22.5 The effect of an increase in the angle of side (as for the left front compared with the right) is to lower the segment top (relative to the eye) and to reduce the vertex distance

power of the addition and on the segment size. It can be shown that the field of view becomes smaller as the power of the addition increases.

22.2.2.6 The vertex distance
The greater the vertex distance, the lower the segment top appears to the wearer (Fig. 22.4). The smaller the vertex distance, the larger the field of view, both through the distance and the near portions (Fig. 22.4). Increasing the angle of the side will have the same effect for the near portion because it too reduces the vertex distance (Fig. 22.5).

22.2.2.7 The STP of an established multifocal wearer
If a patient is happy with their present multifocal lenses, it is unwise to change anything but the power of the addition. The dispenser should only

consider changing one aspect or another when the wearer complains about it. Any change should be preceded by a discussion of the exact nature of the problem, and the possible solution(s) available. Brooks & Borish (1979) and also Dowaliby (1988) call attention to this point.

22.2.2.8 Eye posture
Holmes *et al.* (1958) noted that some people seldom look directly into another person's eyes, maintaining their gaze considerably below eye level. He suggested that, for them, segments should be placed as low as possible.

22.2.2.9 Head turners and eye turners
Some patients tend to turn their heads more than their eyes. This applies usually to higher hyperopes, because of the restricted field of view imposed by the spectacle lenses, while progressive lens wearers may be taught to benefit from deliberate head movements for intermediate and near vision purposes, thus avoiding the lens areas with aberrations. This may possibly be experienced by patients wearing 'soft' design progressive lenses. Other patients tend to move their eyes more than their head.

Head turners may be quite happy with relatively small segments since they turn their heads to cover the area of regard with the segment. The dispenser should note whether they also tilt their

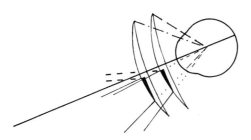

Fig. 22.4 The greater the vertex distance, the lower the apparent segment top position and the smaller the field of view through both distance and near portions

head down for reading. If yes, the segment top can be placed relatively high.

Eye turners tend to fixate objects without much head movement. Because their near visual points must fall within the segment at all times during near vision, they will need larger segments. When they use multifocal lenses mainly for desk work, the segment top should be set rather high.

22.3 Basic Segment Top Positions

Two quotations that touch upon the question 'what is the correct segment top position?', are: 'Experience has shown that in cases of doubt it is always better when the segment top lies 0.5 mm lower rather than higher' (Fleck *et al.*, 1960); and '... it is better to err on the segments being too high than too low' (Sasieni, 1962). Sasieni adds in the same paragraph: 'spectacles do sometimes slip down a little in wear – they never slip upwards'. This is certainly true; it may even be an understatement. Drew (1970) went so far as to write that 'bifocals are usually fitted too low'.

Of the different parts of the eye that can be used as references point for the STP, namely the pupil centre, and the 6 o'clock positions along either the pupil edge, limbus or lower lid, only the last two have commonly been employed because the positions of the former two are too uncertain, or variable (see Section 22.5 (12)). The segment height is usually measured from the limbus or lower lid, to the lowest horizontal tangent to the lens (that is, into the groove of the rim; see Section 22.4). However, because the STP should be specified with respect to the horizontal centre line, the segment height (Fig. 22.6) must then be subtracted from half the boxed vertical lens size of the frame (where a 'negative' value indicates that the segment top will lie above the horizontal centre line). However, for frames that have no upper or no lower

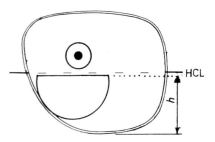

Fig. 22.6 The segment height h of a bifocal lens. HCL, horizontal centre line

rim as such (Supra and semi-rimless frames), the measurement must be taken from the reference point for the segment top to, respectively, the lowest or to the highest tangent of the lens (Fig. 22.7). This must be specified unambiguously because it is not the conventional way of presenting the STP.

The STPs shown in Table 22.2 and Fig. 22.8 are conventional positions for these multifocal lenses.

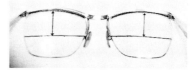

Fig. 22.7 A Polymil front fitted with E-style bifocal lenses. Each arrow indicates the distance between the highest horizontal tangent to the spectacle lens, and the segment top

TABLE 22.2 Segment top positions for various segmented multifocal lens types

Type	STP
Round	At limbus level
Curved top	1 mm below limbus
D-segment	2 mm below limbus
E-segment	2 mm below limbus
Trifocal	2 mm above limbus
Smart segment	2 mm above limbus

Note: (1) the fitting cross of progressive lenses normally lies in front of the pupil centre; (2) the STP of bifocal lenses for aphakics normally lies 2 mm above the limbus.

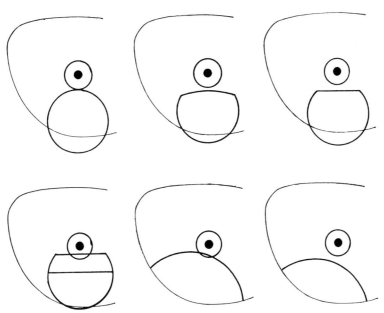

Fig. 22.8 *Conventional segment top positions for various multifocal segments. From left to right, top row: round segment, curved top and D-segments; bottom row: trifocal, invisible solid and visible solid segments*

22.4 Determining the Segment Top Position

The STP must be measured with the selected frame adjusted on the patient's face. A millimetre rule is then held vertically against the front.

Dowaliby (1988) made the point that plastics rules designed for ophthalmic use, or segment height gauges (see below) should be used: inexpensive flexible rules may give a false reading and when a metal rule slips it may injure the patient.

With the dispenser's eye level with that of the patient, the distance between the 6 o'clock position along the limbus and the lowest tangent to the lens shape is measured (allow 0·5 mm for the depth of the rim of metal fronts, and 1 mm for plastics fronts). This is the segment height (Fig. 22.9). The lowest points of limbus and lower lid usually coincide. However, when the lower lid sags (as in an ectropion) or covers up the limbus (as in an entropion), the lowest limbus point should be taken as reference point.

In BS 3521, Part 1 (1991) it is suggested that the STP of all types of segmented multifocal lenses and the progression height of progressive lenses are specified with respect to the horizontal centre line. It may be recorded as 'x below', 'on centre line' or as 'x above' where 'x' is given in

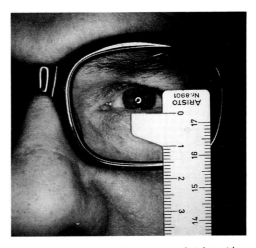

Fig. 22.9 *Measuring the segment height with a plastics rule*

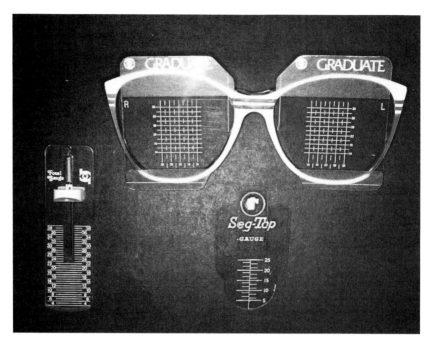

Fig. 22.10 *A selection of segment height gauges. Above: a pair of self-adhesive platelets fixed to a front; below: a spring-loaded gauge (left) and one with a forked top which holds the upper rim*

millimetres. This has the advantage that, provided the bridge width remains unaltered, when a lens size is required other than the one of the front at hand, the recorded measurement is still correct, because the horizontal centre lines of the fronts will coincide. If a front with the correct bridge width is not available the rule-of-thumb is to add 1 mm to the segment height for every 2 mm increase in bridge width. This applies to pad bridges only. For saddle bridge type fronts account must be taken of any difference in bridge height.

It is far from unusual to measure different monocular STPs in a pair of eyes (see Section 3.2.3). If the segment top is visible to the onlooker (as in E-type multifocal lenses), it is wise not to specify different STPs for a pair of lenses: onlookers, such as relatives, will ask the wearer why the straight segment tops are not level. They will assume that there is something

wrong with the glazing, and the wearer will have to explain the situation (if possible, or be embarrassed). One solution is to place the segment tops halfway between the two STPs measured. If that is unacceptable to the wearer, the segment tops should be placed at the lower STP. In this way the segment will not interfere with the field of view of the 'lower' eye. If it is necessary to specify different STPs, it may be wiser to use a type of multifocal lens where the segment top is less obvious. Progressive lenses have no visible dividing lines and so the problem does not arise.

A selection of segment height gauges is shown in Fig. 22.10. These gadgets have one feature in common in that they can be fixed in or on the lens aperture of a rimmed front; some come in pairs and have one or more millimetre scales printed or embossed on them. When a pair of segment height gauges has been fixed to a front, the frame is placed on the patient's face.

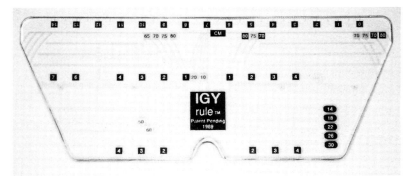

Fig. 22.11 *The multi-purpose IGY rule*

The position of the reference point (for instance, lower limbus edge) is then read off the scale while the dispenser ensures to be at eye level with the wearer's eyes. A more versatile gauge, the IGY Rule, available from Datum Optica, 13 Station Road, Ainsdale, Southport PR8 3HN, UK is shown in Fig. 22.11.

DeHaan (1982) wrote that the segment top of bifocals used by pilots should be level with the highest instrument on the forward instrument panel. Individually designed multifocal spectacles for civil aviation pilots were discussed by Backman & Smith (1975).

Shapiro (1994) warned about the problem of progressive lens wearers who have a head tilt. They may complain that one eye's retinal image is always blurred whether looking into the distance or at a near object. On re-examining (refraction) the patient *monocularly* no problem is encountered, which is confusing to both the patient and the practitioner. Therefore, it is prudent to ascertain whether there is a head tilt during reading or distance vision. The use of a $\frac{1}{2}$ prism dioptre prism, base vertical, may be sufficient to realign the head. However, because of 'prism thinning' of the lenses, unwanted differential vertical prism may be present, particularly in anisometropic corrections.

Having carefully positioned the frame on the head, ask the patient to follow a fixation target in the reading position, and estimate the head tilt (if any). Determine the progression height and required inclination of the progression itself. This can be done by specifying a particular monocular near centration distance. Take care when applying this to an astigmatic lens: if the axis is not adjusted for this purpose, the patient may still complain about blurred vision!

22.5 A Different Approach

The following steps to determine the monocular centration distances, progression heights or STPs may appear complicated. However, they provide accurate measurements and can be taken quite quickly.

(1) Ask the patient to hold a small light source (for instance, a pentorch) at the required viewing distance. The dispenser places their preferred eye above the light source and observes the light reflections in the patient's corneas.

(2) Place a PD rule in the patient's spectacle plane, and measure the distance between the light reflections. This represents the near visual axes distance (VAD). Now, by measuring from one reflection to the midline of the nose, one near monocular VAD is obtained. Subtract this value from the near

VAD, to find the other near monocular VAD. Remove spectacle frame from the patient's head.

(3) Since the near monocular VAD has been determined, 2 mm must be added to each to obtain the distance monocular VADs. Record these values as the R and L MCDs (Section 21.1.1) required to order progressive lenses from a prescription house. For most segmented multifocal lenses it is sufficient to specify the distance centration distance and either the near centration distance of the lenses, or their inset (Section 21.10). For high-powered lenses the distance or near MCDs should be given so that the patient may enjoy the best retinal image quality.

(4) If the front is not fitted with demonstration or dummy lenses, place a strip of self-adhesive transparent tape vertically over each lens aperture.

(5) Using a frame rule and pen, mark the R and L VADs with a vertical line, on the lenses in the front.

(6) Place the frame on the patient's face. Verify that the VAD lines fall within the pupils of the eyes. If not, repeat the previous steps, except (4).

(7) The dispenser should ensure that she is at eye level with the patient.

(8) The dispenser holds the light source to one side of his head, at eye level (Fig. 22.12), and instructs the patient to look at the light source.

(9) Observe the corneal light reflection in the patient's right eye and mark the *level* of that reflection, on the dummy lens, etc. If the lens aperture of the front is fitted with a segment height gauge, the level may be read off the scale. This represents the level of the fitting cross. The progression height, relative to the horizontal centre line, can now be measured.

(10) Repeat for the other eye; it is not usually necessary to move the light source to the other side of the head.

(11) Check that the marks are at level with their respective pupil centres. If not, repeat from (8) onwards. For progressive lenses, go to (15).

(12) Remove frame from the patient's head and place it on the frame rule. Draw a horizontal line 5 mm (because the vertical iris diameter is about 10 mm) below each level mark and long enough to show its position below the vertical VAD line (Fig. 22.13).

(13) Replace the frame on the patient's head and check whether each line is level with their respective eye's limbus. If it is, the line represents the level of the basic segment top position for segmented bifocal lenses.

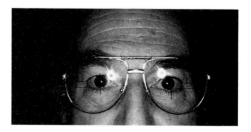

Fig. 22.13 The upper line is drawn level with the corneal reflection while the patient wears the frame. Having removed the frame from the patient's face, the lower line is drawn 5 mm lower and will lie level with the bottom of the limbus, as for this right eye. However, the lines for the left eye are then more than 1 mm too high. This can now be rectified and then checked

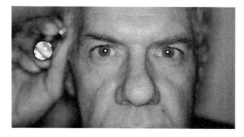

Fig. 22.12 While the dispenser holds a light source to the side of his head, he can see the corneal reflections of the light source in the patient's eyes

(14) Use the frame rule to cover the lens below the STP. The patient's distance vision should not be hampered. Next, cover the lens above the STP. Now the reading area should be unobstructed. If necessary, adjust the STP.

(15) Check with the patient standing that the STPs or progression heights are at the correct level while the patient looks at a distant object. Make any necessary adjustments.

(16) To arrive at the STP or progression height to be recorded, place the frame on the frame rule and read off the position(s) relative to either: (a) the horizontal centre line, or (b) the segment height.

Because the centre line is not a physical mark on the front, it may be preferable to measure the vertical boxed size of the lens, divide the number found by 2, and subtract the measurement according to (16b). If the position is above the centre line, add the word 'above'.

Note that BS 2738 (1991) allows a tolerance of ±0.5 mm per glazed lens.

22.6 Instructions for Multifocal Lens Wearers

22.6.1 SEGMENTED MULTIFOCAL LENSES

First-time segmented multifocal lens wearers should be instructed in their use. The following approach may be taken. Having adjusted the spectacles to fit on the head, give the patient some reading matter in hand and

(1) instruct the patient to look straight ahead – not at the reading matter;
(2) then instruct the patient to glance down at the reading matter without moving their head;
(3) now allow the patient to adjust their head position so that they will be reading comfortably;
(4) remind the patient consciously to make these

adjustments just for the short period it will take for this routine to become a habit.

22.6.2 PROGRESSIVE LENSES

First-time progressive lens wearers must be shown where aberrations will affect their vision. Use the following sequence. Having adjusted the spectacles to fit on the patient's head, give him some reading matter in hand, and

(1) instruct the patient to look ahead at a distant object; this should be seen clearly;
(2) instruct the patient to glance down at the reading matter, which should also be seen clearly;
(3) let the patient move their head slowly from side to side without changing the fixation point or the position of the reading matter; they will notice that the reading matter will become less distinct outside the reading zone and will get an idea of the size of that zone;
(4) repeat this demonstration with reading matter of appropriate size, held at an intermediate distance and the patient looking at it through the progression. The patient will notice that the progression has a smaller 'clear vision' width than the reading zone.

22.6.3 GENERAL

Very tall patients and first-time multifocal wearers with a relatively high addition should be warned and shown that on looking down, the floor/curb/stairs will look blurred. It is also possible that the distance to these objects will be misjudged. However, they should be assured that they will soon adapt to the new condition.

22.7 Vertical Adjustment of Glazed Multifocal Lenses

The segment top position of segmented multifocal lenses or the progression height of progressive lenses may be altered by:

(1) Increasing the angle of the side. As a result, the segment top or fitting cross is lowered a little (Fig. 22.5).

(2) Increasing the vertex distance (of low and medium power prescriptions) results in a lowering of the segment top or progression height, as the frame will come to rest lower on the nose. If this method is used with higher prescriptions the back vertex power of the lens(es) will have to be altered. This may defeat the object of the exercise.

(3) Increasing the distance between the pad centres of metal pad frames will make the pads rest on a lower part of the nasal flanks, thus lowering the segment top or fitting cross. Note that the effect will be larger for noses that have a small angle between the nasal flanks than for those that have a larger angle (Fig. 22.14). This result can also be achieved with plastics pad frames when the bridge width is increased by filing away some material in this area, or stretching the bridge after heating (Section 16.4.1).

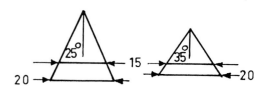

Fig. 22.14 *Increasing the distance between pad centres makes the pads rest on a lower part of the nasal flanks. The larger the angle between the flanks, the smaller the effect*

The segment top and fitting cross may be raised by reducing the angle of the side, decreasing the vertex distance (if possible), or decreasing the distance between pad centres. Reducing the bridge width (by cementing some additional plastics material onto the pads) or the crest height of a saddle bridge frame (achieved by cementing material onto the crest) will also raise the position of the segment top and progression height with respect to the eyes.

REFERENCES

Abel, P. (1952). *Die Grundlagen der Brillenanpassung*, p. 153. Düsseldorf: Verlag W. Schrickel.

Backman, H.A. & Smith, F.D. (1975). The design and prescription of multifocal lenses for civil pilots. *Am. J. Optom. Physiol. Optics* **52**, 591–599.

Brooks, C.W. & Borish, I.M. (1979). *System for Ophthalmic Dispensing*, pp. 76, 127. Chicago: Professional Press.

BS 2738 (1991). *Spectacle Lenses. Part 3: Specification for the Presentation of Prescriptions and Prescription Orders for Ophthalmic Lenses.* London: British Standards Institution.

BS 3521 (1991). *Terms Relating to Ophthalmic Optics and Spectacle Frames. Part 1: Glossary of Terms Relating to Ophthalmic Lenses.* London: British Standards Institution.

Darras, C. (1982). *La Tête et ses Mesures*, 3rd edn, p. 132. Paris: Centre de protection oculaire.

DeHaan, W.V. (1982). *Optometrist's and Ophthalmologist's Guide to Pilot's Vision.* Boulder, CO: American Trends Publ. Co.

Dowaliby, M. (1988). *Practical Aspects of Ophthalmic Optics*, pp. 48, 62. New York: Professional Press Books/Fairchild.

Drew, R. (1970). *Professional Ophthalmic Dispensing*, p. 276. Chicago: Professional Press.

Epting, J.B. & Morgret, F.C. (1964). *Ophthalmic Mechanics and Dispensing*, p. 269. Radnor, PA: Chilton Book Co.

Fleck, H., Heynig, J. & Mütze, K. (1960). *Die Praxis der Brillenanpassung*, pp. 33–35. Leipzig: VEB Fachbuch Verlag.

Fonseka, C.M.R. & Obstfeld, H. (1995). The effect of the constringence of afocal prismatic lenses on monocular acuity and contrast sensitivity. *Ophthal. Physiol. Optics* **15**, 73–78.

Hill, S.G. & Kroemer, K.H.E. (1986). Preferred declination of the line of sight. *Human Factors* **28**(2), 127–134.

Holmes, C., Jolliffe, H., Gregg, J., Cameron, I.S. & Blyth, R. (1958). *Guide to Occupational and Other Visual Needs.* Los Angeles: Anderson, Ritchie & Simon.

Reiner, J. (1972). *Auge und Brille*, p. 76. Stuttgart: F. Enke Verlag.

Sasieni, L.S. (1962). *The Principles and Practice of Optical Dispensing and Fitting*, p. 309. London: Hammond, Hammond & Co.

Shapiro, I.J. (1994). The effect of facial asymmetry and head tilt on fitting progressive addition lenses. *Optom. Update, Israel* No. 2, 13–15 (in Hebrew; transcript from author at P.O.B. 1282, Pardes Channa, Israel).

Uhlmann, K.-H. (1969). Neue Nahteilformen. *Süddeutsche Optikerz.* **24**(6), 374–176.

CHAPTER 23

Care and Protection of Spectacles

23.1 Introduction

Spectacles are worn, but not continuously. During wear, they may make contact with another object and get damaged. While not being worn, they should be kept in a safe place. Two questionnaires dealing with these aspects were distributed by Hill (1979) among the general population. Forty-six completed forms were returned about damaged spectacles, and 240 forms about care of spectacles. Both samples matched fairly well the female to male population ratio of people over the age of 16, in England and Wales. However, this was not the case with respect to age groups in that there were relatively few people included whose age was over 60 years.

The following sections contain a mixture of details gathered by Hill (1979) and commentary from other sources.

23.2 Damaged Spectacles

Hill's (1979) survey revealed that 40% of all reported accidents concerned spectacles belonging to the group aged between 20 and 40 years, and that 60% involved glasses owned by females. Scrivener (1973) found that the largest percentage of accidents occurred in the 20–40-year-old group, and in younger age groups.

Most cases of damage occurred while the spectacles were not being worn (60%). This figure was almost equally divided between being dropped and being sat or trodden on. Two individuals reported that their spectacles broke during cleaning, and another two while trying to adjust them. The causes of damage that occurred during spectacle wear were divided into three major groups, namely due to a blow (33%), due to a collision (44%) and due to 'other types' of accidents (22%). Five individuals reported that their spectacles 'just fell apart' for no apparent reason. Most frequently damaged were the sides (46%), followed by the bridge (40%) and the rims (12%) (cf. Section 13.9). Only 13% of the respondents tried to make the repair themselves; 87% of wearers took their spectacles to be repaired or replaced within 1 week of the damage occurring, and of these 37% had the frame repaired, the same percentage replaced the damaged appliance with a new pair, and 13% had the old lenses placed into a new frame.

While many people have never had an accident with their spectacles, some have had many, often minor accidents that led eventually to a breakage. Several people returned more than one form; others stated that the details referred to their 'last' accident. Hill (1979) estimated that some 15% of the spectacle wearing population will incur damage to their spectacles which is severe enough to impair the function of the appliance.

23.3 Injuries caused by Spectacles

Damage to spectacles can lead to eye injuries. Estimates of the incidence of serious eye injuries caused by broken spectacles vary. Such injuries are rare among children, and trauma in adults due to broken glasses and resulting in enucleation is equally rare (Duke-Elder, 1954). Buchanan (1921, quoted by Duke-Elder, 1954) reported two such cases out of 61 eyes that had to be enucleated after trauma, adding that they had been caused by a direct blow by a stone which would have destroyed the eye irrespective of wearing spectacles. Such injuries are usually due to a spectacle lens fracturing. Keeney *et al.* (1972) concluded that all the injuries they reported could have been prevented, that heat-tempered glass lenses offered greater protection than non-tempered glass lenses, and that plastics lenses offered greater protection still. One may also speculate that if polycarbonate lenses had been fitted in these frames fewer eyes would have been injured. However, the frame itself may have caused injury to the facial structures surrounding the eye, in particular if the back plane of the front included protruding metal parts.

Scrivener (1973) reported on 1443 cases of ocular trauma where only 51 patients, or 3·5%, were spectacle wearers. Of the broken spectacles 28 cases (55%) caused ocular trauma. All of these were caused by broken lenses. The other interesting aspect is that the majority of accidents (16 cases) occurred during leisure activities. Loran (1992) found that more than 15% of spectacle- and more than 20% of contact lens-wearing squash players had experienced eye injuries, while the 'overall' percentage was just under 15%. Scrivener (1973) encountered only two cases that were due to domestic accidents. Höfling (1974) reported two cases where injury of a child's temple had been caused by a metal spectacle side as a result of a fall.

As most eye injuries are caused by fractured spectacle lenses, it is appropriate to add a note about the relationship between spectacle frame materials and lens breakage. Keeney & Reynaldo (1975) used the drop ball test (defined in BS 3521,

Part 1, 1991, as 'a means of testing for robustness in which a specified ball is dropped upon the lens from a stated height'; specifications vary from country to country and between standards). They found that the force required to fracture lenses in a plastics frame, was twice that needed to fracture the same strength lenses in a metal rimmed frame. The lowest fracture and posterior dislocation rates were found for industrial plastics frames which had a lens-retaining lip. However, plastics frames may be weakened by incorrect handling (Drew, 1970). Breakages are caused by stresses created during manufacture and dispensing, particularly when insufficient heat is applied during a bending process (Figs 13.7 and 23.1). Such weaknesses and rough handling may cause the frames to snap. Bewley (1970) referred to the danger of a reduction of the field of view caused by spectacle frames (Section 5.2.7).

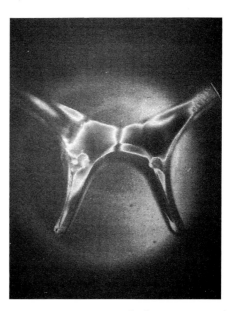

Fig. 23.1 *Stress in spectacle frame parts can be demonstrated with a strain tester or polariscope (Section 24.5 and Fig. 24.10). This photograph shows stress in the bridge of a Supra frame. Stress is greatest where bright and dark areas meet, such as in the centre of the bridge. See also Fig. 13.7*

23.4 Spectacle Cases and Other Devices

Patients should be made aware that a pair of spectacles is a relatively delicate, precision optical appliance and that it should be treated as such. This awareness should help to prevent damage to the spectacles and extend their life. Every pair of spectacles should have its own spectacle case.

The purpose of a spectacle case (Hill, 1979) is to protect spectacles, when not worn, against damage of the frame, and of the lens and frame surfaces, from dirt, and against deformation of the spectacles. Hence, a spectacle case should be hard on the outside and soft on the inside. Davies (Gibbs, 1990) added further criteria: the type of case should depend on the spectacle wearer's occupation (an office worker requires a different case from someone doing heavy industrial work); and the case must remain serviceable as long as the spectacles (say, 3 years).

Some manufacturing details were described by Hardy (1989).

Of the respondents to Hill's (1979) second questionnaire 41% indicated that they possessed more than one pair of spectacles. Most kept their second pair in a spectacle case (70%), others kept them loose in a drawer or in the glove compartment of their car (15%). Hence, almost 30% of the additional pairs were not protected when not in use.

More than 85% of participants indicated that they had a spectacle case. The types and distribution of spectacle cases is shown in Table 23.1.

Hard-bodied cases (Fig. 23.2) should be used because they provide maximum protection. Soft cases (Fig. 23.3) do not give protection against breakage and deformation of the frame. A spectacle frame placed in such a case and kept in the pocket of a dress or jacket can easily be broken when the wearer leans against a hard object. The slip-in type of case is normally open on one side. Hence, it does not protect against dust and dirt.

TABLE 23.1 *Distribution of spectacle cases by type*

Type	%
Plastics/fabric covered metal body, spring shut	**49**
Plastics/leather slip-in	**25**
Plastics/leather purse	**19**
Others	**7**

Moreover, lenses may become scratched when the spectacles are slipped into the case (Fig. 23.3B). However, the dispenser has to cope with conflicting aspects and interests (e.g. available space in women's handbags): a hard case will give protection, but occupy more space while soft cases give less protection and usually occupy less

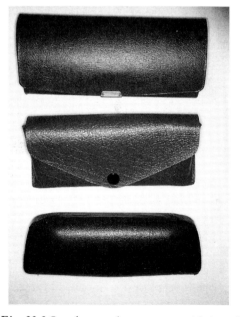

Fig. 23.2 Sample spectacle cases: a case with a metal base and semi-rigid flap (above), an imitation leather case with a rigid plastics centre which supports the casing and centres the frame in the case (centre), and a case with a metal body and sprung lid covered with an imitation leather material (below)

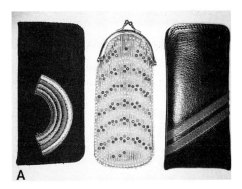

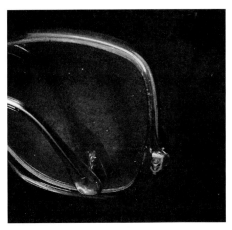

Fig. 23.4 *The drop of sides attached to a front with a very large lens size, has scratched the back surface of the lens while the spectacles were being placed in their case*

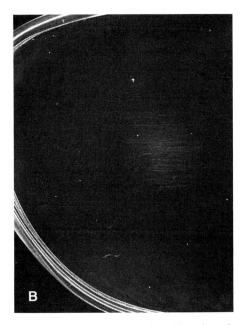

Fig. 23.3 *Soft spectacle cases. A, neither the nylon slip-in case (left) nor the purse-type case decorated with beads (centre) gives any protection against impact; the slip-in case on the right has a hard base. B, a plastics lens showing scratches caused by the tight-fitting, hard base of the slip-in case of A (right)*

space. This applies in particular when frames that have large lens sizes are fashionable. The back surfaces of plastics lenses fitted in some large fronts are likely to be scratched when the drops of the sides move over them (Fig. 23.4). A spectacle case should be large enough not to deform the frame when closed and small enough for the

frame not to move around too much inside it when shaken.

Old spectacle cases should be checked to ascertain whether the hinges and fastenings are worn, and for cleanliness. When the patient proposes to use an old case for a new pair of spectacles, the case should be inspected for cleanliness otherwise dirt particles in its lining may cause scratches. If the case is too small for the new spectacles, they will be deformed during storage. It is, therefore, wise to let each new pair of spectacles be accompanied by a new case. After all, the cost of a case is usually only a fraction of that of the new spectacles.

Less than half the respondents (44%) indicated that they always returned their spectacles to its case, and another 20% did this only occasionally. One-third indicated that they never put their spectacles back into their case. Of the latter category, the spectacles were then most likely to be left on a table or chair, and less frequently on the bedside table, or in a handbag or pocket, or just somewhere convenient (end of the bath, under the bed, etc.). One solution, originally

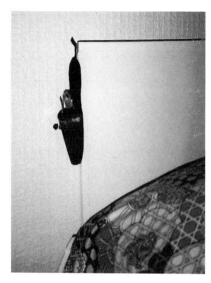

Fig. 23.5 *A slipper attached to the headboard of a bed serves as a decorative spectacle case*

seen in Switzerland, may be suitable for a bedroom if not elsewhere: see Fig. 23.5.

Only 6% of respondents owned a spectacle chain or brooch (Fig. 23.6), and only 1% of spectacle wearers regularly used such an accessory. This demonstrates that neither provides a satisfactory answer to a problem. Neither device protects spectacles against dirt, dust, impact and abrasive effects. In addition, the spectacles may dislodge and drop. Spectacle chains provide ready access to the spectacles, and they can be taken off and 'dropped' quickly, whereupon they hang on the chain. This can be important to presbyopic shoppers and to others who 'use' (that is, play with) their optical aid for psychological purposes, for instance, to impress another person or to 'collect their thoughts'. However, when leaning over a table top the spectacles may swing out and hit the table, or the lenses may become scratched by the tables surface.

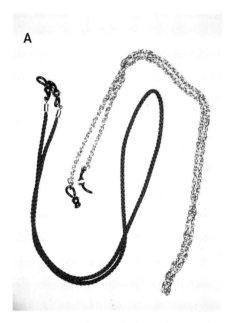

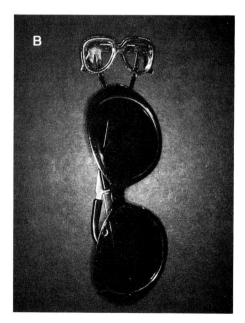

Fig. 23.6 *A, a metal spectacle chain (above) and one made out of cord. Note the black plastics grips at the ends which slide over the sides of the frame. B, a spectacle brooch in the form of a miniature frame. The brooch is attached to the wearer's clothing. One side of a pair of sunglasses is slipped through a hook attached to the miniature frame, which makes for easy removal*

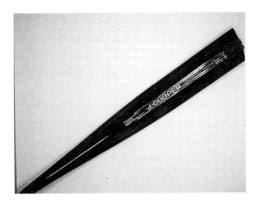

Fig. 23.7 A side engraved with the owner's name

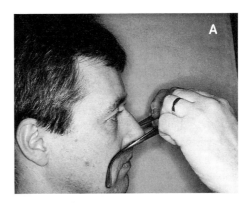

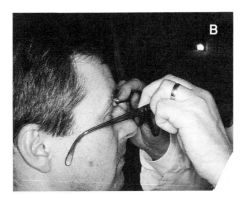

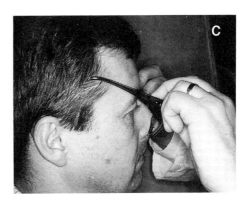

Fig. 23.8 A, the dispenser should hold the frame in such a way that it is made to approach the patient's face with the sides pointing downwards; B, the sides have been advanced to just in front of the ears; C, the front should be rotated so that the drop-ends can be moved over the ears. The front can now be placed on the nose, and the drops behind the ears

Spectacle sides may be engraved (Fig. 23.7) with, for instance, the owner's name. This helps to identify the owner if the appliance is lost, and may prevent theft. Some manufacturers have started to provide frames with serial numbers to prevent theft of expensive and/or designer frames. Some optical practices used to emboss their practice name in a side.

Sides can be engraved with a pantographic engraving machine (Fig. 10.8). An embossing tool may consist of a template containing a symbol or desired lettering, which is then impressed with a pair of pliers or similar device, on a portion of the frame.

23.5 Handling Spectacles

Teaching a patient how to handle their spectacles starts by setting a good example. The dispenser should not take off and put on his spectacles with one hand, nor should he place them on a surface with the convex lens surfaces downwards.

A dispenser should always place a spectacle frame on the patient's face with both hands. The frame should be made to approach the patient's face with the sides pointing downwards (Fig. 23.8A) so that they cannot possibly enter the wearer's eyes. When the drops have been advanced to just in front of the ears (Fig. 23.8B), rotate the front so that the drop-ends can be moved over the ear points (Fig. 23.8C). The front can now be placed on the nose, and the drops behind the ears.

Wearers should be instructed to remove and replace their spectacles using both hands. If this is not done, the angle of let-back of, usually, the contralateral side, will gradually be forced open further than is suitable for a well-fitting pair of spectacles. When certain items of clothing are removed, such as a pullover, before the wearer's spectacles have been removed, the glasses may be removed simultaneously and may fall on the floor and may break.

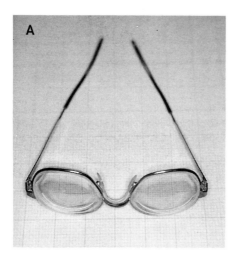

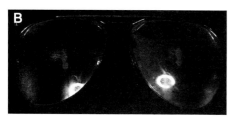

Fig. 23.9 *A pair of spectacles (A) placed upside-down to rest and (B) a front with lenses showing surface abrasions caused by resting the frame on its front*

To prevent damaging the lenses spectacles should be placed on any surface with the sides folded and the convex lens surfaces uppermost, or with the sides opened and 'upside-down' on the surface, so that the front is almost vertical (Fig. 23.9). Spectacles fitted with heavy lenses tend to tip over so that they come to rest on the convex lens surfaces, if placed 'the right way up' on a horizontal surface.

23.6 Visits for Adjustments

All spectacles need to be adjusted from time to time. French *et al.* (1978a,b) found that although patients will return if their spectacles do not fit after the final fitting and collection visit, they may not return several months later to have them checked and adjusted. Stimson (1971) thought this to be for the following reasons:

- they thought that the dispenser was no longer interested in their spectacles

- there had been delays during the original dispensing procedure and the patient might not like to experience another delay

- indifference on the part of the patient

- technical inadequacy of the spectacles.

Technical problems and delays can be dealt with only by the dispenser. However, patient education will help to dispel the fallacy that the dispenser is no longer interested in the patient and their spectacles, beyond the time of collection. More experienced patients know that adjustments are not normally charged for. Because people often tend to think that 'what is free is not worth having', it should be pointed out that the after-service charge is included in the original charge for the dispensing of the spectacles.

Older pairs of spectacles should be especially carefully examined. If any flaws or weaknesses,

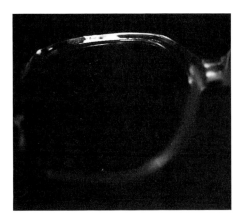

Fig. 23.10 The bright area in the top rim of a front is a hairline crack which shows up with transillumination. Other types of cracks may be seen on inspection against a bright background

23.7 Cleaning Habits

Table 23.2 shows the frequency with which wearers cleaned their spectacles. Note that

TABLE 23.2 Frequency of cleaning of spectacles

Frequency	Wiping (%)	Thorough cleaning (%)
Several times a day	13	
Two to three times per day	28	
Once a day	28	24
Once a week		29
Only when too dirty to see through	32	37
Never		10

TABLE 23.3 Methods of cleaning and drying of spectacles

	%
Cleaning	
Dry method:	
Wipe on –	
Tissue	40
Handkerchief	36
Special cloth	21
Any available cloth	12
Moisture method:	
Breathe on lenses and wipe on –	
Handkerchief	35
Tissue	35
Special cloth	16
Any available cloth	10
Wet method:	
Wash with –	
Soap and water	29
Plain water	21
Special fluid	8
Any other fluid	8
Drying	
Wipe lenses dry	55
Let them dry naturally	5

such as hairline cracks in the material (Fig. 23.10), are discovered, a note should be made on the record card and the defect should be pointed out to the wearer. This prevents accusations of the dispenser having caused the damage. The dispenser should also inform the patient when they feel that they are taking a risk in adjusting or repairing a frame. Only when the patient understands the possible consequences should the adjustment or repair be carried out. The patient should also be informed when to return for any further adjustment.

Patients should not be encouraged to adjust spectacle frames or to effect repairs themselves, except in emergencies. Self-made adjustments are more likely to cause further problems rather than solve them, while a self-made temporary repair may make it more difficult to carry out a permanent one.

Patients who cannot effectively operate without their spectacles should be advised to have a spare pair. Observation appears to indicate that those who are more likely to need such a pair are less likely to have one. This appears to apply in particular to high hyperopes, any remaining aphakics and high myopes.

'cleaning' refers more frequently than not to the cleaning of the lenses rather than the frames, or both. The frequency and methods of cleaning and drying are summarized in Tables 23.3.

Myopes tend to keep their spectacle lenses clean while hyperopes tend not to do so. This may be associated with the position of the first focal plane of their eyes and the retinal image formation (Obstfeld, 1982). The spectacle lens plane of myopes lies close to, or coincides with their eyes' first focal plane. Hence, a dust particle or a grease mark on a lens will be projected as a blur on the retina, and may thus be noted. However, the first focal length of the hyperopic eye may be greater than the vertex distance. Although a dust particle on the hyperope's lenses will also be imaged on the retina of his eye, it will be several dioptres out of focus, giving rise to a larger, low-contrast image which is less likely to be perceived.

23.8 Advice

When questioned whether they had received advice on the care of their spectacles, 80% of respondents answered 'no'. The type of advice received by the other 20% of spectacle wearers is summarized in Table 23.4. Some received advice on more than one aspect. Two patients were advised to return periodically to have the fit of their spectacles checked. Only one person was given a booklet; however, he did not mention whether he had read it.

TABLE 23.4 Advice on care of spectacle

Advice	%
Cleaning	52
How to put down spectacles	39
Putting on and taking off	17
Type and use of spectacle case	15
Given a special booklet	2

23.9 Cleaning Spectacles

Spectacles may be cleaned using a non-abrasive, liquid detergent, rinsed with clean, warm water, and dried with a soft, dust-free and lint-free cloth. Silicone-treated paper and so-called wet-strength tissues should not be used. Some chemical cleaning materials can affect the mechanical properties or clarity of the material(s) from which eye protectors are constructed (BS 7028, 1988).

Several specially formulated cleaning fluids for spectacle lenses and frames are available. Vinegar has been suggested as cleaning fluid, however, a more suitable and less odorous substance is contact lens cleaning fluid.

Rain spots should be removed from lenses before they dry and leave evaporation marks. This applies particularly to multi-anti-reflection coated lenses and others given 'high-tech' treatments such as an anti-mist coating (BS 7028, 1988).

Care must be taken when cleaning plastics frames at higher temperatures because of the different coefficients of expansion of plastics lens materials and their coating; the latter may split from its substrate at temperatures greater than 60°C.

Ultrasonic cleaning instruments (Fig. 23.11) are employed to clean frames and lenses, but their

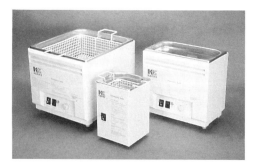

Fig. 23.11 Some ultrasonic baths suitable for the cleaning of spectacles (courtesy Kerry Ultrasonics Ltd, Hitchin, Herts, UK)

mode of action may damage lens coatings. The equipment produces ultrasound waves of frequency greater than 20 kHz (Jarratt, 1992). The wave energy is transmitted through liquids, usually contained in a vessel made of stainless steel. As a result, a very large number of tiny bubbles forms in the liquid; when these burst their impact has a cleaning effect on the surface of the lens and/or frame immersed in the liquid. This process of cleaning spectacle frames reaches intricate parts that other processes cannot reach.

Young (1989) advised against using soap-containing creams-soaps because they leave a deposit on the lens surfaces; acetone or caustic solutions should not be used either as these are known to damage anti-reflection-coated lens surfaces. Salt and bead frame heating baths (Section 24.6.2.3) may also cause minute crazing of the coating.

Spectacle frames used for display purposes that may be 'tried on' by prospective wearers should be cleaned for hygienic reasons (RAL-RG 915, 1961). This applies equally to trial frames.

23.10 Cleaning Cloths

Spectacle lens cleaning cloths were formerly made of a soft leather referred to in French as 'chamois' and in colloquial English as 'shammy leather'. Now, conventional cloths are usually made of cotton fibres which measure 20–30 μm in diameter. They remove dust particles, and can be impregnated so that they act as a degreasing, anti-misting and anti-static agent (Tyckner, personal communication, 1993).

Microfibre cloth is made of synthetic material such as polyester and nylon/polyester mixtures and woven to give it 'capillary action'. The size of the fibre is said to be 2 μm diameter. It acts like a twin-bladed razor, mopping up oils and other deposits in the gaps between the fibres. The

cloths, which have not been treated with silicon or other chemicals and are relatively expensive, can be washed with detergent in water of up to 40°C (Anonymous, 1989, 1992). Cloths finished with a hemmed edge tend to be manufactured in Asia; less expensive cloths are given a serrated edge.

23.11 Cleaning Solutions

The formulations of proprietary cleaning solutions for spectacle lenses are a closely guarded secret (Tyckner, personal communication, 1993). Mild detergents, such as washing up solutions and contact lens cleaning solutions, have proven to be suitable alternatives provided that they do not leave, after rinsing, a residual film on the spectacle lens. The lens should be dried with a soft, dust-free and lint-free tissue or cloth.

23.12 Provision of Information

There is a certain demand by patients for information about the care of spectacles (French *et al.*, 1978; Hill, 1979) which was also recognized by the compilers of RAL-RG 915 (1961). This demand resulted in the inclusion of a clause in BS 7394 (1994), entitled 'Marking and instructions for use'.

The following is the text of an information and advisory leaflet for spectacle wearers (after Hill, 1979, modified in view of the recommendations of BS 7394, 1994). Dispensers should decide for themselves whether they wish to provide as much detail as set out below (it may be used as a basis, and modified).

GETTING THE MOST FROM YOUR SPECTACLES

Date_____ Reference_____

Patient's name_____

The purpose of the spectacles:
[ ] general use
[ ] distance vision
[ ] intermediate vision
[ ] for use with Visual Display Units in accordance with the Health & Safety (Display Screen Equipment) Regulations, 1992
[ ] near vision/reading
[ ] sunglasses
[ ] sports glasses
[ ] eye correction and protection
[ ] other use(s)_____

The lenses are:
[ ] not 'break resistant'
[ ] 'break resistant' (according to BS 7394, 1994) and suitable for general or street wear
[ ] of increased robustness and suitable for low hazard activities
[ ] the lenses and frame together constitute 'low energy impact resistant spectacles' and are suitable for moderate hazard actitivites in accordance with BS 7394, 1994
[ ] photochromic
[ ] polarizing

The lenses have been given the following coating(s):
[ ] abrasion resistant
[ ] anti-reflection
[ ] anti-mist
[ ] anti-static

The luminous transmission of the lenses is approximately_____%

They are not suitable for use
[ ] in poor lighting conditions
[ ] during driving at night
[ ] other(s)_____

Follow this advice to keep your spectacles in good condition:

- use both hands to put on and take off your spectacles so as not to deform them
- when removing them temporarily, fold the sides and put them down with the front surface upwards
- keep your spectacles safely in a hard bodied spectacle case when not wearing them
- use a soft, clean cloth, or one specially designed for the purpose to wipe your spectacles. Hold them by the rims when you clean them
- to keep the frame and lenses clean, wash them regularly in a mild, liquid detergent. Dry on a soft, clean cloth or lint-free tissue
- we shall be pleased to adjust your spectacles. So, please come and see us
- if you are unlucky and suffer damage to your spectacles, we shall be pleased to advice you about repair or replacement. May be we can put it right quicker than you might have thought

Presented by ....

(Much of the contents of this chapter is based on the work of Miss A.M. Hill (1979).)

REFERENCES

Anonymous (1989). Cleaning up the accessories market. *Opt. Management* February, 40.

Anonymous (1992). Toraysee lenscleaner van Friedrichs. *Oculus, Amsterdam* **54**(6), 40.

Bewley, L.A. (1970). Spectacle frames cause traffic hazards. *J. Maryland Optom. Ass.* **3**(3), 8–10.

BS 3521 (1991). *Terms Relating to Ophthalmic Optics and Spectacle Frames. Part 1: Glossary of Terms Relating to Ophthalmic Lenses.* London: British Standards Institution.

BS 7028 (1988). *Guide for Selection, Use and Maintenance of Eye-protection for Industrial and Other Uses.* London: British Standards Institution.

BS 7394 (1994). *Complete Spectacles. Part 2: Specification for Prescription Spectacles.* London: British Standards Institution.

Drew, R. (1970). *Professional Ophthalmic Dispensing.* Chicago: Professional Press.

Drew, R. (1975). Care of lenses. *Ophthal. Optician* **15**(19), 882.

Duke-Elder, S. (1954). *Textbook of Ophthalmology, vol. VI: Injuries.* London: Kimpton.

French, C., Mellor, M. & Parry, L. (1978a). Patient's view of the ophthalmic optician, part 1. *Ophthal. Optician* **18**, 784–787.

French, C., Mellor, M. & Parry, L. (1978b). Patient's view of the ophthalmic optician, part 2. *Ophthal. Optician* **18**, 857–842.

Gibbs, A. (1990). A case in point. *Optician* **200**(5264), 22–24.

Hardy, S.C. (1989). D.H. Hall and Company. *Dispensing Optics* **4**, 16–18.

Hill, A.M. (1979). Care of spectacles. Final Year Project. London: City University.

Höfling, G. (1974). Verletzungen durch Brillengestelle. *Augenspiegel* **20**(2), 82–84.

Jarratt, T. (1992). Ultrasound cleaners. *Optical World* **21**(154), 15–20.

Keeney, A.H., Fintelmann, E. & Reynaldo, D. (1972). Clinical mechanisms in non-industrial spectacle trauma. *Amer. J. Ophthal.* **74**, 662–665.

Keeney, A.H. & Reynaldo, D.P. (1975). Impact resistance of ophthalmic lenses of various strengths and influence of frame design. *Canad. J. Ophthal.* **10**, 367–376.

Loran, D. (1992). Eye injuries in squash. *Optician* **203**(5344), 18–26.

Obstfeld, H. (1982). *Optics in Vision*, 2nd edn, pp. 56–57. London: Butterworth Scientific.

RAL-RG 915 (1961). *Gütebestimmung im Augenoptikerhandwerk. Individuell angepasste und handwerklich fertiggestellte Korrektionsbrillen.* Berlin: Beuth-Vertrieb GmbH.

Scrivener, A.B. (1973). Impact-resistant spectacle lenses. *Br. J. Physiol. Optics* **28**, 26–33.

Stimson, R.L. (1971). *Ophthalmic Dispensing.* Springfield, IL: Thomas.

Young, J.M. (1989). Surface preparation for AR coating. *Optical World* **18**(120), 8–12.

CHAPTER 24

Workshop Practice

24.1 Introduction

The following sections deal in some detail with a number of workshop techniques and processes. However, they do not cover every possible aspect. Some other details and techniques not described below may be found in Chapter 10 (see also Index). It should be noted that a great deal is to be learned from colleagues and from experience.

It is useful to keep up to date with new equipment, gadgets and replacement parts. Reviews of workshop equipment appear in the professional press. Some wholesalers specializing in workshop equipment will organize practical demonstration sessions; their catalogues can be very useful sources of information on available tools and spare parts. For a review of optical pliers see Crundall (1971).

24.2 Angling

This refers to adjusting the angle of the side (*temple*) (BS 3521, 1991). Many modern spectacle joints (*hinges*) are designed such that angling can be done by hand (Fig. 24.1). Such joints almost invariably have three charniers (*barrels*) (Fig. 24.2) and are often concealed (*hidden*) in the lug (*endpiece*) area of the front, and attached to, or are part of the side wire (the metal insert of a reinforced side; *core*).

Having altered the angle of the side, the angle of let-back is usually found to be smaller than before. On inspection it will be noticed that,

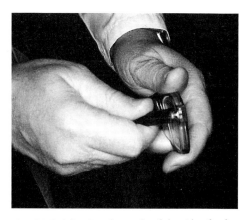

Fig. 24.1 *Adjusting the angle of the side of a frame with a three-charniers joint. Note that the side must be partially closed during the adjustment*

whereas lug and side were in apposition along the whole of the vertical extent of the side, they now only touch at a point, and that there is a gap either above, below, or on either side of the point of

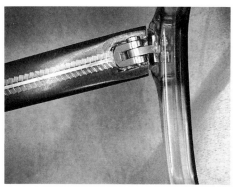

Fig. 24.2 *Close-up of a three-charniers joint. The half-joint to the front is concealed in the lug, and the two-charniers half-joint to the side has been welded to the side wire*

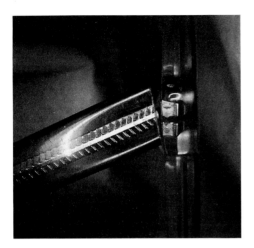

Fig. 24.3 Now the angle of the side has been increased, a gap appears between the back plane of the front and the side

touch (Fig. 24.3). To restore the angle of let-back, apply a few file strokes to the butt-end until it matches the lug again and the desired angle is produced. This method is also used to increase the angle of let-back (Section 16.4.3). The angle of let-back can best be increased while the joint is supported on a special tool (Fig. 24.4).

It is practically impossible to alter the angle of side of some metal frames (Fig. 16.10). An alternative is to bend the side near the joint or

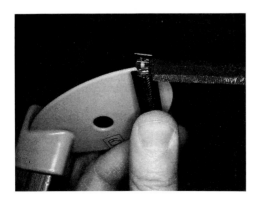

Fig. 24.4 A special support clamped on a table edge (left), and designed for filing out the joint so as to increase the angle of let-back

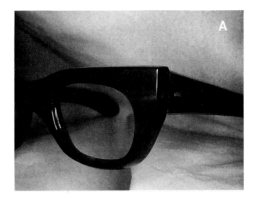

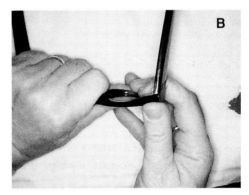

Fig. 24.5 Adjusting the angle of the side of a heavy plastics frame. A, this front has a concealed half-joint to the front and the half-joint to the side is attached with a rivet plate; B, by heating the lug and pushing it over with the thumb, the angle of the side is increased, but the angle of let-back is probably simultaneously decreased, and will need to be re-established

beyond the butt. Adjusting the angle of the side of some heavy plastics frames can be very difficult too (Fig. 24.5). One can heat the lug and then attempt to deform it while altering the angle of the side. Take care not to loosen pinned or concealed joints by overheating. The angle of let-back may have to be restored, as described above.

24.3 Cementing

24.3.1 BONDING AGENTS
Broken frames made of cellulose acetate, cellulose propionate, Optyl and SPX may be

TABLE 24.1 *Solvents for plastics materials*

Material	Solvent/cement
Cellulose acetate	Acetone
Cellulose propionate	Ethyl acetate
Optyl and SPX	Epoxy resin cement

cemented (bonded, glued). Although such repairs should not be considered as permanent, some will be remarkably strong. The common solvents or cements are shown in Table 24.1.

Other materials may also be cemented. However, those mentioned do not need special skills or knowledge, unlike those required for the use of the solvent of polymethylmethacrylate, or the splicing of tortoiseshell (Section 6.2.1.3; Mac-Gregor *et al.*, 1992).

24.3.2 METHODS

24.3.2.1 Cellulose acetate and propionate bridges

To repair a broken bridge, start by preparing a place on a work surface where the frame can be left undisturbed. Place a small amount of the appropriate solvent in a shallow glass or metal container (a deep negative glass lens could be used, or a Petri dish). Hold the broken surfaces of

the bridge in the solvent while steadying the hands on the work surface (Fig. 24.6). The older the material the longer the time required: 1–3 min.

It is usually best to let the frame rest upside down (Fig. 24.7) with a wooden support under the bridge. Place the parts carefully together on the support. Check that they are aligned in all planes. Ensure also that the front is appropriately bowed. Hold the parts together for at least 1 min. Then leave the frame undisturbed for 12 h, or overnight.

It is possible to reinforce the bridge during the repair. Take a metal pin, such as those used for repinning a joint, a little shorter than the bridge width of the front and about 1 mm diameter. Drill a hole in the middle of the broken surface of the bridge, parallel to the horizontal centre line. Use a drill of the same diameter as the pin (or a little smaller), and make the depth of the hole equal to half the length of the pin. Insert the pin

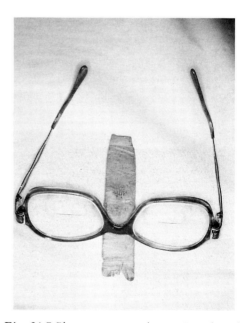

Fig. 24.7 Place a support, such as a piece of wood, underneath the broken bridge of a front that has been cemented and is drying

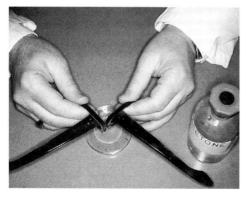

Fig. 24.6 The broken bridge of a cellulose acetate front is held in acetone prior to being cemented

into the hole. To facilitate insertion, warm the bridge and pin with the frame heater.

Use the pin to mark the other broken surface of the bridge, and drill a hole on that side. Insert the pin. If the broken surfaces do not meet, warm the bridge and push the two halves together so that they are in contact. Separate the bridge portions a minimal distance and, using a small brush, moisten the two opposing surfaces several times with the solvent. Having pushed the halves together again, leave to dry.

Another way to reinforce the broken bridge is the following. Having cemented the bridge but without the use of a pin, select a thin, but large enough, preferably crystal-clear, piece of cellulose acetate. A lens former such as those used with automatic edging machines and made of a suitable plastics material might be used for this purpose. Cut it down to size with cutting pliers and file to the required shape. Warm it with a frame heater and form it to follow the bridge's curve by pressing it carefully against either the front or the back surface of the bridge. Brush the facing surfaces several times with the solvent, and place reinforcement and bridge together. Use a clothes peg as clamp. Leave to dry.

When such a repair is inspected the following day, it is likely that a thin white film will have been formed in the area treated. This can be removed by careful polishing. It may also be necessary to fashion this area using a small file and sandpaper, thus removing any excess material and blending the parts. Finally, carefully polish the area of the former break.

24.3.2.2 Broken rim

Remove lens from front. If lens edging equipment is available, edge away a little material from the lens on the 'corners' on either side of the break. If the break is on a corner, edge away lens material in that area. Insert lens into rim and check whether the two broken surfaces can be pressed together with the fingers, using minimal force. If not, continue edging a little material away until the rim sections can be brought together. Remove the lens from the rim.

Apply solvent to the break several times at short intervals. Using finger pressure, determine whether the material has become 'sticky'. If necessary, apply more solvent. When the material has become 'sticky', insert lens, and wrap a strong elastic band around the rim so that its pressure will ensure that the broken surfaces are in touch. Leave to dry.

The break may be reinforced and cleaned as described in the last part of Section 24.3.2.1.

24.3.2.3 Optyl and SPX

Both Optyl and SPX may be repaired with epoxy resin cements such as Araldite or two-part UHU according to the instructions provided. Use only a minimal amount of the cement. See Section 24.3.2.1 above for the type of support required when repairing a broken bridge.

24.4 Cresting

This refers to shaping the arch of a plastics bridge to provide an angle of crest (BS 3521, 1991). While holding the front horizontal, use a frame rule or protractor to incline a semi-cylindrical file at the required angle of crest (Fig. 24.8). Having formed the crest through filing, apply sandpaper to remove surface roughness. The finish is effected with a polishing mop or by buffing.

24.5 Fitting Lenses Into and Removing From Metal Rims

The prime requirement for any lens to fit well into a metal rim, is for the lens to be of the correct shape and size. If the shape is correct but the size is too large, one cannot fully close the closing block. This can be remedied by removing a little

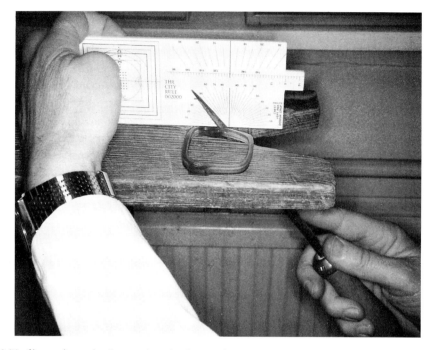

Fig. 24.8 *To file out the angle of crest, place the front with its back plane upwards, on the filing block. Using a protractor, place the cylindrical portion of the semicylindrical file at the required angle (here about 45°) with the back plane. Having removed the protractor, move the handle forwards and backwards and rotate it simultaneously*

more lens material all around, thus reducing the lens size. Repeat the process until the closing block can be fully closed. If the lens is too small the lens will fall out of the rim, even if the closing block is fully closed. By inserting a length of 'packing' (thin, V-shaped plastics material; Fig. 24.9) between lens and rim, this may be remedied. The packing should be cut to the required length (experience will tell which length is required), and both ends given a V-shape with an enclosed angle of about 30°. Self-adhesive packing is also available. To prevent dethreading and facilitate smooth turning of the closing block screw, put a drop of light oil on it before the closing block is finally closed. Remove any excess oil.

Lenses fitted into a metal rim should always be inspected with a strain tester (also called polari-

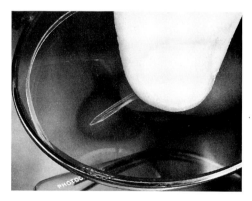

Fig. 24.9 *A piece of packing emerges from the space between the metal rim and a lens. Note that the end of the strip of packing has been cut to an enclosed angle of about 30°*

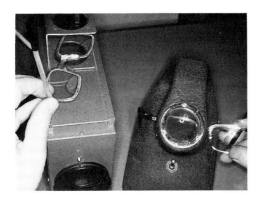

Fig. 24.10 *Strain testers. On the right is a conventional model; on the left is an instrument which includes an iris diaphragm (below), with which lens surface blemishes can be made visible by projection on a screen*

scope) after fitting (Fig. 24.10). The instrument consists of a polarizer and an analyser with their planes of polarization at right angles. Where the material is under stress, it becomes birefringent and will show up tight points along the lens' circumference as bright and dark fringes (see also Fig. 23.1). Glass lenses that show such pressure points may break on receiving an impact. Plastics lenses may become deformed, especially when held in a stainless steel or titanium rim. Deformed spherical surfaces tend to assume a toric shape; deformed toric surfaces tend to assume different surface powers and/or axis directions. However, the back vertex power(s) of the lens, measured with a focimeter, are unchanged. However, the shape factor(s) (see Obstfeld, 1982) which is (are) affected by the, now toric or altered, front surface power(s), will change. A few wearers who are sensitive to shape factor changes may then complain about aesthenopia (Obstfeld, 1988).

Edging away a sliver of material at tight spots will alleviate the problem, but checking with the strain tester remains a necessity. To reduce the problem, manufacturers have sometimes provided the inside of the metal rim with a pliable plastics (nylon, silicone) layer (Fig. 4.11B). This allows a greater tolerance of lens size, and provides a shock-absorbing medium around the lens.

To remove a lens from a metal rim, unscrew the closing block screw (see Table 11.5). It is often unnecessary to unscrew the screw fully. Take care to prevent the lens from dropping onto a hard surface: glass lenses may break, and plastics lenses may scratch. Note that some closing block screws may have been secured by a tiny, auxiliary screw (see Table 4.11A).

24.6 Heating Spectacle Frames

24.6.1 INTRODUCTION

The rims of most plastics fronts need to be heated before the lenses can be inserted into them. However, certain fronts or rims made of polyamide or carbon fibre-reinforced polyamide material are provided with a closing block containing a screw. Lenses should then be fitted as in fronts with metal rims. Lenses may also be sprung in 'cold' in SPX frames. Some polyamide rims should be fitted with lenses that are up to 0.5 mm larger than the actual lens aperture size, and sprung in cold. However, if heating is needed, only very little should be applied because polyamide is likely to shrink if overheated (>100°C). Cellulose propionate frames must be heated to about 70°C. Cellulose acetate and cellulose nitrate will shrink when cooled suddenly, for instance, in cold water.

Polymethylmethacrylate and Optyl must be heated until it can be deformed by minimal pressure. Optyl should be thoroughly warmed to about 90°C before the lens is sprung in. Because a cold lens will almost instantly reduce the temperature of the material it touches, it is recommended that the lens is warmed. Note that anti-reflection coatings on plastics ophthalmic lenses may develop cracks and deformations caused by differences in the thermal coefficients of expansion of the two materials when heated. Avoid heating these lenses, particularly above about 70°C.

Having sprung in the lenses, some dispensers warm the frame again so that the molecules may realign themselves. This reduces any strain in the material and prevents it from becoming brittle and breaking more easily.

Some frames require special treatment. Manufacturers generally attach a label with instructions which should be followed carefully. This applies, in particular, to frames encrusted with imitation precious stones or similar materials.

24.6.2 FRAME HEATERS

24.6.2.1 Introduction

Some older types of heater are no longer allowed under health and safety legislation because of their inherent dangers. These include the radiant heater, because of the risk of burning oneself or the frame against the metal cylinder surrounding the electric heating element, and also the methylated spirit and the gas jet heaters, because both have an open flame. Steam was sometimes used to soften tortoiseshell and cellulose nitrate frames.

24.6.2.2 Fan heaters

These type of heaters are in common use (Fig. 24.11) and provide, almost instantly, air of the required temperature. The housing contains a small fan and an electric heating element, just like a hair dryer (Fig. 24.12). Thanks to the fan, which propels air over the heating element, the latter does not reach a temperature where it starts to glow. Various models are available. Most

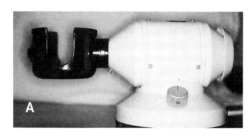

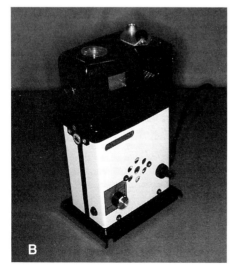

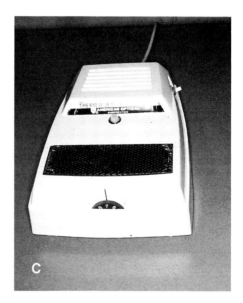

Fig. 24.11 *Various frame heaters. A, this type has a cup-like extension on the left and a dial with which the operating temperature can be altered; B, this model has several openings and regulators, and also a thermometer; C, this model is usually employed with a funnel placed over the black grid so that the hot air may be directed at a given part of a frame. It operates silently*

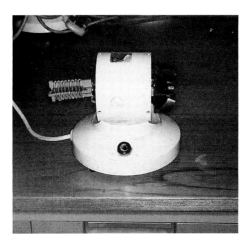

Fig. 24.12 *The main parts of a frame heater (see Fig. 24.11A). On the left is the heating element, in the middle the casing containing the fan motor, and on the right the fan*

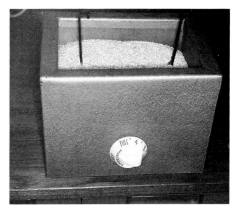

Fig. 24.13 *A bead bath frame heater. It consists of a casing which conceals an adjustable electric heating element, and the bead 'bath' in which the frame is placed during heating*

have an integral cup-like extension into which the hot air is blown and in which the frame can be placed or held. Some have an adjustable aperture which concentrates the hot air flow on a small part of the frame such as a pad or the bridge. There are thermostatically controlled heaters; others have switches whereby the heating element may be switched off so that the instrument will produce cold air once the element and its casing have been cooled by the air stream. Some instruments have a switch which activates a second heating element while another variety has a dial that facilitates a gradual temperature change. There are quiet and also noisy fan heaters.

24.6.2.3 Bead heaters

This type of heater (Fig. 24.13) is used in workshops or under circumstances where a large number of frames need to be heated, and therefore the instrument will be in constant use. It does not provide 'instant' heat and takes some time to warm up. It consists of a tray containing either salt or glass beads, 1–2 mm in diameter, that is heated from below by an electric element.

It is particularly suited to warm whole fronts since these can be immersed amongst the beads. Hence, the front is evenly heated, which is preferred by some for springing-in work. Ensure

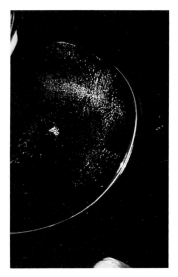

Fig. 24.14 *A crazed lens coating made visible by transillumination. The crazing was not visible under normal lighting conditions. The wearer complained about increased halos around lights at night when looking through certain parts of the lens. This lens may have been damaged during (over)heating with a bead heater, before insertion into the spectacle front*

that no beads are stuck in the rim before attempting to insert a lens. Some coated plastics lenses develop minute crazing of their coating (Fig. 24.14) after emersion in a bead heater.

24.6.2.4 Infra-red heaters

These heaters are only used in places such as sunglass manufacturing plants, where there is continuous use for the instrument. Its casing contains either an infra-red lamp or element. The radiation penetrates the plastics part and heats throughout. There are industrial heaters that warm the frame or front while the latter passes underneath on a continuous belt.

24.6.2.5 Miscellaneous comments

Spectacle frame heaters with an integral temperature gauge, or a means of selecting known air temperatures are now available. In view of the various temperatures required for different spectacle frame materials (see Table 7.3) they are a welcome addition to the range of heaters.

Camau (1985) speculated whether or not it would be useful to specify on the spectacle frame the temperature that should be used for adjustments. With the proliferation of plastics materials that has taken place since the mid-1980s, this would be useful. Take as an example Ceroid, a plastics frame material introduced in 1993 in the UK. From the description of the manufacturer (Optinova, undated) it would appear to be a material akin to cellulose propionate. However, whereas the latter can be adjusted at a temperature below 70°C, it is advisable to heat Ceroid to 100–110°C.

24.7 Lens Insertion in Plastics Fronts

If at all possible, lenses should be sprung-in or inserted into the rim from behind. If one inserts a lens from the front, it is possible to mark, or even

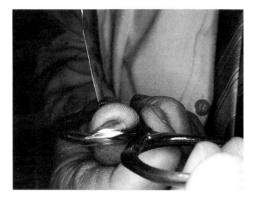

Fig. 24.15 *When the pad has been heated, the thumb is passed through the front's aperture. Thumb pressure against the back surface of the pad is used to reduce the splay angle*

damage the front surface. This will be visible to the onlooker, and can be difficult to make good. However, there are spectacle frames designed specifically to stop lenses from leaving and, therefore, entering the front's rim from the rear. This is usually done for safety reasons: impact on a lens would not result in it striking the eye or its surround, although the lens might break. Pads with a large splay angle, as required in children's frames, may prevent lenses from being sprung-in from the rear. Heating the pads, and reducing the angle through pressure with the thumb (Fig. 24.15), will allow lens insertion from behind.

Many children's frames are not manufactured with the large splay angle required for their wearers' comfort (Section 17.4). This allows lens insertion from behind, which should be followed by an adjustment of the pad (Fig. 24.16) to give the large splay angle required.

To prepare the front's rim for the insertion of a lens, it should be heated evenly. This is easily achieved if the rim is of fairly even thickness. However, some rims and fronts vary substantially in thickness. The heat should then be directed at the thickest part of the rim; avoid overheating lugs containing joints or rivets as this may loosen the latter. By flexing the front or

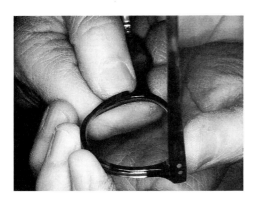

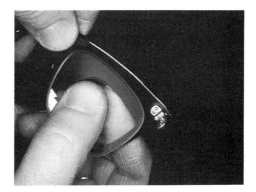

Fig. 24.16 Having heated the pad, thumb pressure is applied to the pad's bearing surface to increase the splay angle

Fig. 24.17 Having heated the rim of the front, lens insertion starts with lining up the sharpest corner of the lens with the corresponding corner of the front's aperture

rim one can test whether the rim is sufficiently pliable to receive the lens.

Taking account of the temperature recommendations, if any, given by the manufacturer, proceed as follows:

(1) Check whether the upper rim of the front has a curvature matching that of the lens (meniscus-shape for most lenses). If not, shape front and rim with your fingers to follow the curvature of the lens' edge.
(2) Hold the lens with your thumb resting on the concave surface, the correct surface facing the front (for most prescriptions, convex surface facing the back plane of the front for rear insertion), and the sharpest corner lined up with that of the rim (Fig. 24.17).
(3) Insert the sharpest corner into the rim first (it is very difficult to force the rim around such corners afterwards). The sharpest corner is likely to be situated on the upper nasal side of the lens shape, but there are exceptions. In such cases it is necessary to study the lens shape carefully, for instance by lining up the lens and lens aperture of the frame. A further complication arises when the right and left lens have identical shape, such as round and PRO shapes.

(4) Force the lens into the upper rim and force the rim with your fingers around the upper temporal corner.
(5) Continue to the lower temporal corner (Fig. 24.18), and the lower nasal corner.
(6) Once the lens has been sprung in, check that the rim has not become deformed or twisted (Fig. 24.19). If it has, remove the lens, apply some heat to the affected portion, and remould it with your fingers, then reheat the front and reinsert the lens. Having originally

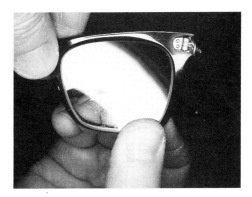

Fig. 24.18 Having inserted that sharpest corner of the lens into the front's aperture, force the lens into the upper rim and the rim around the upper temporal corner of the lens

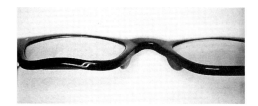

Fig. 24.19. A lower rim deformed as a result of lens insertion

inserted the lens from the back, reinsertion of the lens from the front may twist the rim back into its original shape, but may also mark the front.

24.8 Lens Removal from Plastics Fronts

Lenses are almost invariably removed from the anterior surface of the front. Heat the thickest

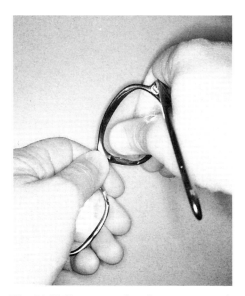

Fig. 24.20 To remove a lens from its aperture, heat the thickest part of the rim, and holding the other half of the front in one hand, press with the thumb of the other on the concave side of the lens, near to the sharpest corner

part of the rim until pliable (see Section 24.7, above). Grasp that half of the front *not* containing the lens to be removed in one hand and place the thumb of the other hand on the concave side at the sharpest corner of the lens to be removed. Press with the thumb on the lens while holding the front with the other fingers of the same hand (Fig. 24.20). The sharpest corner of the lens should slip out first. It is possible that a thin, negative (usually glass) lens will break during this process and it is therefore wise always to have a full record of all lenses that are being handled.

24.9 Pinning

24.9.1 INTRODUCTION

Pinning is the fitting of a half-joint to the front or to a side of a frame. Although few half-joints are still secured by pinning, it is a technique which can be useful when a frame repair needs to be carried out, or when a special frame is made by hand.

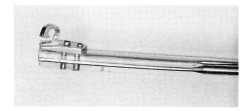

Fig. 24.21 A rivetted half-joint to the side with a damaged charnier

24.9.2 REMOVING AND (RE)PINNING A HALF-JOINT

Figure 24.21 shows a side carrying a half-joint with a damaged charnier. To replace the half-joint:

(1) Remove the domes of the pins by filing them level with the side plate of the half-joint (Fig. 24.22).

(2) Using an instrument such as the Clavulus (Fig. 24.23), line up the pin punch with one of the pins (Fig. 24.24). To release the half-joint from the pin, apply some pressure to the pin by means of the punch. Insure that the punch does not travel much further than the thickness of the joint plate.

(3) Repeat for the second pin.

(4) Remove the joint plate (Fig. 24.25)

(5) Remove each pin using a rivet punch (Fig. 24.26).

(6) Insert new pins in the holes, and place a new joint on these pins (Fig. 24.27).

(7) Use a (double) rivet driver to force the joint plate down (Fig. 24.28A) and the rivets into the countersunk holes of the side (Fig. 24.28B).

(8) Cut off the pins so that about 1 mm of their length protrudes above the joint plate (Fig. 24.29).

(9) File the tops of the pins flat (Fig. 24.30A).

(10) Apply a rivet head maker, to dome the pins (Fig. 24.30B).

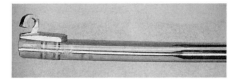

Fig. 24.22 The domes of the rivets have been filed away

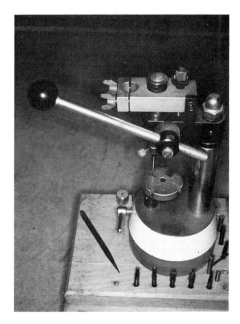

Fig. 24.23 A Clavulus instrument fitted with a punch, and a punch for use with a hammer (left)

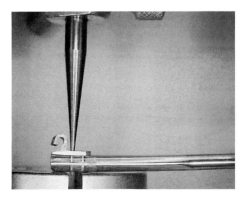

Fig. 24.24 The punch of a Clavulus lines up with a rivet

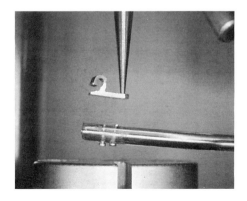

Fig. 24.25 The joint is removed from the side. The joint plate does not always stay attached to the punch

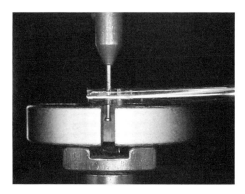

Fig. 24.26 The rivet punch of a Clavulus removes the rivet from the side. Note that the table of the instrument must be adjusted to allow the rivet to pass into the slot

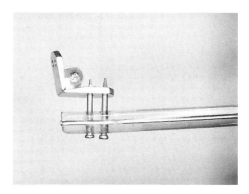

Fig. 24.27 New rivets have been inserted through the holes in the side, and a new joint has been placed on the rivets

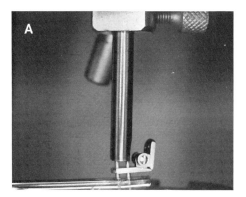

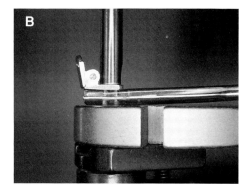

Fig. 24.28 A rivet driver. A, a double rivet driver is placed over the pair of rivets; B, the double rivet driver is applied and forces the joint plate onto the inner aspect of the side and the rivet heads into the countersunk holes on the outer aspect of the side

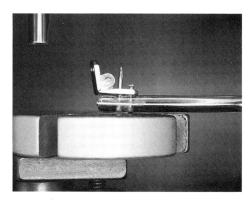

Fig. 24.29 One rivet has been cut so that it protrudes about 1 mm above the joint plate

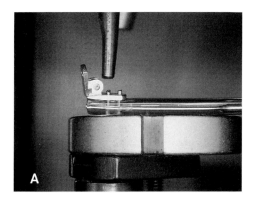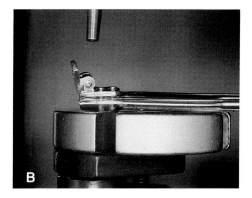

Fig. 24.30 *Doming rivets. A, a rivet head maker is about to be applied to the rivet nearest to the charnier; B, both rivets have been domed*

24.10 Screws

24.10.1 INTRODUCTION

BS 3172/EN ISO 11381 (1987) specifies the screw threads, taps and gauges to be used for and with spectacle frames (see Section 4.2.3).

Two main problems arise with screws: they may be lost from frames and, more seriously, they break.

24.10.2 LOST SCREWS

When a screw is 'lost' from a frame, it must be replaced. The question is then which screw will fit? By removing the screw from the contralateral side, one can inspect it and select an identical screw. Estimate the diameters, length of head and shank, and the pitch (the distance between successive threads of a screw) as this will help during the visual part of the selection process. Boxes containing a selection of spectacle screws may be purchased from suppliers of workshop accessories. Manufacturers may also supply screws and other spare parts for their frames.

Although the problem of lost screws is a long-standing one, a satisfactory solution appears to have eluded designers. The reason is twofold: one must be able to remove the screw, but it should not come out on its own. This applies particularly to joint screws, where the joint is continually being opened and closed. Efforts to solve this problem have included a plastics sleeve inside the charnier (*barrel*) of the joint (Fig. 4.6), and fitting a lock nut (Fig. 11.18). The latter solution sometimes backfired – patients have reported that the lock nut was missing and requested that it be replaced.

Joint screws are often manufactured with a dimple at the bottom of the shank (Fig. 4.7). Application of peening pliers (Fig. 4.7) to the screw will spread the bottom so that it will extend over the charnier (*barrel*). Hence, it will not work loose and be lost. However, if the screw needs to be removed the spread metal needs to be filed away. To seal a screw in its charnier, place a drop of a proprietary adhesive such as Lock-tite, or clear nail varnish, in the charnier. This should not be necessary when the charnier contains a polyamide insert.

24.10.3 BROKEN SCREWS

Screws other than joint screws and closing block screws seldom break. Earlam (1985, 1986/87) gave two reasons for spectacle screws breaking:

(1) Over-tightening, which has the effect of stretching the fine screw threads thus loosening them. As the force is continued the screw stretches and breaks because the threads in the charnier (*barrel*) no longer match those on the shaft. Replacing the screw at an earlier stage may still lead to the same problem: because the thread of the shaft has been abused, the thread of the new screw may jam, as a result of which that screw will break.

(2) The screw has been bent. If such a screw is now tightened, it is likely to break. This applies particularly to closing blocks screws.

Earlam recommends two methods for removing screw remnants:

(1) With a scribe (a pointed instrument for scoring lines) (Fig. 24.31). Owing to abuse it is likely that the remnant will be loose in the charnier, and may be rotated using the very sharp point of the scribe. The broken piece will unscrew and drop out of the charnier without causing damage, whereupon a new screw may be fitted.

(2) With a slotting file. This is a file with a very thin blade carrying file teeth (Fig. 24.31). The file is used to cut a slot into the bottom of the broken screw. One has to accept that it will probably also cut a slot in the bottom of the charnier. The screw can then be rotated with a screwdriver, and replaced.

Other methods include:

(3) Using a screw extractor (Fig. 24.31). This tool looks like a screwdriver. However, instead of ending in a thin blade, it has a jagged bottom. When this is pressed onto the remnant of the screw-head and turned it will take the head along and rotate it.

(4) Drilling out the screw remnant. This is a rather tricky operation requiring a high-speed drill which is bound to 'wander' in-

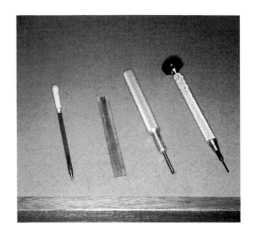

Fig. 24.31 *From left to right: a scribe, a slotting file and two screw extractors*

stead of passing through the middle of the remnant. It will then destroy the thread in the charnier, which will then have to be retapped.

(5) Punching out the screw remnant. This is the method most likely to cause severe damage to the joint. Support the charnier on, for instance, a vice with the jaws slightly open to allow the piece of broken screw to pass through. Select a punch (Fig. 24.26) and position it carefully on the broken piece of screw. The punch is hit firmly with a hammer and, hopefully, the piece will leave the charnier.

There are mechanical punches which combine the effect of punch and hammer. The Clavulus (Fig. 24.23) and similar instruments may also be used for this purpose.

It is necessary to restore the damaged thread of any charnier by retapping it, before an oversized screw is fitted. Unfortunately, it is more usual to be left with a (deformed) joint containing a piece of screw that has broken off flush with the surface. When this happens, it may be necessary to supply a new frame part – assuming that that is obtainable.

Hintermeister (1984) suggested that when a

screw cannot easily be turned, to quickly heat it up with a soldering iron and immediately try to rotate it with a screwdriver. However, one must ensure that the plastics surround remains unaffected by the heat.

24.11 Setting Up

This procedure refers to the adjustment of a spectacle frame at the conclusion of manufacture (BS 3521, 1991), or of the glazed spectacles. The following sequence may be followed:

(1) Ensure that the halves of the front lie in the same plane. If the front is twisted, align it after heating if the front is made of plastics material. If a metal front is twisted, adjusting it may require the use of pliers.
(2) Ensure that the angles of let-back are similar (Section 24.2).
(3) Ensure that the angles of the side are similar (Section 24.2).

In general, all angles and measurements of a frame ready for collection should be nearly identical. However, because no patient's head will be symmetrical, one may follow a pragmatic approach whereby, after general inspection, only gross deviations are rectified. Once the patient has arrived, the frame is adjusted and fitted to the actual head.

24.12 Supra Threading

24.12.1 INTRODUCTION
There are two type of Supra frames, namely those which are fitted with lenses that have a combination of flat and bevel edges, and those fitted with lenses that have just a flat edge (Figs 11.4 and 24.32). The flat edge of both types contains a groove which is about 0.5 mm deep, into which a polyamide cord is fitted; this retains the lens.

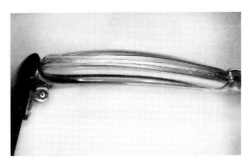

Fig. 24.32 The flat edge of a combination of flat and bevel edged lens, fitted in a Supra front. Note the polyamide cord situated in the middle of the flat edge

During the height of their popularity, in the 1950s and 1960s, 'combination edge' Supra frames were mainly made in Britain while 'flat edge' Supra frames were produced in continental Europe, in France in particular. The latter type was frequently referred to by the name Nylor, a Supra style originally manufactured by a company which is now part of Essilor. Some flat-edge Supra frame styles were manufactured during the mid-1990s. Supra-style half-eye frames of either type have also been marketed. Because polyamide cord stretches, particularly when the ambient humidity is high, Supra frames were never a success in tropical climates.

The combination edge lenses are secured to their plastics front with a polyamide cord, where each end of the cord passes through a small hole. One hole is usually situated on the nasal and the other on the upper temporal side of the front (Fig. 24.33). By convention, holes are countersunk so that the knot at the end of the cord rests inside the hole, where it acts as an anchor. Holes in regular bridge Supra frames are frequently covered with a plug. The bevelled section of the edge of the lens fits into the groove of the front.

Flat edge lenses are secured in a different manner. They are usually fitted to metal or combination frames which resemble semi-rimless frames. However, the shape of the rim is

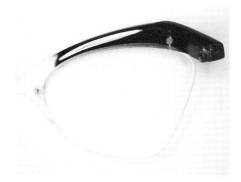

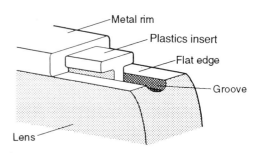

Fig. 24.34 Diagram of the suspension of a flat edge lens in a Supra front

Fig. 24.33 A combination edged lens fitted into a Supra front. The holes in which the polyamide cord is anchored are situated on the back surfaces of the bridge and the upper rim, near the 'swept-back' lug

unlike conventional metal rims in that a T-shaped polyamide ribbon is embedded in it on the lens side (Fig. 24.34). The lower end of the vertical limb of the ribbon protrudes about 0.5 mm beyond the rim, and fits into the groove of

the lens. Together with the polyamide retaining cord, it forms an almost complete ring around the lens. The cord is secured by weaving each end through a pair of tiny holes at each end of the metal rim (Fig. 24.35). Because the distance between the pair of holes is small, a loop is formed. When the lens is fitted, the loops are under stress, as a result of which they act as anchors. Finally,

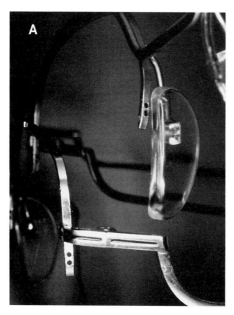

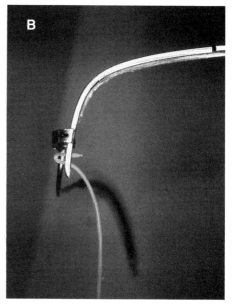

Fig. 24.35 A, the pair of holes on the temporal end of the metal rim of one front (below); another front showing the pair of holes on the nasal end of the metal rim which is often (partly) hidden behind the pad (above); B, a loop is formed when the cord is fed through the two holes at the end of the rim. Note the plastics insert protruding from the lower aspect of the rim

each end of the cord is embedded in the rim, like the ribbon.

24.12.2 REMOVING A CORD

In order to remove the (broken) cord from a combination edge Supra front, take the cord between your fingers or use a pair of flat jaw pliers, and try to push the knot out of the countersunk hole in which it rests. If this proves to be too difficult, destroy the knot. This can be done by either rotating a screwdriver with a blade width equal to the diameter of the hole, or by rotating a drill of such diameter in the hole. If the hole has a plug, first use a drill to remove the plug. Having destroyed the knot, pull the cord out of the hole. It may be necessary to remove remnants of the knot from the hole.

To remove a (broken) cord from a flat edge Supra front, it is usually necessary to use a safety pin to dislodge the end of the cord from the lens side of the metal rim (Fig. 24.36). Next, place the

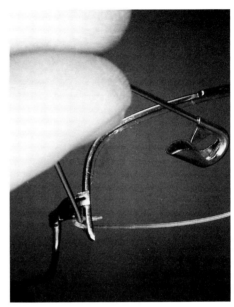

Fig. 24.37 *The safety pin's point is inserted in the loop in order to increase the size of the loop. Now the cord can be removed from the holes. The sharp end of the cord is visible, pointing towards the right*

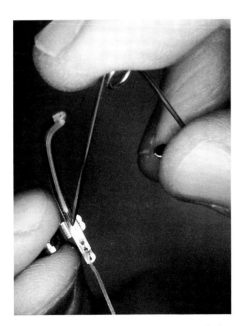

Fig. 24.36 *A safety pin is inserted underneath the end of the cord, to dislodge it from the metal rim. The light line above the pin's point is the plastic insert of the metal rim*

pin in the loop between the two tiny holes, and move the pin about so as to increase the size of the loop (Fig. 24.37). When the loop is several millimetres long, the cord can be removed. A pair of pliers with flat-round or round yaws may be used for this purpose.

24.12.3 FITTING A CORD

Polyamide cord, 0.5–0.7 mm diameter, may be purchased from fishing tackle shops. Supra sunglasses should be fitted with dark tinted cord while conventional prescription lenses should be fitted with clear cord.

To fit a new cord to a combination edge Supra, start with cutting a suitable length of polyamide cord. A length twice the estimated circumference of the lens should be adequate. Using a sharp cutting edge, such as that of a modelling knife, cut diagonally across both ends

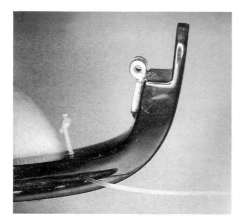

Fig. 24.38 The temporal hole in the upper rim of this plastic Supra starts in the groove and opens out into a countersunk opening in the back plane of the front. When the cord is fitted around the lens, and thus pulled tight, the knot will disappear into the countersunk opening

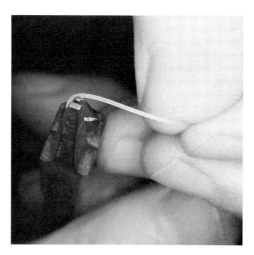

Fig. 24.39 The cord is curled around the conical jaw of a pair of pliers. This will allow the cord to pass through the elbow in the canal

of the length of cord. This will help to guide the cord through the hole in the frame. Many holes consist of two perpendicular parts: one part lies in the plane of the front and opens into the groove, the other opens out onto the back surface, thus forming an elbow-shaped canal. The opening in the back surface is usually countersunk to accommodate the knot (Fig. 24.38).
Proceed as follows:

(1) To enable the cord to pass through the 'elbow', curl the thin end of the cord around the round jaw of a pair of pliers (Fig. 24.39).
(2) With the curl turned towards the back surface of the front, enter the cord into the hole in the groove on the nasal side of the rim. After some manipulation, it will emerge from the opening on the back surface.
(3) Tie a knot and tighten it at a short distance from the end of the cord. Pull the knot into the countersunk hole.
(4) Repeat (1) and (2) for the other end of the cord, which is entered into the hole on the temporal side of the front.

(5) Holding the lens between thumb, index and middle fingers, place its bevel edge in the groove of the front (Fig. 24.40). Guide the cord around the lens with the fingers of the other hand and ensure that the cord lies in the groove of the flat edge. Pull the free end of the cord tight (Fig. 24.41).
(6) Use a marking pen to indicate the point

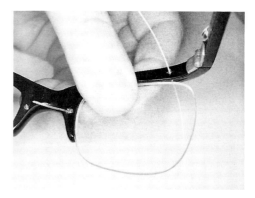

Fig. 24.40 The lens is held between the thumb, index and middle fingers and pressed into the groove of the upper rim. Note the cord protruding from the countersunk hole on the nasal side while the knot has been drawn into it

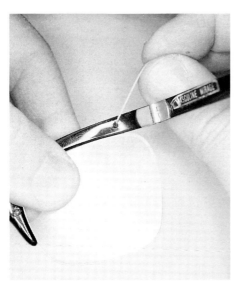

Fig. 24.41 The free end of the cord is pulled tight while the cord lies in the groove of the flat edge

where the cord emerges from the back plane of the front. Remove the lens.

(7) Tie a knot on the frame side about 5 mm away from the mark. Tighten the knot. The greater the circumference of the lens, the greater the distance between mark and knot should be.

(8) A thread-free or polyamide ribbon, about 0.5 cm wide, is looped around the cord and held tight between thumb and index finger.

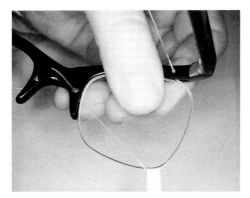

Fig. 24.42 The white ribbon (below) is used to guide the cord into the groove of the flat edge

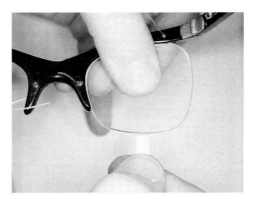

Fig. 24.43 The white ribbon has been pulled to a flat part of the lens shape

Holding the lens as in (5), use the ribbon to guide the cord into the groove. It is usually best to start on the temporal side where the sharpest corner of the lens shape is likely to be and to move the ribbon towards the nasal side (Fig. 24.42).

(9) When the cord snaps into the groove so that the lens is secured against the front, hold the ribbon in the plane of the front and, if necessary, pull it to the nearest flat part of the lens shape (Fig. 24.43). To remove the ribbon, grip the edge of the lens with two fingers of the free hand and pull the ribbon in the plane of the front (Fig. 24.44). This ensures that the cord will slip back into the groove. Any threads left under the cord may be removed by pulling each one individually.

(10) Remove excess cord by shaving it off with a sharp blade in the back plane of the front, taking care not to disturb the knot.

To check whether the cord is sufficiently tight, hold the front in one hand and the lens in the other. Try to rotate the lens out of the plane of the front. When this is difficult, the cord has the desired length and tension. When the lens comes away, shorten the cord by placing a second knot within the one on the temporal side of the front.

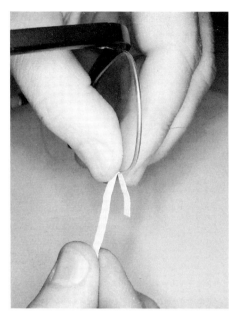

Fig. 24.44 *While gripping the lens edge and the ribbon, pull it in the plane of the front to free it from the cord*

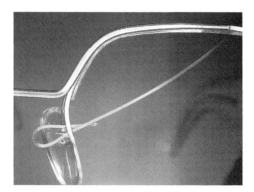

Fig. 24.45 *The cord has been looped through the pair of holes on the nasal side of a metal Supra front*

The cord should now be sufficiently tight. Remove the protruding cord end (see (10) above).

Fitting a new cord to a Supra which takes a flat edged lens also starts with cutting a suitable length of cord and cutting points at its ends. Proceed as follows:

(1) Insert a pointed end of the cord from the lens side, into the hole situated nearest to the nasal end of the rim. Pull several millimetres through the hole, and insert the end into the second hole (Fig. 24.45).
(2) Pull a few millimetres of cord through the hole. Using a pair of flat plastics-jawed pliers, squeeze the cord into the groove on the lens side of the rim. This end has now been secured (Fig. 24.46).
(3) Insert the other end of the cord from the lens side into the hole on the extreme end of the rim.

(4) Holding the lens between thumb and index finger, place its groove against the rim so that the T-ribbon fits into that groove. Guide the cord around the lens so that it lies in this groove. Pull the free end of the cord tight.
(5) Mark the point where the cord emerges from the hole, with a marking pen.
(6) Remove the lens, and cut the cord obliquely at the mark.
(7) Follow the instruction described in (2).
(8) Follow the instructions in (8) and (9) on p. 289 for the fitting of the cord of a combination edge Supra.

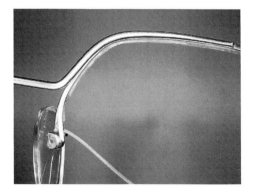

Fig. 24.46 *The end of the cord has been secured in the groove so that it becomes almost continuous with the plastics insert. The insert protrudes from the rim*

24.13 Surface Treatment

24.13.1 INTRODUCTION
It is always worthwhile to prepare carefully any object for surface treatment because it gives a better end result and one which can sometimes also be achieved quicker.

24.13.2 THE VICE
A vice is an instrument with two jaws (Fig. 24.47). The jaws may be tightened to hold an object firmly. Before clamping an object in a vice, ascertain whether the internal surfaces of the vice's jaws are smooth or furrowed. If they are furrowed, they are likely to mark some of the objects held between the jaws. By placing L-shaped thin metal plates or polyamide covers over the jaws (Fig. 24.47), the object is protected. When treating the surface of a spectacle part it is more efficient to clamp it in a vice rather than holding that part in one's hand when both part and hand are certain to move. Vices used in spectacle frame workshops tend to be either fixed to a workbench (Fig. 24.47) or have a universal ball joint so that they can be adjusted in any direction (Fig. 24.48).

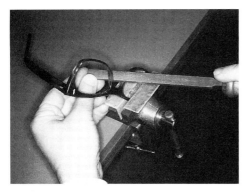

Fig. 24.47 A small vice clamped on a workbench edge. The jaws are covered with thin, L-shaped metal plates. These protect the frame surfaces from the furrows on the surfaces of the jaws

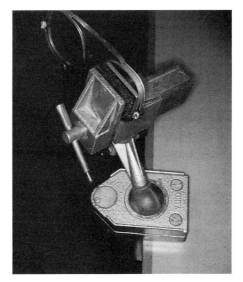

Fig. 24.48 A vice on a universal ball joint

24.13.3 FILING
A distinction may be made between coarse and fine files (instruments with sharp-edged furrows for smoothing or rasping materials). Their effects may vary from producing a very rough to a nearly polished surface. Coarse files are used to remove large quantities of material. Files are available in a great many shapes and sizes (24.49). Note that some have one or more non-cutting surfaces or edges which should be placed adjacent to any surface not to be treated.

Make certain that the handle of a file is securely attached to the file itself. If this is no longer the case, and provided that the handle is made of wood, proceed as follows. After removal of the handle, heat (on a gas ring) the pointed end of the file until almost red hot. Holding the cold end of the file, insert it into the hole in the wooden handle. Then, hit the wooden handle's flat end several times on a solid surface such as a concrete floor, to drive the pointed end into the wood of the handle. Let the metal cool before use. Note that there are also large files with integral, plastics handles available.

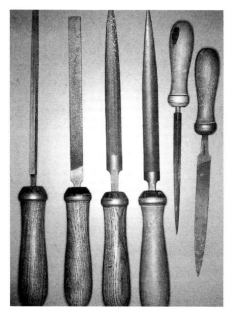

Fig. 24.49 Various files. Note the difference in surface coarseness of the two middle tools. The furthest left file shows a narrow, smooth edge and is about 30 cm long

Very small files (needle files) (Fig. 24.50) have an integral handle which is an extension of the file itself. It may be more effective to use emery boards (see Section 24.13.5) instead.

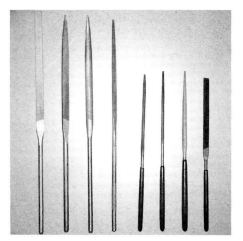

Fig. 24.50 Two sets of needle files. The longer files are about 15 cm long

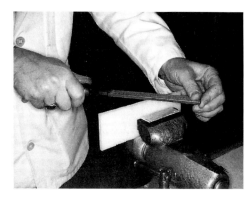

Fig. 24.51 Coarse files are best used while standing because this provides better control over a file. Because greater pressure can be exerted on the file, a greater quantity of material can be removed with each stroke

Coarse files are best used while standing, with the object clamped in a vice (Fig. 24.51). This allows better control over the file and allows the exertion of greater pressure. It is more efficient to use the whole length of the furrowed portion of the file making long strokes away from one's body, rather than fast and/or short strokes. With plastics materials care should be taken not to remove too much material. A good quantity is often removed after just two or three file strokes. Check the result after each couple of strokes to avoid removal of too much material.

Because of the nature of plastics the furrows of files may rapidly become clogged. To remove the material either run a finger over the file, apply a brush (not a metal brush because this may blunt the cutting edges of the file's teeth), or run a piece of brass across the furrows so that the file cuts furrows in the brass (Fig. 24.52). The crests between the furrows will then clean the furrows of the file when the piece of brass is run over the latter.

Small, fine furrowed files are best used seated. One can remove only minute amounts of plastics material with them and they clog rapidly; they are more efficient on metals.

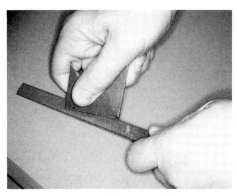

Fig. 24.52 Moving a thin piece of brass across the narrow portion of the file cleans the furrows

24.13.4 SHAVING

Plastics surfaces may be smoothed and/or shaped by shaving off thin layers. There are special tools, but one can also make one's own (Fig. 24.53), provided that the right type of thin metal plate is available. It is best to clamp the object to be treated in a vice. It is also necessary to angle the tool with respect to the surface to be shaved, and determine by trial and error which angle produces the best result. The tool is drawn, with

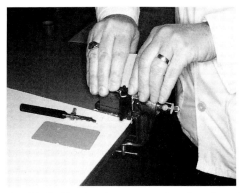

Fig. 24.53 Shaving the narrow edge of a piece of plastics to give it a curved shape. In the foreground are two shaving tools. The flat blade tool is identical to the one in use and is made of mild steel. The other tool (made by Breitfeld & Schliekert GmbH, of Bad Vilbel, Germany) can be used to produce a steeper and a flatter curve, an angled flat surface, and also the groove in the rim of a front

hand pressure, over the surface from which thin slivers of material are to be removed.

24.13.5 SMOOTHING

This is done with abrasive material. The abrasive material itself is, for this purpose, fixed to a base such as paper or fabric. It is available in sheet form. The abrasive materials commonly used are crystals of aluminium oxide and silicon carbide (carborundum). They are available in various hardnesses. The larger the particle size, or the smaller the number of particles per unit area, the coarser the effect.

Smoothing can be done by rubbing the surface with a portion of the abrasive sheet while applying hand pressure. However, it is more effective to cover a portion of a tool with the sheet. This can be done by folding the paper around a piece of wood similar in shape and size to a file. Greater and more evenly distributed pressure may be applied, particularly on a flat surface, when the object to be smoothed is clamped in a vice. Having used a relatively coarse type of abrasive paper, repeat the process (at right angles to the first) with smoother and progressively finer paper (again, at right angles to the previous). Note that fine abrasive paper has a limited life and must be replaced frequently.

Applying an emery board with a flexible wooden centre, as used by manicurists, is a most effective and speedy alternative. Such boards make it possible to control accurately the quantity of material to be removed. The surface quality produced is such that a good polish is easily achieved without further preparation. The boards can be cleaned by washing in warm water.

24.13.6 POLISHING

This should only be undertaken when the surface is free of grooves visible to the eye. A number of precautions should be observed. Wear suitable

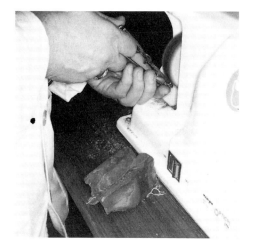

Fig. 24.54 *The frame's front is held tangentially to the polishing mob. In the lower foreground is a block of polishing compound*

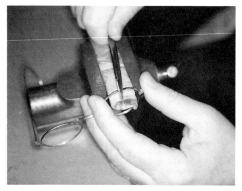

Fig. 24.55 *A burnishing tool being rubbed over the soldered part of a rim to restore its polished appearance*

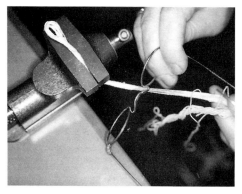

Fig. 24.56 *Awkward corners can be polished with cotton threads*

protective eye wear and tuck away long hair, tie, necklace, bracelet, etc. so that it cannot be caught by the rotating mop (Fig. 24.54) or motor axle. Protective clothing should be worn over normal clothing, to protect and keep these clean. If the motor by which the mop is driven is powerful, a safety switch should provide instant interruption of the electricity supply.

Do not hold the object to be polished stationary while the polishing mop rotates: this will cause removal of material on one spot, and may 'burn' plastics materials.

In general, metals should be polished at a greater mop circumference speed than plastics. Final polishing should be done at an even greater speed, using a finer polishing compound.

Different polishing compounds are available for different materials. One should apply only one compound to any one mop. Seek advice from the supplier as to which combination of motor speed, polishing compound, mop material and mop diameter to use. See 'buffing' in Section 10.2.1.

Soft metals can also be polished with a burnishing tool (Fig. 24.55) which is rubbed over the part to be treated. The latter must be held against a suitable support. Finally, the metal part can be polished by hand, with cotton threads (Fig. 24.56) and polishing compound.

24.14 Sides

24.14.1 LENGTHENING A SIDE
A plastics side cannot usually be lengthened because there is not sufficient material to do so. Ordering a longer side is the proper solution. Unfortunately, a longer plastics side may not be available.

A metal side that has a drop covered with an end cover (*tip*) can be lengthened as follows. Warm the end cover (*tip*) with a frame heater, straighten the side and pull the end cover off the side. Choose a new, longer end cover from the selection of workshop accessories (available from workshop accessory wholesalers). Warm the longer end cover a little and push it on to the end of the side. Having warmed the end cover sufficiently, place the ear point at the required length to bend. When cooled, place the spectacles on the wearer's head and check whether further adjustments, including the downward and inward angles of drop, need to be made.

If a longer end cover is not available, try to use the old end cover, which may be fitted as follows. Warm the end cover a little, and straighten the side. Move the end cover away from the butt by a length equal to the desired increase in the length to bend. Warm the end cover and place the ear point. Because the tip of the end cover no longer encloses a metal wire it will be fragile and should be heated only minimally; great care should be taken while adjusting the inward angle of drop. If heated too much, the plastics end cover may collapse or the end of the wire may protrude through it.

24.14.2 SHORTENING A SIDE

If a plastics or metal side has a pinned half-joint, it may be possible to repin the half-joint (Section 24.9). Alternatively, heat the ear point area and straighten the side. Having measured the length to bend beforehand, mark the desired position of the ear point, and place the bend. If the length of the drop is excessive, that is longer than about 45 mm, it is necessary to shorten the drop. Cut the excess length off the tip of the drop, and fashion the drop with a file. Then smooth the material, and polish it. Alternatively, file the excess material away, then smooth and polish the tip. Either way, try to ensure that the side wire remains covered by a layer of plastics material.

Metal sides covered by an end cover may be shortened as follows. Warm the end cover a little, straighten the side and remove the end cover.

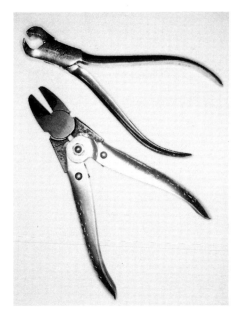

Fig. 24.57 *Two pairs of cutting pliers*

Note that the end of the side is pointed. Shorten the side by a length equal to the reduction in the length to bend by cutting it with cutting pliers (Fig. 24.57). Using a file, fashion the end of the side to a point. If the original end cover is to be used, shorten it by the same length as the side by cutting off a section on its open end. (If the butt of the side is wider than its bend and the end cover is not shortened, it may split when fitted.) Use a file to refashion that end; smooth and polish it. Warm the end cover a little and fit it on to the side; next, warm the end cover sufficiently to place the ear point. If a shorter end cover is available, use this to replace the original.

24.15 Workshop Accessories

24.15.1 INTRODUCTION

In this section mention is made of both equipment and accessories which can be of use in the adjustment or modification of spectacle frames.

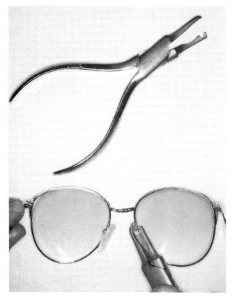

Fig. 24.58 A pair of pad adjusting pliers (above) and how it grips the pad. See also Fig. 16.7

They are given in no particular order and the contents are not exhaustive.

24.15.2 SPECIAL PURPOSE PLIERS

- **Pad adjusting pliers** (Fig. 24.58)   These are indispensable for the easy and accurate adjustment of the pads of metal frames.
- **Peening pliers** (Fig. 4.7)   These vary in shape and size. They spread (*flare*) the bottom of a screw thus securing the screw in the barrel of the charnier. The consequence may be that it is difficult to remove the screw, when required. It will then be necessary to file away the peened screw bottom.
- **Joint angling pliers/side angling pliers**   These are used to alter the inclination of a joint or of a side (*temple*) respectively. There are different types for plastics and for metal frames.
- **Side adjusting pliers**   These are used to straighten or bend sides (*temples*).

- **Stamping pliers**   These are provided with a block in which, for instance, the name of the practice is engraved. The pliers are used to stamp spectacle frames with this name to prevent theft, etc. (Section 23.4; Fig. 23.7).

There are many pliers for more general purposes. Jaws are usually flat or conical and made of plastics or metal, or one of each. A pair of cutting pliers should be present in every workshop.

24.15.3 SCREWDRIVERS

No practice can be without a set of screwdrivers. However, they are often abused, as a result of which blades may break. When applying a screwdriver to the head of a screw, ensure that the width of the screwdriver blade matches the diameter of the head of the screw. If the blade is narrower, it may bend or break.

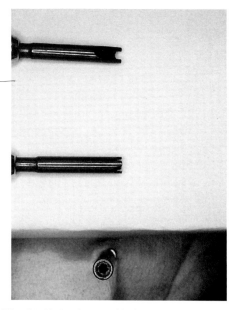

Fig. 24.59 A selection of locknut spanners: for use with (top) a slotted locknut where the slot in the spanner's blade accommodates the bottom of the screw, (middle) a crown-shaped locknut and (bottom) a hexagonal locknut

A spectacle frame may sometimes be produced fitted with Phillips cross or hexagonal head screws. Perhaps manufacturers can be persuaded not to use such screws; they do not conform to standards for spectacle frame screws (Fig. 11.18). Locknuts have occasionally been used to secure screws. A locknut should be turned with the appropriate locknut spanner (Fig. 24.59).

24.15.4 REPLACEMENT AND CONVERSION PARTS

Endcovers (*tips*) can be used either to replace a damaged part, or to extend the drop of a metal side (*temple*) by fitting one that is longer than the original.

Auxiliary plastics pads made out of cellulose acetate, can be cemented onto existing pads to build them up and reduce the distance between pads or rims. Pads made of plastics foam tend to have a short life since they soon become dirty from perspiration and dust. Self-adhesive pads (Fig. 24.60) tend to suffer the same fate.

Auxiliary silicone endcovers are slipped over the existing endcover and, because of the nature of silicone, increase the friction between drop and the wearer's head thus preventing the frame from slipping. There are also plastics covers that can be slipped over a curl side. When heated, they shrink to form a flexible and permanent cover.

Plastics curls are also available suitable to convert a plastics or metal drop end side into a curl side.

A spectacle frame with a conventional plastics pad bridge does not normally fit on a nose with a negative crest height. Replacing the pads with a metal-reinforced silicone bridge fastened with screws (Fig. 24.60) into the bridge of the frame may well solve the problem.

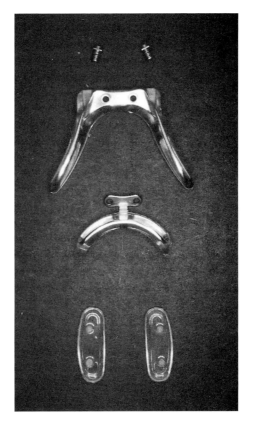

Fig. 24.60 *Bottom: self-adhesive silicone pads; middle: a silicone-clad curved auxiliary bridge that can be screwed onto the plastics bridge of a front; top: a silicone-clad saddle bridge used for the conversion of a metal pad bridge*

It is sometime possible to convert a metal pad frame into a saddle bridge frame using a similar fastening method (Fig. 24.60). Likewise, plastics pad frames may be converted into a frame with pads on pad arms where the latter are screwed into the rim of the plastics front (Fig. 19.6B).

REFERENCES

BS 3172 EN ISO 11381 (1987). *Screw Threads for Spectacle Frames.* London: British Standards Institution.

BS 3521 (1991). *Terms Relating to Ophthalmic Optics and Spectacle Frames. Part 1: Glossary of Terms Relating to Spectacle Frames.* London: British Standards Institution.

Camau, R. (1985). L'indication du matériau est-elle utile sur les lunettes. *Opticien-Lunetier* No. 379, 46.

Crundall, E.J. (1971). A guide to optical pliers. *Optician* **162**(4196), 10–19.

Earlam, R. (1985). Removing a broken screw. *Optical Receptionist, London,* Spring Issue, 8.

Earlam, R. (1986/87). Removing and replacing a broken screw. *Optical Receptionist, London,* Winter Issue, 27.

Hintermeister, H. (1984). *Feinmechanische Arbeitstechniken.* Pforzheim: Verlag Bode.

ISO 11381 (1994). *Optics and Optical Instruments – Ophthalmic Optics – Screw-Threads.* Genève (CH): International Standards Organisation.

MacGregor, R.J.S., Orr, H., Davidson, D.C. & Eadon–Allen, S. (1992). Real tortoiseshell. *Ophthalm. Antiq. Int. Collectors Newsletter (UK)* No. 41, 3–8.

Obstfeld, H. (1982). *Optics in Vision,* 2nd edn. London: Butterworths.

Obstfeld, H. (1988). General considerations in prescribing. In: Edwards, K. & Llewellyn, R. (eds) *Optometry,* p. 465. London: Butterworths.

Optinova (undated). Ceroid. Optinova, Italy. (brochure).

INDEX

Note: Main entries pertain to British Standards definitions rather than North American.
Abbreviations used: CD, centration distance; PD, (inter)pupillary distance